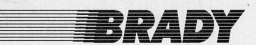

**Fourth Edition**

# Being A Homemaker/ Home Health Aide

D1551019

## Elana D. Zucker, RN, MSN

**Executive Director, Nursing
and Chief Nursing Officer
Overlook Hospital
Summit, New Jersey**

*SYLVIA SERRIES*

**BRADY
Prentice Hall
Englewood Cliffs, New Jersey 07632**

*Library of Congress Cataloging-in-Publication Data*

Being a homemaker / home health aide / Elana D. Zucker, editor.—4th ed.
     p.     cm.
    Includes index.
    ISBN 0-89303-018-X
    1. Home health aides. 2. Home care services. I. Zucker, Elana
D., 1941-   . II. Title: Being a homemaker home health aide.
    [DNLM: 1. Home Care Services. 2. Home Health Aides. WY 115 B422
1996]
    RA645.3.B45  1996
    610.73'43—dc20
    DNLM/DLC
    for Library of Congress                95-16239
                                          CIP

To Brian without whom nothing would be possible and the world and our family would be poorer.

---

### NOTICE

It is the intent of the author and publishers that this textbook be used as part of a formal Homemaker/Home Health Aide course taught by a qualified instructor. The procedures presented here represent accepted practices in the United States. They are not offered as a standard of care. Home health care is to be performed under the authority and guidance of qualified supervisory personnel. It is the reader's responsibility to know and follow local care protocols as provided by the medical advisors directing the system to which he or she belongs. Also, it is the reader's responsibility to stay informed of home health care procedure changes.

---

Director of Manufacturing and Production: Bruce Johnson
Project Manager: Janet McGillicuddy
Acquisitions Editor: Barbara Krawiec
Editorial/production: Proof Positive/Farrowlyne Associates, Inc.
Interior design: Laura Ierardi
Cover design: Miguel Ortiz
Cover photo: © Bill Losh/FPG International
Manufacturing buyer: Ilene Sanford
Photography: Michael Heron
Composition: Carlisle Communications
Printer/Binder: Webcrafters

 © 1996, 1991, 1988, 1982 by Prentice-Hall, Inc.
A Simon & Schuster Company
Englewood Cliffs, New Jersey 07632

Printed in the United States of America

10  9  8  7  6  5  4  3  2

ISBN 0-89303-018-X

Prentice-Hall International (UK) Limited, *London*
Prentice-Hall of Australia Pty. Limited, *Sydney*
Prentice-Hall Canada Inc., *Toronto*
Prentice-Hall Hispanoamericana, S.A., *Mexico*
Prentice-Hall of India Private Limited, *New Delhi*
Prentice-Hall of Japan, Inc., *Tokyo*
Simon & Schuster of Southeast Asia Pte. Ltd., *Singapore*
Editora Prentice-Hall do Brasil, Ltda., *Rio de Janeiro*

# Contents

## Chapter 19  Common Diseases You Will See    349

## Chapter 20  Emergency Procedures    375

## Procedures

# Preface

*Being a Homemaker/Home Health Aide* has been compiled by a multidisciplinary team of practicing home health care professionals. It is formulated to teach homemakers/home health aides to be efficient, caring members of the health care team. This manual provides a simple, clear, and concise framework for learning. It can be used both as a primary learning tool and as a mechanism for future review of procedures and theoretical information.

The content includes material to guide the beginning aide and to expand the knowledge base of the more experienced worker. It is also designed to be a reference for aides as they work in the community. Information is presented within the context of the home and the community. Further, all material is designed to assist students in defining their role within the home health care system.

Vital aspects of home health care are thoroughly covered, including:

- *Anatomy and Physiology*, as they relate to the home health setting
- *Children Under Stress*, both as clients and as family members
- *Geriatric Clients*, both in the home and the community
- *Terminally Ill Clients*
- *Disabled Clients*
- *Rehabilitation in the Home*
- *Mentally Disabled Individuals*, both as clients and family members
- *Diseases Commonly Seen in Clients*
- *Nutritional Information*
- *Emergency and First Aid Procedures*
- *Communication*
- *Infection Control*
- *Postpartum Care*

Each chapter is divided into short, manageable sections. To further encourage learning, each section includes:

*Objectives*—tell students what they will learn in the section.

*Introduction*—serve as a general introduction to specific topics.

*Guidelines*—list pertinent points to guide students on the job.

*Procedures*—give a logical, step-by-step approach to the tasks that must be performed in the work setting.

*New Words*—are printed in color and immediately defined in the text.

*Topics for Discussion*—end each chapter and serve as a review and stimulus for further learning, for both the instructor and the student.

*Abbreviations*—listed as a special section at the end of the text.

*Glossary*—combines all new words presented in the text, and includes related health care terms and their definitions.

*Notes Column*—provides ample space for students to jot down notes.

The authors, reviewers, and numerous advisors who contributed to this book have endeavored to produce a comprehensive, thorough, yet enjoyable text for the fastest growing segment of the home care industry—the homemaker/home health aide.

## Contributors

Joan B. Kane, BS, RPT
> Registered Physical Therapist, Private Practice, New Jersey

Theodosia T. Kelsey, OTR
> Occupational Therapist, Private Practice, New Jersey

Janne Litzelman, MS CCC
> Speech Pathologist, Private Practice, New Jersey

Elaine Muller, MA
> Private Practice, New Jersey

Patricia Taboloski, RN, MSN
> Research Assistant, University of Rochester School of Nursing, New York (Family Health, Nurse Clinician Practitioner)

Eleanor Bannon, RN
> Enterostomal Therapist, Overlook Hospital, Summit, New Jersey

Gloria J. Bizjak
> The Maryland Fire and Rescue Institute at the University of Maryland

## Acknowledgments

A special thanks to the many people who were supportive and insightful throughout the process of writing this book. First, to all the homemaker/home health aides who have written to me with suggestions and encouragement. Thank you. I have tried to incorporate your ideas and meet the needs you expressed. Secondly, to the instructors who have taken the time to write with comments and detailed letters and calls. I appreciate your time and honest counsel.

No book such as this becomes a reality without professionals who work behind the scenes to edit, proofread, and produce a finished product. To Barbara Krawiec, my editor and lifeline to the publishing world, thank you! You were always available and always supportive. Thanks also to your right hand Louise Fullum, who mailed, called, and kept us both on track. It is still a wonder that she can remember all the details she does.

To my new friends at Proof Positive/Farrowlyne Associates, Inc. in Illinois, who transformed the typed manuscript into the wonderful book you hold in your hands, I can only say, "Thank You." It has been a pleasure and an honor to work with you, to learn from you, and to have you part of my latest endeavor. If there is a reason to write again, you are it. Dan Weiskopf and Ann Lindstrom were always there and always a friendly voice on the phone. I do not know what fate put us together on this project, but I am thankful for the experience.

Lastly, to my husband, who mailed, helped type, and helped me with my computer, thank you. Your love and support have always been part of my life and has contributed to my growth as a professional nurse.

# Introduction

Welcome to *Being a Homemaker/Home Health Aide.* You are, or will be, working as part of the home health care team. This team cares for people who need skilled, professional health care in the home.

You will work with nurses, doctors, and technicians; speech, physical, and occupational therapists; and nutritionists. You can take pride in your work. The most important person in the health care system is the client. Everyone strives to meet the needs of the client and his family.

## How to Use This Book

This book has been written to help you do well in your job. The first step is to learn how to use it efficiently so you will be able to get the most out of it. This manual is designed to guide you. It is a learning tool, a reference book, like a dictionary. Use it in classes for taking notes. Look at it whenever you have a chance. Use it at home for studying and reading before class. Use it during your work, to review the procedures. Study the pictures. They will help to make things clear.

All of the tasks described in this manual are listed in the table of contents. Use it to find the page number of any procedure you might want to review.

Most chapters are divided into sections. This makes it easier for you to learn the many and varied tasks of your job.

Though this is currently an occupation held mainly by women, more and more men are entering the home health field. We welcome them! But for convenience and ease of presentation, the text will normally refer to the supervisor as "she" or "her" and to the client as "he" or "him."

## Objectives: What You Will Learn to Do

The Objectives serve as realistic goals for you to reach as you go through each section. Objectives tell what a successful student is able to do at the end of the section.

## Introduction

Under the **Introduction** you will find the reasons behind each procedure you will be doing. Knowing why you are doing something will help you to prepare for and carry out the procedures in the best possible way.

## Guidelines

Often there are basic principles, ideas, and methods that must be remembered for the overall care of a client. As an example, you will always treat the client with courtesy, kindness, and sympathy. Such a principle does not make up a full procedure, but it is important for you to remember. In some situations the order in which the tasks are done doesn't matter. Your instructor will tell you this and discuss these guidelines. These are not true procedures and so they are put in this section.

## Procedures

A task is an assigned duty, something you are expected to do. In this manual, each task has been divided into a logical, orderly series of actions or steps. The full set of steps is a procedure. In health care agencies, procedures are done according to a set method. Several procedures will be somewhat different in different agencies, but the underlying principles or ideas are always the same. Only the sequence or style for a task may be different. Be sure you know the methods, the policies, and the style of the agency where you are working. Usually, however, the way things are done will be very similar to the series of steps given in this manual for a procedure.

## Procedure: Sample Procedure

1. Assemble all necessary equipment.
2. Wash your hands.
3. Ask visitors to step out of the room if appropriate.
4. Tell the client what you are going to do.
5. Do the procedure at the correct time, as instructed.
6. Discard all disposable equipment and supplies as soon as the procedure is completed. Put the material in the proper containers.
7. Clean the reusable equipment and put it in the proper placc as soon as you have finished the procedure.
8. Report what you have done and how the client tolerated the procedure. Report your observations. Record the necessary information as is consistent with agency policy.

## Things to Remember

You will be working under the supervision of the nurse, team leader, or therapist. They are not necessarily the same person. We will use the term *supervisor* to refer to the person who supervises you with that particular procedure.

■ If you don't know how to do a procedure, ask your supervisor for help. If you are not sure of yourself, tell her. It is better to get help than to do something wrong.

■ Use this book. Read the procedures until you remember every step. Check the Glossary in the back for the meanings of words you don't know.

## Notes Column

Use the blank space on each page to make notes or underline the important information on each page. Writing things down helps you to remember them. Keep a pencil in hand as you study. Jot down key words and "thought clues." They will come back to you later when you need them. As your instructor goes over each procedure with you, he or she will explain things that are done differently in your setting. Taking notes is a good way to record these differences.

## Glossary and Abbreviations

New words are tools for communication. In your work, you will be introduced to medical terminology. You should increase your vocabulary as much as you can so you always understand what the supervisor tells you. Besides, it is a personal achievement. Learning new words can help to make you more self-confident.

When you are reporting to your supervisors, you must make yourself clearly understood. It is important you accurately communicate information about the client and his or her situation or condition. The text marginal glossary and the end of the book Glossary and Abbreviations List will help you to understand the meaning of many words and terms used in health care. Some new words will appear in the text in boldface. Those words will appear in the marginal glossary for extra clarity. You can look up other new words in the end of book Glossary.

## Topics for Discussion

These subjects are ones that you should think about. Discuss them with your classmates. Discuss them with your instructors. There are no right or wrong answers to any of these questions. They are placed in this book to help you become familiar with your feelings and ideas.

**Elana Zucker**

# Chapter 1

# Orientation to the Home Care Industry

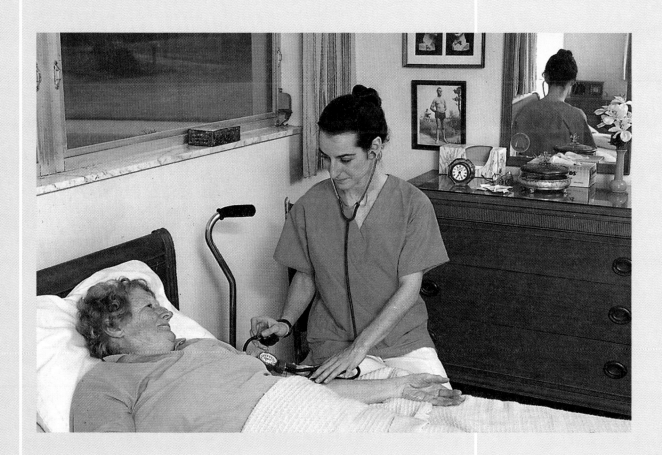

# Section 1  The Home Health Agency

## Objectives: What You Will Learn to Do

- Explain the purpose and organization of a home health agency.
- Discuss some of the changes health care reform has had on home health care.
- Identify the responsibilities of members of the health care team.
- Define the meaning of the word *policy.*
- Identify the agency credentials.
- Discuss various methods of paying for home care services.

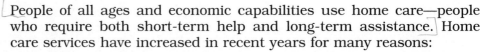

### Introduction: Home Health Care

During your orientation period, your instructor will give you the names and titles of personnel in key positions in your home health care agency and those agencies with which you will work. A home health care agency is one that delivers care and services to people within their home. There are many different types of home health care providers. Some agencies deal mostly with the delivery of services to people; some agencies concentrate on the delivery of equipment to be used in the home; some agencies deliver specialized care, such as respiratory services or counseling. You will come in contact with all types of agencies, and your instructor will tell you what policies are in effect as you relate to these agencies. It is important to know what you, as a member of the health care team, can expect from each type of agency and where you fit into the entire health picture.

### WHO USES HOME HEALTH CARE?

People of all ages and economic capabilities use home care—people who require both short-term help and long-term assistance. Home care services have increased in recent years for many reasons:

- People prefer to be cared for at home in familiar surroundings where they can take an active part in the planning and implementation of their care, rather than in an institution.
- Hospital stays are shorter than in years past.
- Home care is usually less expensive than hospital or institutional care.
- Sophisticated services, once available only in hospitals, are now available at home.
- As people live longer and the elderly population grows, the number of people requiring some type of assistance is increasing.

### HEALTH CARE REFORM

Within recent years, there have been many changes in health care. Various groups have tried to streamline and control costs by making changes. These changes have affected the way people get health care, as well as how they use it and pay for it. In addition, different people are now involved in the client's care.

Insurance companies review the care of each client and may offer suggestions for changes in that care. These suggestions will be communicated to you through your supervisor. The reviewers, however, may also visit the house, ask questions, or talk to the client. Discuss with your agency how you should handle these inquiries. Be sure to let your agency know if the insurance company calls the client, asks to visit, or sends papers for the client to complete. If an insurance company asks you direct questions, be polite and refer them to your supervisor.

The way in which people get health care has also changed. In some cases, the insurance company may have identified doctors, hospitals, and vendors that the client is referred to for care and equipment. If the client goes anywhere else, his coverage may be less. You are obligated to use the designated vendors so that the client will continue to receive coverage of the needed service. Do not suggest that the client go to another more familiar doctor or vendor without first consulting your supervisor. Some insurance companies also designate hospitals and rehabilitation services for use. Only in emergencies can a client go to another facility.

## CASE MANAGEMENT

**case manager** coordinates care for the client with all caregivers

Insurance companies and other payors coordinate and organize the care of a client. A **case manager** is employed to review the care provided by all members of the health care team, ensure there is no duplication of services, and ensure that the client is progressing according to the original plan of care. If changes occur in the client's status, the case manager will change the plan of care. Your supervisor will discuss changes with the case manager. The case manager may or may not visit the client. The records you keep and the observations you make will always be part of the review. It is very important that you write accurately and objectively your observations of the client's status and the effect of the plan of care.

## MANAGED CARE

This is the term used to describe many of the insurance industry's different payment options. Usually the client prepays the company providing care a sum of money each month. When care is needed, the company provides the care for the fees already paid and the fees the client has agreed to pay in the coming months. Each company has clear and strict rules for each insurance option. Assist your client in following these rules. The coverage by the insurance company may depend on these details. If you have questions, call your supervisor or advise the client to call the insurance company directly. Always have the client write down the name of the person with whom he speaks.

## CUSTOMER

This is a term that means that one person receives a service from another person for some sort of payment, meeting of a need, or gain. Each of us has many customers and is a customer to many people. Your health care agency has many customers: the client, the doctor, the insurance company, and yourself. Each has different expectations of the agency, all of which must be met. Because it is not possible to meet the needs of all customers all of the time, an agency and the people who work there identify their key customers. This way they can concentrate their effort on meeting the needs of these customers first. Ask your agency who it lists as its key customers. If you do not agree, discuss it with your supervisor.

## PATIENT RIGHTS

Every patient or client has certain rights and expectations of those agencies and people who care for them. Your agency has a published list of these rights. Carry them with you. Share them with the client when you first meet. Although the format and wording may be slightly different, the document will contain at least the following:

- The right to civil and religious liberties
- The right to voice complaints without fear
- The right to refuse care
- The right to have an active part in establishing the care plan
- The right to be treated with respect
- The right to be free of physical and mental abuse
- The right to be free of chemical or physical restraints
- The right to privacy
- The right to communication with family, friends, and medical care providers

## AGENCY CREDENTIALS

**credential** a letter or certificate indicating that a right or privilege has been attained or that a position of authority may be exercised

Most states require health care agencies to conform to standards and submit to periodic inspections and surveys. This process assures the public and the agency's employees that the agency is operating within minimum standards. The documents indicating that the agency has achieved these standards are called **credentials.** As you learn more about the agency, ask for the agency's credentials just as it asks for yours. The following are some agency credentials that may be displayed:

1. *Licensure.* The agency has met minimum standards set by the state. Some states do not have this procedure, and some states require that only certain types of agencies apply and receive a license.
2. *Certification.* All states must certify to Medicare and Medicaid that their minimum standards have been met so they are eligible for Medicare and Medicaid reimbursement. You will be asked to provide certain documents so that your agency can conform to the standards of certification.
3. *Accreditation.* Several professional organizations will investigate and accredit an agency. This is a voluntary process and indicates that the agency has met the standards of the organization.
4. *Bonding.* The agency pays a bond, or insurance policy, so that, if it is sued due to an employee's actions, any damages can be paid to the consumer.

## FUNCTIONS OF HOME CARE AGENCIES

1. To provide care for the ill, disabled, or injured within their homes and communities

2. To become involved in preventive community health care
3. To promote individual and community health
4. To provide an opportunity for the further education of health workers
5. To promote research in the health care professions

## PAYMENT FOR SERVICES

There is a charge to someone or some insurance company for your services. These charges are collected by the home health agency and eventually make up your salary. Payment for home health care services can come from many sources. Medicare, Medicaid, and private insurance companies are all sources of payment. These payments vary from state to state and from year to year. Refer all questions to your supervisor.

Some of the time your client or his family will pay the agency directly for your service. Your agency has a **protocol** (set of plans or procedures) for deciding the method of payment that clients will use. Payment sources and amounts are arranged by your supervisor and the client before you are assigned to the case. It is not wise to discuss payment with clients. If clients have questions, refer them to your supervisor.

**protocol** rules directing the actions of specific people

### Sources of Payment

| | Eligibility | Services Covered |
|---|---|---|
| *Medicare:* federally financed health plan | Over 65 years old: disabled more than two years, persons on dialysis; must be home-bound under medical supervision, need intermittent skilled nursing, physical, occupational, or speech therapy; must obtain services through a certified home health agency | Nursing, PT, OT, ST, MSW, HHA, some supplies and equipment |
| *Medicare hospice:* federally financed program providing care to terminally ill patients | Eligible for Medicare, use certified hospice, the relinquishing of usual Medicare benefits, six-month prognosis | All necessary services with some copayment |
| *Medicaid:* state health care for low-income persons | Financial eligibility differs from state to state; services must be provided under MD supervision | Part-time nursing, HHA, medical supplies/equipment, possible coverage for PT, OT, ST, audiology, personal care, day care, transportation |
| *Health insurance:* Private | Individually purchased coverage | As per policy |
| *Special* | Worker's compensation, auto insurance | As per situation |
| *HMO* | Prepayment health | As per plan |

## HOME HEALTH AGENCY PERSONNEL

### *The Homemaker/Home Health Aide: Part of the Team*

The goal of the home health team is to provide care so the client can function optimally—to help him be the best he can. If he is ill, the team will assist him with recovery. If he is disabled, the team will assist him with adapting his everyday needs so that he can function in society and his own home environment. As a homemaker/home health aide, you are an important member of the health care team. As part of the team, you will be assigned to care for a specific client in his home. Teamwork means that everyone knows what he is supposed to do and does it to the best of his ability with a spirit of cooperation.

The agency that employs you will assign a supervisor to your case. This person may be a professional nurse or another professional member of the health care team. All these people recognize the homemaker/home health aide as a valuable worker and member of the team. Your supervisor will help you learn and understand your job. If you have a question about one of your tasks or something that happens in your client's home, ask the professional member of the team who assigned the job to you.

### Home Health Agency Professional Personnel

| | |
|---|---|
| Community health nurse (public health nurse) | A registered nurse (RN) with a college degree, licensed by the state to practice nursing. She applies her knowledge to the promotion and preservation of health. |
| Registered nurse | Has a license from the state to practice nursing. |
| Licensed practical nurse or licensed vocational nurse | Has a license from the state to work under the direction of a registered nurse, physician, or dentist. |
| Physical therapist | Licensed to practice physical therapy by the state; concerned with restoring function and preventing disability following disease, injury, or loss of a body part. |
| Occupational therapist | Graduate of an approved occupational therapy curriculum and granted a certification/license from the state; concerned with patient's ability to perform essential daily living tasks. |
| Speech pathologist | Graduate of an approved speech pathology program and granted a certificate of clinical competence; treats persons with speech disorders caused by physical defects or mental disorder. |
| Respiratory therapist | Graduate of an approved respiratory therapy program and granted license/certificate from the state; Concerned with evaluating breathing, assisting with prescribed breathing treatments/regimes, and equipment. |
| Nutritionist | Applies the science of food consumption and utilization to the growth, maintenance, and repair of the human body. |
| Social worker | Has formal education required to treat individuals, families, groups, or communities with social and/or psychological problems. Coordinates community resources to meet client and/or family needs. |

*emphysema develops due to smoking — chronic obstructed pulmonary disease (COPD)*

*wheelchair, special bed etc.*

# Section 2  Your Job as a Homemaker/Home Health Aide

## Objectives: What You Will Learn to Do

- List the responsibilities the home health agency has assigned to you.
- List the tasks you will be doing on the job.
- Be familiar with qualities that are desirable in a homemaker/home health aide.

**job description** written document listing the parts of employment, such as the tasks one is responsible for

**responsibilities** those tasks one has to execute and for which one is held accountable

**role** one's function

## *Introduction: Tasks and Responsibilities*

The tasks and responsibilities expected of you are summarized in your **job description.** It is very important that you understand this and agree to it. Then there will never be a misunderstanding later as to what you are expected to do. **Responsibilities** are trusts that are expected of you. Everyone you work with will have a set of responsibilities and expectations. By being very familiar with the responsibilities and expectations employers, clients, and team members have of you, you will be able to act in the proper manner and feel more comfortable. Your **role** will be slightly different in each house, but your overall function will be spelled out in the job description.

### WORKING IN A CLIENT'S HOME

You will be caring for people in their homes. Until they get to know you, you will be considered a stranger. Many people are afraid of strangers and have fears about letting them into their home. They are often afraid you are there to "make order." It will be an important part of your first meeting with the client and his family to assure them that you are in the home to help and to abide by their routine as much as possible (Fig. 1.1). Although your agency trusts you and knows you are an honest and considerate person, the client does not—yet. There will be a brief period when you, the client, and his family will have to get to know each other. Besides relating with the client, you will also relate with the

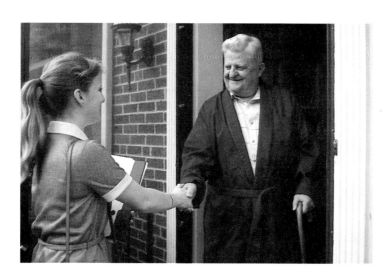

*FIGURE 1.1* First impressions set the stage for future interactions.

**principal care person.** This is the person in the family who has been designated as "being in charge" of the client's care. Here are some helpful hints to decrease the fears clients may have about you as a new person:

- Wear your uniform. It identifies you as a member of the health care team.
- Wear your name pin and any identification your agency requires. This tells the client you are who you say you are.
- Introduce yourself immediately in a clear, quiet voice. Identify your agency and your job title. Write down the information if they ask you to.
- Discuss with the client your responsibilities, tasks, and hours of work. Assure the client you are there to work in his home in a manner that is comfortable for him. You are not there to change everything.
- Ask the client if he has any questions. If you cannot answer his questions, refer him to your supervisor.

## RESPONSIBILITIES OF THE HOME CARE AGENCY TO ITS EMPLOYEES

The agency that employs you has many responsibilities. When you are given a job, the employer assumes the responsibilities of paying you for your work, providing a safe and meaningful working environment, providing supervision, providing periodic evaluations of your work, and treating you with respect.

During your orientation period, you will become familiar with many agency personnel policies. These explain what the agency considers its responsibilities and what it considers your responsibilities. These policies deal with such topics as health examinations, salaries, uniforms, evaluations, documentation, communication, vacations, assignments, and hours of work. It is most important that you review and understand these policies, for these are the rules under which you will work.

You will always work under the supervision of a registered professional nurse or other health professional. It is that person's responsibility to plan the client's plan of care and to assign tasks to you in an understandable manner.

## EMPLOYEE'S RESPONSIBILITIES

It is your responsibility to do only those tasks that are assigned and to do them to the best of your ability. You are expected to care for your clients with thought, consideration, and respect. If you do not know a procedure, ask! It is also your responsibility to be a contributing member of the health care team. Share your ideas, your thoughts, and your knowledge. The clients will benefit, your fellow employees will benefit, and the agency will benefit.

## EQUIPMENT

It is always necessary to have the proper supplies and equipment to perform your tasks. When you accept your assignment, ask your supervisor the following questions:

- What equipment is needed for the client's care?
- Who will obtain the needed equipment? Will the family buy it? Will the nurse bring it? Will it be delivered?

Are the necessary tools and equipment to keep the house clean available? Can they be borrowed from neighbors? Will the family purchase the needed equipment?

You may be asked to work with the supplies that are already in the client's home instead of purchasing new ones. In many cases you will have to improvise by using an item for a task for which it was not originally designed. An example of an improvisation is the use of a tablecloth as a draw sheet on a bed. It is important to take good care of the client's equipment. Families often judge your attitude toward them by the way in which you care for their belongings. Respect for their possessions indicates your respect for them as people.

Think through your tasks before you do them. This exercise allows you to note the items you will need for a particular job. In this way you will be able to assemble all the needed equipment before you start a job and not have to stop in the middle of it to get the required tools. By planning your work and the supplies you need, you save your energy and decrease the number of times you leave the client in the middle of a procedure.

If you find that the needed supplies to care properly for your client and his home are not available, discuss your needs with your supervisor and arrangements will be made.

## WHAT YOU WILL DO IN YOUR JOB

When you have finished your training, you will be able to:

- Report useful information objectively to your supervisor.
- Assist clients with personal care, toileting, and grooming.
- Make a bed and keep the client's environment clean, orderly, and safe.
- Assist with various phases of rehabilitation, such as positioning, ambulation, therapeutic exercises, and learning household tasks.
- Understand people's basic needs including the client's and his family's.
- Understand the needs of clients with various diagnoses and the impact on their families. Some groups you will discuss in class are cardiac, diabetic, geriatric, pediatric, and postpartum clients.
- Understand the needs of the dying client and his family.
- Measure vital signs.
- Assist the client with preparation of his therapeutic diet or nutritional supplements.
- Perform procedures, such as simple dressing changes; measure intake and output; and assist with the collection of specimens.
- Care for equipment necessary for the client's well-being and safety.
- Give basic care in an emergency.

## MOST EFFECTIVE QUALITIES TO SUCCEED

You have decided that you want to be the best! You want to do the best possible job. What kind of person makes a good homemaker/home health aide? Certain traits, attitudes, and habits are often seen in people who are successful in the health care field. Some of these traits are built into one's personality. This means you have had them since you were young. Other traits can be learned through practice. Then they become part of one's improved personality.

Read through this list, review those qualities you have already, and then check those you think you could learn and use in your work and personal life.

- ✓ You are a person who can be trusted.
- ✓ You are a person upon whom others can depend.
- ✓ You enjoy working with others.
- ✓ You get along well with others.
- ✓ You are sensitive to the feelings and needs of others.
- ✓ You are a good listener.
- ✓ You try to be courteous.
- ✓ You get satisfaction from helping others.
- ✓ You show sympathy and patience with others.
- ✓ You always try to control your temper.
- ✓ You believe you are doing important work.
- ✓ You want to improve your skills.
- ✓ You try not to let your private life interfere with your work.
- ✓ You do not discuss your personal problems while at work.
- ✓ You maintain client confidentiality.
- ✓ You are comfortable meeting and working with people from cultures different than yours.

### Dependability

Your agency is organized to function efficiently when a certain number of people are on the job. If you are not there, a client may be deprived of needed care. Your absence may cause your fellow workers to have an overload of work. It is very important that you arrive promptly every day, unless you are ill. If you are sick, call your office as you have been instructed by your agency. Your clients can then be assigned to another homemaker/home health aide.

Dependability means more than coming to work every day and coming in on time. It means that your supervisor can rely on you to do things at the proper time and in the proper way.

### Accuracy

As part of the health care team you will be concerned with human lives and feelings. What might appear to you to be a tiny mistake or oversight could affect the recovery of your client.

It is important for you to follow your supervisor's instructions exactly. Be accurate when you are recording a temperature. Be careful in making a bed. If you make a mistake, report it. If you do not understand something, ask again. Always remember: There is a reason for every step of the client's care.

### Following Directions

Everybody follows instructions and goes by rules. Otherwise, jobs would never get done. Even supervisors and administrators have rules to follow. These rules—policies and protocols—are made to give everyone guidelines for their work. They are made up with professional, ethical, legal, and practical relationships in mind. If you do not understand a rule or protocol, ask!

Here are some good rules to remember in your work. They can help to make you a better homemaker/home health aide and can help you in your relationships with your fellow health care workers.

- Be accurate to the best of your ability.
- Follow carefully the instructions of your supervisor.
- If you do not understand something, ask your supervisor.
- Report accidents or errors immediately to your supervisor.
- Keep information about clients to yourself, except when it might affect the client's health.
- Do not waste supplies and equipment.
- Be ready to adjust quickly to new situations.
- Try to get things done on time—use a systematic work schedule.
- Report all complaints, no matter how small, to your supervisor.
- Perform all your duties in a spirit of cooperation.

## ETHICS

**ethics** system of moral behavior and beliefs

**Ethics** is a code of rules set up to govern behavior. Although homemakers/home health aides do not take an oath of ethics as nurses and doctors do, it is assumed they will work within an accepted set of rules (Fig. 1.2).

- Do your job correctly to the best of your ability. This means you should ask for assistance when you are unable to do an assignment correctly.
- Be honest with your clients and their families.
- Respect the rights of clients and their families.
- Do not discuss your personal problems with clients.
- Honor the responsibility of the agency that employs you.
- Do not discuss client information with relatives or friends of the client, with fellow workers except when it is client related, or with your family.
- Do not discuss one client with another client.

---

**DO NOT DISCUSS CLIENT INFORMATION WITH**

- One client about another client
- Relatives and friends of the client
- Representatives of news media
- Fellow workers, except when in conference
- Your own relatives and friends

---

FIGURE 1.2 Confidentiality is an important part of client care.

## LEGAL CONSIDERATIONS

Laws concerning clients and workers in the health care system are written to protect both the client and the worker. Each state has its own laws governing which procedures a homemaker/home health aide may and may not do. You should be familiar with the laws and how they affect you and the clients under your care. Clients must be cared for properly and within the law. When you accept this job, you also accept this responsibility.

The agency that employs you assumes the legal responsibility for your actions as long as you work within its guidelines. It is your duty to know what tasks you have been assigned and to carry them out according to instructions. If you have any questions, ask! If you are in doubt as to what to do, report the situation to your supervisor. It then becomes your supervisor's responsibility to interpret the situation and tell you what to do.

Your agency has policies and procedures to guide you and your coworkers in your jobs. They are written to give everyone the same framework for work. When you come to work, you agree to live by these policies and procedures. If you do not agree with them, discuss this with your supervisor, but do not just ignore the rules. If you do not follow the policies, you leave your agency and yourself open for question by the client, the doctor and, if something unplanned happens, the law.

Negligence is a legal term meaning the failure to give proper care, when you know how to do so, which results in physical or emotional harm to the client. Your agency will discuss with you how to protect yourself from any question of negligence.

### INCIDENTS

An incident is an event that does not fit the daily routine of the home or agency where you are working. It may be an accident or an unusual happening. Types of incidents are:

- Client, visitor, or employee accidents
- Accidents that happen to you any time while you are on the job
- Accidents occurring on the outlying property of the client's home, such as sidewalks, parking lots, or entrances

Whenever an incident occurs, a report must be made (Fig 1.3). Careful, prompt reporting is important to the safety program of the agency and for the protection of all health care workers. For the agency to be prepared for possible liability suits or damage claims, report promptly all facts related to any incident or accident.

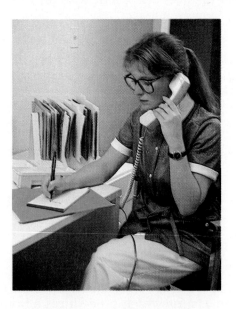

**FIGURE 1.3** Reporting incidents protects you, the client, and your employing agency.

### PERSONAL PRACTICES

All members of the home health team are teachers by the example they set. They influence each other, their clients and their families. The practice of good personal hygiene becomes a teaching tool (Fig. 1.4). Remember:

- Dress properly and neatly. Follow the dress code of the home health care agency where you work.
- Bathe daily.
- Use an unscented deodorant.
- Keep your mouth and teeth clean and in good condition.
- Keep your hair clean and neat.
- Wear clean clothes every day.
- Wear comfortable low-heeled shoes with nonskid soles and heels.
- Repair rips and replace missing buttons on your clothing.
- Do not wear jewelry such as earrings, bracelets, pendants, or large rings.
- Keep your nails short and clean.
- Wear conservative makeup.
- Do not use perfume or scented sprays.
- Keep yourself in good health by eating properly.
- Get plenty of sleep—be alert when you come to work.
- Polish your shoes—be sure the laces are clean.
- Always wear your name pin and agency badge.
- Always wear a wristwatch with a second hand.
- Always carry a pen and a pad of paper.

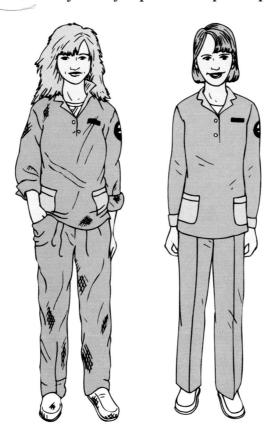

*FIGURE 1.4* Taking pride in your appearance says you respect yourself and those with whom you come in contact.

![bar] *Topics for Discussion*

1. You are working with a person who displays qualities you feel are inappropriate in the work setting. What do you do?
2. A fellow worker who is late all the time asks you to falsify her time sheet. What do you do?

3. The client tells you that his usual doctor is not covered by his insurance company and that is the reason he does not follow up with physician visits. What do you do?
4. The insurance company telephones and asks you questions about the client's condition and his ability to be alone. What do you answer?

# Chapter 2

# Communication Skills

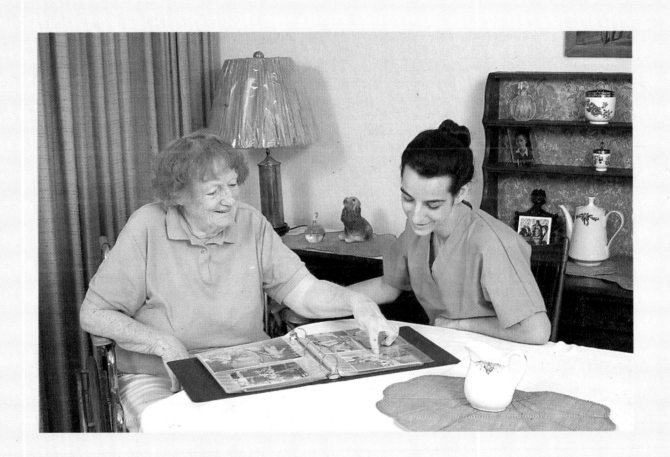

| Objectives: What You Will Learn to Do | ■ Know what is meant by communication. |
|---|---|
| | ■ Recognize the three basic ways of communicating. |
| | ■ Become aware of what we communicate. |
| | ■ Become familiar with the basic rules of communication. |

## *Introduction: Communication*

**communication** exchange of information

**Communication** means exchanging information with others. We exchange information about feelings, opinions, or facts. People let others know how they feel or what they want all day and even during the night. You can tell if your friend, supervisor, or client is happy, in pain, sad, or bored. And they can tell the same about you. You can tell if a sleeping client is in pain or resting comfortably. Communication takes place in several ways: through verbal exchange, through written words, and through body language or nonverbal methods. Communication is necessary so that people can function together—in other words, so they can "get along." Developing the ability to get along with people—clients, visitors, fellow workers—is a very important part of your job. Being a good communicator is a basic activity in your job.

When you work in people's homes, they often ask your opinion. If you are not sure or you think your opinion will be upsetting to the client, you might say, "This is your house and here it is more important how you feel about this situation than how I feel."

### VERBAL COMMUNICATION

Verbal communication is the exchange of ideas or information through the spoken word. When your supervisor tells you about an assignment or you say, "Good morning" to your client, that is verbal communication. The tone of your voice, the speed at which you speak, your inflection, and your actual choice of words are all part of the verbal picture you paint as you speak.

### WRITTEN COMMUNICATION

Anytime you write or draw, you are communicating through writing. Each time a nurse leaves instructions for you in a home or you write a note describing your activities with a client, you are exchanging facts. The way in which you write tells a great deal about you and how you feel about the subject and your activity. The neatness, the legibility, the choice of words, and how you give the written work to the reader sets the scene for how it is received.

### NONVERBAL COMMUNICATION

**body language** gestures that function as a form of communication

People have many ways of telling each other how they feel, that is, if they are happy or sad to be in a certain place or if they are doing a task willingly or unwillingly. One way is by saying what we feel. The other way is with our body. This is called **body language** (Fig. 2.1). No words are spoken, but the message is given and received by others.

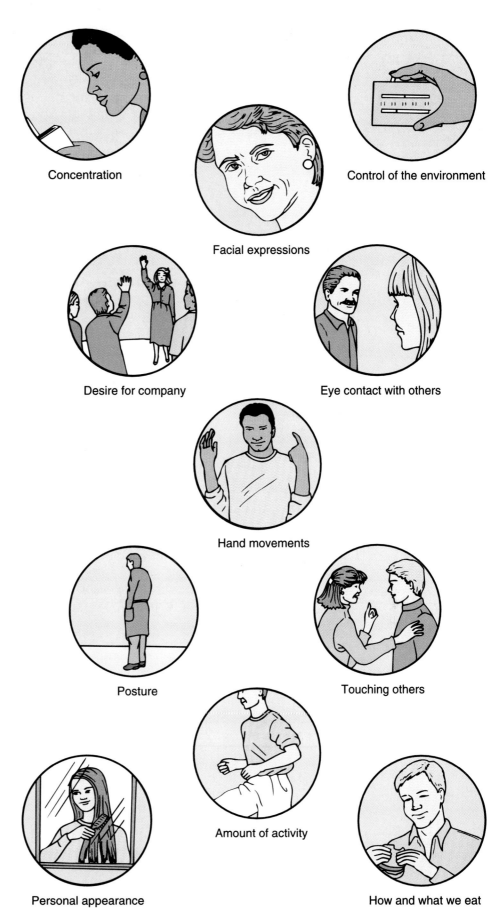

**FIGURE 2.1** Body language gives silent clues to others about how you feel and what you want other people to do.

Concentration

Facial expressions

Control of the environment

Desire for company

Eye contact with others

Hand movements

Posture

Touching others

Personal appearance

Amount of activity

How and what we eat

As a homemaker/home health aide, you will notice clues and other signals that tell how a client feels. These signs will tell you a great deal about the client and the care you are giving. Report your observations accurately to your supervisor so that she can help you interpret them and plan the client's care accordingly.

Be alert to your body language! Your client will know how you feel about giving him care by the way you carry yourself and interact with him.

## ANSWERING WHEN THE CLIENT CALLS

Every client needs a way to signal to other people. You will have to devise a system for your client to call you. A hand bell, a stick used to bang on the bed or the floor, or a voice signal are possible methods of communication. Use whatever method is most appropriate in the house where you are working. By giving the client a way to call for assistance, he will feel he is participating in his own care. He will know he is not alone and helpless.

Answer the client's call as soon as you hear it. Every minute seems like an hour to the person waiting. When the client signals, go to the client and ask him what he would like. Do what he asks as long as it is correct and safe. If you are not sure, call your supervisor and discuss the situation.

## BASIC RULES FOR COMMUNICATING

### Be a Nonjudgmental Observer and Listener

**nonjudgmental** accepting communication without stating a personal opinion

It is important to learn to receive information in a **nonjudgmental** way; that is, in an accepting manner without expressing your opinions. It is necessary that you develop the skill of recognizing when your opinion is important and when you should not express your judgment but rather, be nonjudgmental. Often a client, family member, or coworker wants to express an opinion and have it accepted rather than have it commented upon. Often a person wants to be accepted for the way he looks without comment or change (Fig. 2.2).

### Be a Careful Listener

Always listen when someone speaks to you. Listen to what the person says. Listen to what information is left out of the conversation. Listen for the tone of voice of the speaker and his breathing pattern. Is it fast? Is it slow and slurred? Does it make sense? Is it appropriate to ask questions? Listen to what the speaker says, not what you think he says (Fig. 2.3).

Sometimes it is helpful to write down important information as you hear it. Do not always trust your memory.

### Be Sensitive

There are times when the client does not want to talk. Respect his moods. At times, saying nothing may have more meaning than any words or facial expressions on your part. Sometimes a pat on the shoulder or hand means more to a client than anything you could say. Simply being near the client in a moment of trouble may be the most comforting message of all.

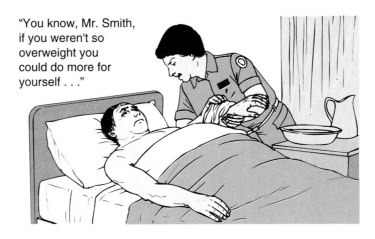

"You know, Mr. Smith, if you weren't so overweight you could do more for yourself . . ."

*FIGURE 2.2* Present your ideas in a nonjudgmental way so as not to offend your client.

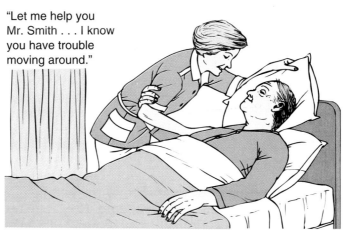

"Let me help you Mr. Smith . . . I know you have trouble moving around."

*FIGURE 2.3* Listen and observe carefully as people speak. Be sensitive to what is said and what is not said.

**TO RELATE AND COMMUNICATE WITH PEOPLE YOU MUST:**

• Be courteous

• Be emotionally in control

• Be tactful

• Be a nonjudgmental listener

• Be a careful, nonjudgmental observer

### Be Courteous

Courtesy means being polite and considerate and cooperating with others. You should be courteous at all times. Never be critical or impolite in your contacts with clients. If you feel like being impolite, try to understand why you are feeling or acting the way you are. By reviewing the situation, you may be able to prevent it from happening again.

Courtesy is important in your relationships with your fellow workers. Your supervisor and instructors will be giving you advice and directions. Your coworkers will be sharing information with you. Show them you are willing to hear what they have to say.

If you are not clear as to what you have heard, you can summarize what you *think* you heard and ask the speaker if that is so. For example, "I heard you say that John was going to the store, then coming home and fixing you dinner before he went to the doctor's. Is that correct?"

When the speaker is talking and you have nothing to add, but you think the speaker is not really clearly communicating to you, you could try a technique called reflection. This allows the client to know what you see and provides an opportunity for him to clarify it. For example, "You seem in pain today." "I'm not, but it is cold in here."

## EMOTIONAL CONTROL

Sometimes a client or a visitor can upset you. You feel like making a rude or nasty remark. Don't do it! Remember that the client is worried about himself, his illness, his family, or his job.

Sometimes a client will be rude or difficult. Often the client is unable to determine exactly what is causing him to feel badly and act in a difficult or unpleasant manner. Tell him you know that he has many things on his mind. Offer to listen to him or get another member of the health care team to listen to his problem.

The stress level of a client or members of the family may affect their ability to communicate and listen. Be sensitive to this. Speak in simple terms. Do not be upset if you have to repeat yourself several times. Be understanding if the client or family member repeats himself too.

Learn to take constructive criticism and accept suggestions from your supervisor and coworkers. You may get angry when somebody tells you that you are wrong. But, remember, your supervisor and your coworkers want to help you give the best possible care. If you do not agree with what is said to you, answer in a polite, courteous manner. Discuss the criticism, not the person who is giving it.

### Tact

**tact** knowing the proper thing to say; a sensitive skill in dealing with people

Try to be as tactful as you can. **Tact** means doing and saying the right thing at the right time. Before you make a remark to a client or his family, think! Is this the right time? Is this the right word to use? Think! Do not speak within hearing distance of the client if you do not want him to hear you, even if you think he is asleep, under the influence of medication, or unconscious.

## RELATIONSHIPS WITH CLIENTS

You are very important to the client and his family. You may spend more time with the client than does any other member of the health team. You perform necessary personal tasks that permit the client to remain at home in a safe, comfortable, clean environment. Clients and their families come to depend on you and share their feelings and thoughts. Often you are the only person a client will see all day.

Always listen. Be a good listener. Listen to what the speaker says and what he does not say. Listen to the way he says it. Always listen when a client makes a complaint or brings up a problem. The client may ask you a question about his doctor or his diagnosis. Do not lie to the client! Do not tell him you do not know when you should be aware of the information. If you lie, the client may find out and never trust you again. It is no shame to say you do not have the information readily at hand. But if you say you do not know, you close the conversation. Tell the client you will get him an answer. Then call and talk to your supervisor. Plan an answer with her. When you promise to get an answer for a client, do it! Do not go back on your word!

## Family and Visitors

Visitors are often the highlight of the day for clients who must remain at home. A client usually feels better when he knows his family and friends are concerned and make the effort to see him.

Visitors, however, may be worried and upset over the illness of your client. They, too, need kindness and patience. Pleasant comments, privacy, and polite, efficient manners are the things that will make them feel at ease.

If it appears that visitors are upsetting or tiring your client, you may have to point this out tactfully and suggest that the client rest. Remember, you are in the house to care for the client, not to wait on or socialize with the visitors. If they leave a mess or dirty dishes and expect you to clean up, speak to your supervisor. The two of you can find ways to deal with this situation.

You will find the following hints helpful to remember:

- Listen to the visitors and family members. Whether it is a suggestion, a complaint, or "passing the time of day," listen. Some suggestions by visitors can be very helpful. Some complaints may be valid, others not. When a complaint is first presented, you probably will want to get more information. You might ask, "Where did this happen?" or "What did you do?" Offer to report the problem to your supervisor, and then do so.

- Try not to get involved in family affairs. Never take sides in a family quarrel.

- If visitors have questions you cannot answer or you are not sure you should answer, tell them you will get the information. Then contact your supervisor. You also may want to discuss these questions with your client to be sure he wants the information given to his visitors.

- If a visitor or family member asks how he may help, give some suggestions.

- Visitors may arrive at the house and give you orders: "While I'm here to watch Mama, you clean the bathroom." Be open about your responsibilities. Explain that your supervisor sets up the plan of care and that you will discuss all changes with her.

- Report the role family and visitors play in the life of your client. It is important to use the talents and energy of family and friends in setting up a plan of care. Often these family members will have to assume the client's care when you are out of the house. Therefore, the more comfortable they feel with the care and the more they know, the better your client will feel when you are gone.

- Report changes in the family function, relationships, and roles both as you observe them and as the client relates them.

# Section 2 Client Observation, Recording, and Reporting

## Objectives: What You Will Learn to Do

- Use your senses of sight, touch, hearing, and smell to observe your clients.
- List some of the observations you will make and when you will report them.
- Demonstrate the difference between subjective and objective reporting.
- Discuss the importance of reporting your observations.

### Introduction: Observing, Reporting, and Recording Your Observations

**observation** gathering information about a client

Get into the habit of observing the client during all your contacts with him. These contacts include bathing, bed making, mealtimes, and any other time that you are with a client. Observation of the client is a continuous process. Observing begins the first time you see a client. **Observation** means more than just careful watching. It includes listening to the client, talking to him, and asking questions. Be extra alert to any unusual things when you are with a client. Changes in the client's condition or appearance are most important. Watch also for changes in the client's attitude or moods and the way in which he interacts with other people. Pay attention to complaints of pain or discomfort or to complaints that do not seem to have a reason. Be alert when the client relates events that took place in your absence. Observation of the client's family and friends is also important and may have great implications for the client's future care.

You are the health care team worker who will spend the most time with the client. You will often be the first to notice a change in the client's condition. This change may be for the better, or it may indicate a worsening of his condition. Observations are useful only if they contribute to the total care of the client. Therefore, it is an important part of your job to report these changes to your supervisor. Then the client's total care plan can be revised.

#### METHODS OF OBSERVATION

Use all of your senses when making observations:

- You can see some signs of change in a client's condition. By using your eyes, for example, you can observe a skin rash or swelling of the feet.
- You can feel some signs with your finger—a change in the client's pulse rate, puffiness in the skin, skin temperature.
- You can hear some signs, such as a cough or wheezing sounds when the client breathes.
- You can smell some signs, such as an odor in the client's urine.
- Listen to the client talking for other changes in his condition. Some changes can be felt and described only by the client himself. Examples are pain, nausea, dizziness, a ringing in the ears, or a headache.

Making useful observations is one of the most important things you will do in your work. Learning how to make useful observations will give you great satisfaction (Fig. 2.4).

**OBSERVATION**

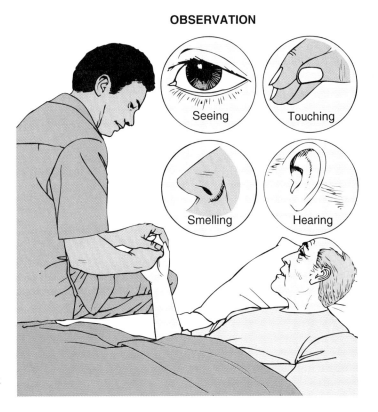

FIGURE 2.4 Use all your senses as you observe and report your client's condition.

You learn by doing. Health care team workers never stop learning more about observing clients and about how to use the information to continually improve the care of clients.

The following chart is a summary of general observations you will make every day with every client. The method of recording and reporting of these observations varies from agency to agency. It is your responsibility to be familiar with the recording and reporting system in use in your agency.

## General Client Observations

| Body Area | Observations |
| --- | --- |
| General appearance | Has it changed? If so, in what way? Is there a noticeable odor or smell in the client's room? Does he always complain about the heat or cold? |
| General mood | Describe the client's actions rather than your interpretation of them. "The client threw a shoe at her daughter" rather than "The client was angry at her daughter." Has it changed? Does he talk a lot or very little? Does he make sense? Can he report things to you accurately? Does he hallucinate (see or hear things)? Is he oriented (know where he is, who he is, and who you are)? Is he anxious, calm, excited, or worried? Does he talk about pain? Does he speak rapidly or slowly? Does he look at you when he speaks? Can he be understood when he speaks? Can he remember? Is he confused or forgetful? |
| Sleeping habits | Have these changed? Is he a quiet or restless sleeper? Does he complain about lack of sleep? Does his report agree with your observations? How many pillows does he sleep with? How much does he sleep? |
| Pain | Where is the pain? How long does the client say he has had it? Is it new pain? How does he describe it? Is it constant? Does it come and go? Is it sharp, dull, or aching? |

| Body Area | Observations |
|---|---|
| | Has he had medicine for the pain? Does the client say that the medicine relieves the pain? Is there any activity that brings on the pain? |
| Daily activities | Does the client dress himself? Does the client walk with or without help? What kind of help? |
| Personal care | Can the client bathe himself? Can the client brush his teeth, comb his hair, go to the bathroom, or wash his face? Does he ask for assistance? |
| Movements | Does the client limp? |
| Skeletal system | Pain, limited movement, swelling in joints, warm tender joints, unusual positioning of any body part, redness in joints |
| Muscular system | Painful movement, swelling, limited movement, color of skin over painful areas. Does he lie still? Does he change position frequently? What is his favorite position? |
| Skin | Temperature, texture, moisture, bruises, healing of bruises, incision appearance, mouth condition. Has it changed? Is the client's skin unusually pale (pallor)? Is it flushed (red)? Are his lips or fingernails turning blue (cyanotic)? Is there any swelling (edema) noticeable? Are there reddened or tender areas? Where are they? Is the skin shiny? Is there any puffiness? |
| Circulatory system | Chest pain; swelling of fingers, toes, feet, ankles, around the eyes; pulse rate and quality; color of lips, nails, fingers, toes; headaches; pain in legs when walking |
| Respiratory system | Pain while breathing, rate and quality of respirations, cough, sputum (color and consistency), wheezing, shortness of breath, color of fingers and toes |
| Digestive system | Pain, appetite, flatus, vomiting (color of vomitus), feces (color, amount, frequency, odor), discomfort before or after eating. Can he control his bowels? Have his eating habits changed? Does he complain he has no appetite? Does he dislike his food? What and how much does he eat? Is he always thirsty? Does he seldom ask for fluids? Is it difficult for him to eat or swallow? |
| Nervous system | Painful areas of body, twitching, involuntary movement, inability to move, inability to feel stimuli  *seizures* |
| Urinary system | Pain during urination; ability to control his urine; urine color, odor, amount, frequency; blood in urine; pain in kidney area |
| Eyes | Pain, discharge, redness, sensitivity to light, vision change |
| Ears | Pain, discharge, hearing change |
| Nose | Pain, discharge, bleeding, smell |
| Female genitalia | Menstrual periods (frequency, amount of flow, pain), vaginal discharge (color, odor, amount), breasts (lumps), discharge, soreness, parasites, draining sores *signs of cancer* |
| Male genitalia | Pain, discharge, parasites, draining sores  *signs of prostate cancer* |

## Reporting

### OBJECTIVE AND SUBJECTIVE REPORTING

It is very important for you to understand the difference between objective reporting and subjective reporting.

**Subjective reporting** means giving your opinion about something or what you think might be the case. One might report, for example, what he or she thinks is the cause of a change in a client's condition or what might be the proper treatment. When you report your opinion to your supervisor, be sure you say it is your opinion. Your opinion could be very important to the care of your client. An example of subjective reporting would be: "Yesterday, Mrs. C. and her landlady were talking in loud voices. I just know they were fighting."

**subjective reporting** giving your opinion about what you have observed

**Objective reporting** means reporting exactly what you observe— that is, reporting what you see, hear, feel, or smell. The homemaker/home health aide must always use objective reporting unless it is clear that the information is an opinion.

Here are some examples of objective reporting:

1. Mrs. Smith's breathing has changed since yesterday. She is breathing 20 times a minute and complaining of chest pain. Yesterday she had no pain and her respirations were 12 per minute.
2. Cindy Jones says that she has a pain in her right upper abdomen.
3. Every time John takes the pain pill, he gets very quiet and then says that he sees horses on the ceiling.

## WHEN DO YOU REPORT?

Each agency has a protocol for homemaker/home health care aides to communicate with their supervisor. It is your responsibility to be familiar with this protocol and use it (Fig. 2.5).

Is it by telephone? By calling the correct phone number and asking for the correct person, you will save time for yourself, the client, and the person in the agency. Is it by mail? By sending the correct information to the right person, you will save time and postage. You may be expected to make specific observations at a specific time of day. Be sure you know what to do with the information you collect.

## WHAT DO YOU REPORT?

The importance of reporting the proper information at the proper time cannot be overemphasized. Each agency has a policy as to what a homemaker/home health care aide reports in writing and what is reported verbally. There are two types of client information:

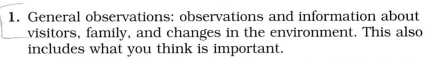

- Is there a special time for me to call the office?
- Is there a special telephone number to call to reach my supervisor?
- If my supervisor is not in the office, who can help me?
- Can I call from the client's home? If not, where is the nearest telephone?
- What information does the agency give by telephone, and what is given in writing?

**FIGURE 2.5** Know what to report, when to report, and to whom to report.

1. General observations: observations and information about visitors, family, and changes in the environment. This also includes what you think is important.

   EXAMPLE: Mrs. Jones's sister came to visit for the first time. She had an opinion about everything we did and the client did. Mrs. Jones couldn't explain why we had set up the routine the way we did. Mrs. Jones started to cry.

Before her sister left, she promised to come back with another doctor's opinion. Mrs. Jones said she always takes over and tries to change things. I have never seen the client in this state.

2. Specific information: Observations of particular client behavior or changes. The supervisor will discuss this type of observation with you. She will explain to you what information is needed and when.

> EXAMPLE: When I changed Mrs. Brown's nightgown, I noticed some blood on the sleeve. I asked her where this came from, and she said, "Oh, you know how it is, I hit my hand." Then she pulled her hand away and said, "I don't think you have to report this." This was the first time this happened. She seemed upset. I can't figure out why.

With one client the reaction to medication may be important, but with another client, mental alertness may be the most important observation. Ask your supervisor if there are any particular observations that are important for you to note. In addition to any specific information, you will always report the total client picture.

## Guidelines for Reporting and Recording

When you take an assignment, be sure that you know (Fig. 2.5):

- To whom to report
- Any specific observations members of the health care team need
- The basic observations you should always be aware of as you interact with the client
- What types of information must be written and what should be reported verbally
- If you need to know about the client's condition, ask.

Although each client is different and you will be reporting different observations, there are basic guidelines to be used in all your reporting and recording.

- Be sure about your information.
- Obtain complete information.
- Report objectively. When reporting subjectively, say so.
- Reporting and recording objective observations is important to protect the client and enable the health care team to deliver the best care possible.
- Reporting and recording objective observations protects you from being held responsible for a possible mistake.
- Report all changes in a client's condition.
- Report the events in the order in which they occurred. Include the persons present at the event.
- When reporting, report the condition of both sides of the body— "the left leg is cooler than the right leg."
- Report and record quietly and calmly.
- Report and record soon after the event. You will forget details if you do not write them down.

*basic*
*guidelines*

## Objectives: What You Will Learn to Do

- List five reasons for differences in people's learning.
- Recognize the differences between an adult learner and a child learner.
- Become familiar with your role in the teaching process.

### *Introduction: Teaching Clients*

Teaching clients is an important part of your job. You will teach clients by example, by discussion, or by taking part in activities with the client. You will teach them new skills, help them relearn old skills, and help them gain independence in as many activities as possible. Everybody learns differently, and therefore, you must have a teaching plan individualized to meet their needs. It is necessary for you to be familiar with the teaching plan that your supervisor has established for your client. If you are not sure about your role, ask!

### REASONS FOR DIFFERENCES IN LEARNING

As your supervisor individualizes the client's teaching plan, the following factors will be taken into consideration:

- Past life experiences
- Disease process
- Motivation for learning
- Family dynamics
- Past experiences with learning
- General abilities
- Teaching skills of teacher
- Age

Your supervisor will also teach children differently than adults. Adults can often read some material and then discuss it. They can practice skills on their own. They can also often clearly relate learning a skill to achieving a certain outcome. For example, an adult who understands the reasons for keeping or maintaining a special diet will learn how to cook, how to shop, and how to prepare special foods because he can understand that, if this diet is not kept, he will become ill. A child, however, may not be able to think about the future and relate the activity of eating to the deterioration of his general physical condition. So, even though the outcome will be the same—learning the diet, the teaching method will be different.

### POINTS TO REMEMBER WHEN TEACHING A CLIENT

- Be sure the client is paying attention and is not distracted by TV, a visitor, or other activities (Fig. 2.6).
- Be sure the client wants to learn.
- Be sure you are familiar with the material you will teach him. Do not try to teach something you do not understand.
- Relate the teaching to the client. Do not tell him the skill will help him become a faster runner if he has no interest in running.

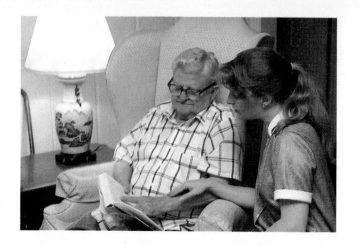

**FIGURE 2.6** A quiet comfortable atmosphere is needed for you to teach and for the client to learn.

■ Speak slowly and clearly—not baby talk, but in words the client can understand.

■ Be able to tell the client the reasons you are doing each step. This will help him understand that it is important to follow your example. It will also assure him that you are not wasting energy or time.

■ Do not try to teach too much at once. Everyone has a different attention span. People who are ill or who are taking certain medication often find it hard to concentrate for long periods. Plan your teaching in small sections.

■ Teach at the time of day most convenient for the client. Some people learn better in the morning, some in the afternoon. Whenever possible, ask the client which he prefers.

■ Use written material so the client will have something to refer to when you are gone.

■ Do not lose patience when you must repeat yourself or show him an activity many times. When the client demonstrates the skill to you, praise him and discuss the positive part of the demonstration before you show him the corrections.

## Topics for Discussion

1. Describe a recent situation. Then write down whether you received your information through verbal, written, or nonverbal communication.

2. Observe a client or a classmate role playing as a client. Write down your observations. Describe which observations you would report and which ones you would not. Why?

3. Report an incident that happened to you yesterday. Do so in a subjective way and in an objective way. Which type of reporting is more appropriate for your situation?

4. Ask classmates how they learn best. Are these the same ways you learn? What are some activities that may affect the way a client communicates? What are some things that may affect the way a client or family members listen? Are you affected by these things too?

5. What effect may improper dress have on the client? On the family? On the way in which you work?

# Chapter 3

# Working with People

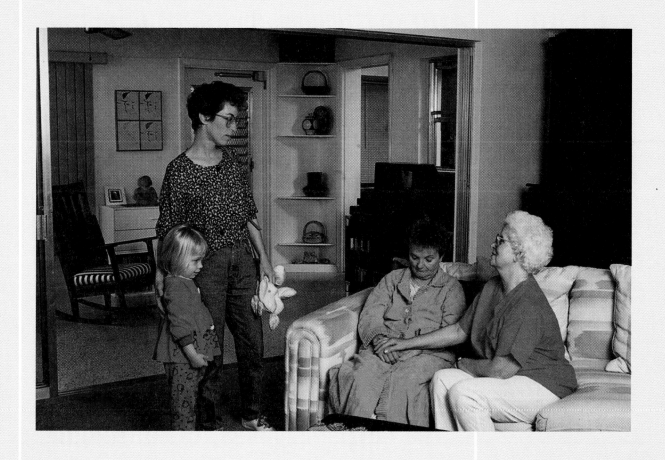

**Objectives: What You Will Learn to Do**

- List the physical needs shared by all human beings.
- List the psychological needs shared by all human beings.
- Distinguish between the needs of the client, the family, and the caregiver.
- Describe actions you can take to meet the basic needs of the client and his family.
- Become aware of behavior that results when basic human needs are not met.
- Describe your role in helping to manage the pain of patients.

## Introduction: Basic Needs

**need** a lack of something

Every person has certain basic needs that must be met so that he can survive. A **need** is a requirement for survival. Sometimes an individual can satisfy his needs himself, and sometimes he requires help. When a person becomes your client, it means he is unable to satisfy all his needs himself. (For example, a person may need help with his meals or he will not be able to meet his need for nourishment.) As a homemaker/home health aide you will help your client meet some of his most basic needs until he is able to meet them without your help.

It is important—and often difficult—to be sure the actions of the health care team are meeting the client's needs. Your knowledge of these needs and your objective observations, will help your supervisor determine whether all the needs in a particular home are being met by the plan of care.

### BASIC PHYSICAL AND PSYCHOLOGICAL NEEDS

All human beings have basic physical needs that must be met in order to live. These needs do not all have to be met completely each day, but the more each person's needs are fulfilled, the better the quality of life (Fig. 3.1).

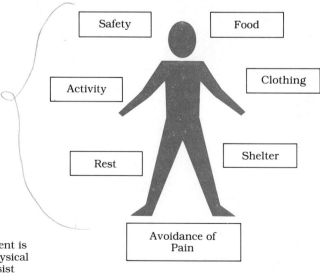

**FIGURE 3.1** When a client is unable to meet his own physical needs, it is your role to assist him.

Safety | Food | Activity | Clothing | Rest | Shelter | Avoidance of Pain

**BASIC PHYSICAL NEEDS**

Psychological needs also must be satisfied to have a healthy emotional and social outlook. As with the physical needs, these do not have to be met totally each day. However, the more completely each need is met, the better the person's emotional state will be. Needs can be met by family, by self, or by someone who is not a family member but is available on an intermittent basis (Fig. 3.2).

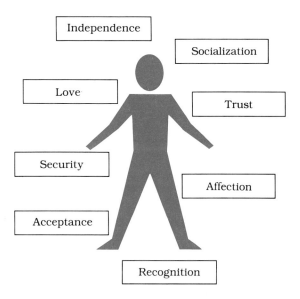

Independence

Socialization

Love

Trust

Security

Affection

Acceptance

Recognition

**BASIC PSYCHOLOGICAL NEEDS**

*FIGURE 3.2* Helping a client meet his psychological needs assists him with living and functioning within his environment.

## BALANCING NEEDS

The needs of children are usually met by family members. During adult years, most people are expected to meet some or most of their own needs. All of these physical and psychological needs overlap and affect each other. Each person determines his own particular balance. When one need is out of balance due to illness, the other needs are also affected. For example, when a person is ill and requires more rest, his food intake must be changed to meet this change in activity. His clothing will change. His weight may change, and his mood may alter. The client is often the one who knows how to restore balance. In this case the client might determine when to eat and what foods to decrease so that he does not gain weight. By consulting the client, you will be more apt to meet actual needs and not guess what they are. Needs can change, so be alert (Fig. 3.3).

Many things can change a client's behavior and attitude during an illness. The client may be frightened, angry, or sad. Some factors or influences may be the diagnosis, seriousness of the illness, age, previous illness, experience, and mental condition. Other things that can make a difference are the client's personality, financial situation, and family relationships.

Each client has different reactions to pain, treatment annoyances, and even kindness. Always treat a person as an individual. Do not compare one client to another. Practice consideration on an individual basis. Encourage the client to take an active part in setting the balance between his activities and his basic physical needs. All behavior has meaning. If you observe a behavior that you do not understand, discuss this with your supervisor. If you notice a change in behavior, report it.

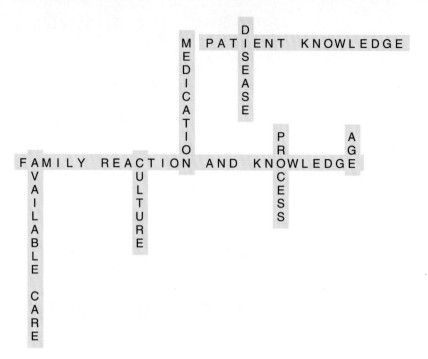

**FIGURE 3.3** The interaction and balancing of many elements provides the background for meeting a client's needs.

## NEEDS YOU HAVE AS A HOMEMAKER/HOME HEALTH AIDE

Homemaker/home health aides have the same basic needs as their clients. It is important that your needs be met, too, but not at the expense of your client's. There are many times your needs will have to be put aside until you leave the client. Discuss with your supervisor both your client's needs and yours. Then a plan will be made so that the needs of the client will be satisfied and you will not feel slighted. Caregivers must be alert to the reasons they do and say things. As you are caring for your clients, be alert and try to identify what basic need you are satisfying and whose it is. Ask yourself these questions:

■ Are you acting because the client's needs must be met or because your needs must be met? For example: Are you giving the client a bath because he will feel better or because you will feel better having done it?

■ Do you perform a procedure with the client because he enjoys having you help him and shows improvement, or because you feel that you must do it?

■ Does helping a client become independent, so he no longer needs your help, make you feel good or useless?

### UNMET NEEDS

When basic needs are not met, human beings show some reaction. If a physical need is not met, the reaction is usually obvious; for example, if the need for food is not met, the person might become irritable or weak. If an emotional need is not met, a person's reactions may be feelings of anxiety, depression, aggression, anger, or a physical ailment without apparent cause.

You will not always be able to decide why a client acts in a certain manner. That is all right. It is necessary, however, for you to report these actions to your supervisor. Often by reviewing client's actions, your supervisor will be able to determine if a need is going unmet. Then, by altering the plan of care, the need will be fulfilled and the behavior changed.

## PAIN

The word *pain* means different things to different people. What is painful to one person may not be to another. It is important to find out how your client reacts to pain and how his family views pain. Many people think that pain is normal and must be tolerated; some feel it is a punishment; some do not want to complain; some people are afraid of medications; and some are afraid that, if they complain, their care-givers will leave them. Some people are afraid to discuss their pain with their physicians because they feel that if the physician could relieve the pain he would do so without asking.

Clients who are in pain are unable to participate in their care, relate to their families, or expend energy on the healing process. Clients who are in pain cannot have a good quality of life.

Pain causes many reactions. Some you can see, and some you cannot see. A client in pain may:

- Have a rapid pulse, shallow and rapid breathing
- Have increased fatigue
- Have increased anxiety
- Have increased stress
- Withdraw and decrease communication
- Decrease food and fluid intake
- Make faces and make gestures with his hands
- Moan and talk in baby talk and cry
- Demonstrate angry behavior

Different cultures treat pain in different ways. Some cultures may hang a charm near the bed; some may say special prayers; some may burn candles; and some may dress the client in special clothes. If these help the client, support the actions even though they may seem unusual to you. Some people do not want to take medication. They are afraid they will become addicted, be questioned by the authorities, or bring shame to their family and to themselves.

The health care team is becoming more and more aware of the many things that contribute to an individual response to pain. Medication is becoming more and more acceptable and available to clients at home who are in pain. When it is prescribed by a physician and given as it is prescribed, no one should be afraid to take it.

Your role as a homemaker/home health aide is to help the client and his family manage the pain. This can be done in many ways:

- Ask the client what usually decreases his pain. Do not change his routine!
- Talk to the client. Explain what you will do and how he may help.
- Allow the client to move at his own pace. Do not rush him.
- Support the medication schedule. Encourage the client to take medication before the pain becomes severe.
- Encourage the family to support the client as he deals with pain.

- Observe the client for any increase of pain. Alter your care accordingly.
- Report to your supervisor if the client's pain changes or if he does not respond to his medication.
- Encourage the client to share his feelings about his pain.
- Encourage the family to share their feelings about the client's pain, his reaction to it, and his medication regime.

# Section 2  Family

## Objectives: What You Will Learn to Do

- Define *family*.
- List the functions of a family.
- Recognize reasons that family structure and function are changing in today's society.
- Become aware of your role working within a family unit.
- Discuss the place of family in decision making.

### Introduction: Family

Most human beings live in some sort of family. It may be an extended family with several generations in the same house. It may be a single-parent family. It may be a unit made up of friends who live together and regard themselves as a family. Different cultures define family in different ways. In the broadest sense, a family is a unit bound together by common interests and working to maintain the well-being, and meet the needs, of all members (Fig. 3.4).

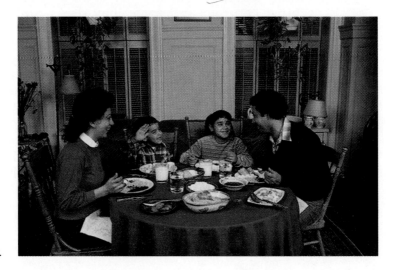

*FIGURE 3.4* Families provide stability, transmit culture, meet individual needs of its members, protect, and teach self-sufficiency.

### CHANGING FAMILY

About 75 years ago it was common to see families made up of several generations. Grandparents, maiden aunts, and orphaned children returned to the extended family home and were incorporated into the functioning family. Families were also bigger, with many more children. With all these members, necessary tasks were divided and everyone benefited. For example, a grandmother might have cared for the young children and folded all laundry. She would also have told family stories and transmitted the family's culture to the younger generation. The mother would have cooked, cleaned, and disciplined the older children. She taught the girls to sew and cook; the older children would have cared for the younger ones, played with them, and assisted with the household chores and caring for the sick. The boys would have worked outside and learned a trade from their father; the father of the household would have worked and earned for the family and provided leadership and protection.

Today, families have changed. Why?

- Families are smaller.
- Women go to work.
- Roles are not as carefully prescribed.
- Family members do not always live near each other.
- People live longer.
- The sick can be cared for in institutions.
- Society now assumes some of the care of the sick and elderly.

Each family has needs and rules of its own. As you enter a family to care for one of its members, you become aware how that family operates. Do they care for one another? Do they punish their members with violence? Do they speak lovingly to each other? Do they stop speaking to one member when they are angry? Do they tease members? As well as you can, it is your responsibility to work and care for your client within the framework of his family. If you change the client substantially and bring in too many new ideas, you will not be welcome and the client will no longer be welcome as a member of his family. Remember, when you leave, the client remains in his family and will have difficulty with the changes you taught him.

## CULTURE AND THE FAMILY

There are many factors that influence the functioning of families: the size, the economic resources, the needs of each member, and the culture of the members and the culture of the country in which they live. Sometimes a family functions within the rules of their native country, but lives in the United States. This may often cause a conflict between the roles of family members and the relationship and expectations of the health care team. The culture of the family has a great impact on their structure, their decision-making pattern, and their reaction to illness, pain, and healing. You will have to be sensitive to these issues as they will affect your client. If you do not understand certain actions or decisions or feel that some actions are not helping your client, discuss this with your supervisor.

## FAMILY MEMBERS AND THEIR ROLES

A role is the part a person has in his family or situation. Each member of a family has a role. Sometimes these roles are learned from older members of the family; sometimes, if there is no role model, the role must be shaped to the best of the person's ability. Family members may each have several roles; for example, a woman may be a mother, daughter, wife, or grandmother. Each role demands different behavior and a different set of responsibilities. The important point is to balance these roles so none of them come into conflict with the others. This is very difficult and often impossible to do. Family members who have difficulty balancing roles often need professional help to accomplish this task. In some families, the male makes decisions; in some families the mother-in-law makes the decisions. In some families, children are important, educated, and cared for, and in others, they are seen as a member of the workforce at a young age.

## GENERATION IN THE MIDDLE

In many homes you may recognize a family situation called "the generation in the middle." This is a woman about forty-five to fifty years old who has the responsibility of caring for her mother or father, who is seventy to seventy-five years old, and of being mother to her own children, who are often teenagers. She may also work and have a husband. This generation is often in need of special understanding and assistance, for they must always balance the needs of others in addition to trying to meet their own needs. In this special situation, as in others, it is important to try to understand the family dynamics and work to maintain them so all members can survive without hurting one another (Fig. 3.5).

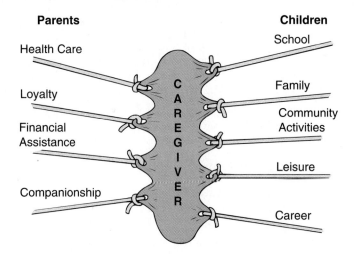

**FIGURE 3.5** Women find themselves in several roles and balancing several sets of demands on their time and their emotions.

## ECONOMICS

All families have some money. All families spend their money according to their own rules and beliefs. Many families will spend on things of which you personally do not approve. You will often find yourself being asked by one family member or another to comment on how their money is being spent: "Do you think my son should have bought that car?" or "How could my daughter pay so much for that dress?" How money is spent may depend on the family history, family needs, culture, and state of the client's disease.

It is most important to act in a nonjudgmental way and not to inflict your opinions about money on the client or his family. (All that you need to say is: "I'm not really in a position to comment on this situation. I suggest that you discuss your feelings with your son.") If you feel that money is being spent in such a way as to injure a family member or cause danger to the family, report your observations to your supervisor immediately.

### *Your Role as a Homemaker/Home Health Aide*

As a homemaker/home health aide, you will be sent into some families where you will not be totally comfortable. At other times, you will be assigned situations in which you are totally comfortable. These feelings may be due to the family or other situations. At this time, speak to your supervisor and discuss your feelings. Are you afraid? Do you understand what is happening? Do the family members have values and actions of which you personally disapprove? Your supervisor will help you become more comfortable with your feelings and understand why these feelings are natural for you to have. It is important to recognize and be honest about your reactions to the client and his family so that these feelings do not get in the way of your good care for him. You may not like a person, but you still must give him the best care you can.

# Section 3  Working with Clients Who Are Ill or Have a Disability

## Objectives: What You Will Learn to Do

- Discuss common reactions to illness.
- Discuss common reactions to disabilities.
- Recognize your feelings concerning illness and disability.
- List broad goals of caring for clients who are ill or have a disability.
- Learn to recognize family support systems.

### *Introduction: Reactions to Being Ill and Dependent*

Every person reacts to illness, being disabled, and being dependent in a different way. Individual reactions are determined by age, family, culture, emotional health, and all the other parts that make up a particular person. Even though there are individual reactions, there are also certain common ways in which most people react to being ill or having a disability. As a homemaker/home health aide, you must be aware of some common behaviors so that you will know what to expect while caring for your clients.

It is important to remember that you bring certain feelings about illness with you when you care for a client. These feelings are part of you. They make you. Sometimes these feelings are helpful to you and your client. Sometimes they are not. The important thing is to identify these feelings and not let them get in the way of your work.

The most useful action you can take as a homemaker/home health aide is to involve the client and his family in the plan of care. Remember, you will leave, but they will all remain in the home. By establishing a routine in which they had a part, they can continue the care of the client after you are gone. Everyone, young and old, regardless of illness or disability, has a right to take part in their care if they want. They also have a right not to take part.

## *The Difference Between Illness and Disability*

**illness** deviation from the healthy state

**acute** state of illness that comes on suddenly and may be of short duration

**chronic** state of disease that lasts a long time

**disability** partial or complete loss of the use of a part or parts of the body

An illness is different from a disability. An **illness** is the absence of good health. An illness usually has pain and discomfort associated with it. This absence of health may be acute or it may be chronic. An **acute** illness starts suddenly and does not last very long. A **chronic illness** is one that continues for a long time.

A **disability** is a condition that produces a physical or mental limitation that may or may not respond to adaptive aids. Usually, a body function that we take for granted is impaired. A disability may be produced by an accident, an illness, or a birth defect. A chronic illness may cause a disability. For example, diabetes, a chronic illness, may cause a person to have poor eyesight. A disability may or may not be painful or cause discomfort. The most important thing to remember about a disability is that it is usually permanent.

### REACTIONS TO ILLNESS AND DISABILITY

**family dynamics** the ways in which family members interact and get along with each other

**support systems** arrangement that gives aid and comfort to a person

Reactions of families to illness, disability, and crisis vary (Fig. 3.6). The unique way in which all members of a family function is called **family dynamics.** This method of functioning has been shaped over many years. **Support systems** are people or actions used to help a person adjust to a new or difficult situation. Families may be able to make the necessary adjustments in their functions and rally to the short-term crisis or acute illness. They may, however, not be able to make the adjustments if the illness is a long-term or chronic situation. Other families are able to make long-term adjustments. Some families are unable to make any changes in their structure and will not be able to cope with any illness or disability.

Ideally, the support systems a family chooses are those that allow them to continue functioning—even in time of crisis. You will recognize many kinds of support systems:

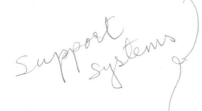

- *Informal systems:* people help one another because they want to—church groups, neighbors, and friends
- *Formal systems:* people help because they are paid to do so and/or they have a particular knowledge necessary and/or an outside agency or government says they must do so—visiting nurse, the homemaker/home health aide, caseworker
- *Support groups:* people gather, usually with a leader or facilitator, to discuss and share similar problems, help each other, and gain knowledge from each other

Your supervisor, along with the family, the physician, and the client, will work together to set up an acceptable support system for the situation. As a sensitive member of the team, your observations as to "what works and what doesn't" are important. Be sure to share your observations with your supervisor.

Often, when the proper help is offered, a family in crisis can make the necessary changes to cope with illness or disability. Remember, the family unit has set up patterns of coping over a long period of time.

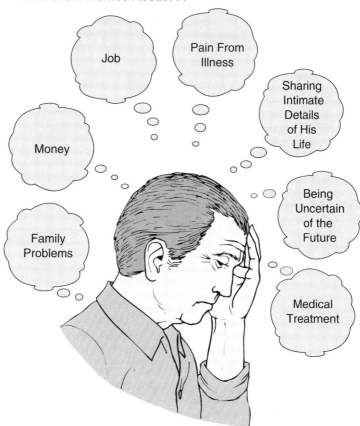

**What a Client Worries About . . .**

Job

Pain From Illness

Sharing Intimate Details of His Life

Money

Being Uncertain of the Future

Family Problems

Medical Treatment

*FIGURE 3.6* Illness and disability cause clients to worry about many temporary and permanent changes in their lives.

You must work with these patterns and help establish a support system that makes the family and patient secure and comfortable.

### DENIAL

**denial** refuses to believe or accept reality

**Denial** is used by some people when they meet a situation with which they cannot cope at the time. They simply say, "This doesn't really exist." They are saying that nothing is wrong. It is very difficult to help a person who denies that a problem exists. Denial is a way that people shield themselves from situations they are unable to face at the time. Sometimes a person will deny an event or situation and then come to accept it at a later time when they are emotionally able to do so. Everyone uses denial at some time. Clients may use denial to help themselves feel more acceptable to themselves and their families.

Often you will be asked to take part in this process of denial. When a person has an illness, the family may wish to keep it from him. They will deny that there is a problem and will ask your help in keeping the secret. You will have to ask your supervisor to assist you with this charade. It is most difficult, and you may become angry that the client or his family is denying the truth and involving you in this lie. Remember, the family and the client have a right to deny a situation if that is their method of coping and the client is not negatively affected. As the caregiver, you must deliver the best possible care within that situation. The important thing to remember is why the client and/or his family find it necessary to deny the situation.

## ABUSIVE WORDS AND DIFFICULT BEHAVIOR

Clients are often impatient. They may show their impatience to one member of the family or only to you. It is important to remain calm and not take the client's words as a personal insult. Often he is angry at the situation, not at you. But you are the closest person with whom he can react. A client may complain that the medicine isn't working, that the exercises aren't working, and that he isn't getting better fast enough. He may complain that you are doing too much or not enough. He may become irritable due to pain, the general situation, or his feeling of helplessness. Remember, remain calm and try to put the client's actions and words into perspective. If you have difficulty doing this, speak to your supervisor and she will help you.

abusive insulting or mistreating

Clients may say things to you that they would not say to their relatives. They may use unpleasant or nasty, **abusive** words. Why? You are not a family member, and therefore, you do not have all the years of family relationship behind you. Because you are paid to care for the client, he may feel that you will return even if he isn't nice because it is "your job." A visiting family member does not have to care for the client, and if the client is unpleasant, the family member may not return. Some clients may say and do things to test you and the limits of the situation. Often clients will be very nice to you but not to their families. This is to make the family jealous and show them that he is still in control of his situation. He can still make people feel good or hurt their feelings. Some clients do or say unpleasant things but are not aware that their behavior is a problem to anyone. If you tell the client that something he does makes you uncomfortable, he will often stop it. Working with a client who is unpleasant to you is very difficult. Remember that there is a reason for such behavior. Discuss the entire situation with the supervisor, and she will assist you in dealing with it.

If you are really uncomfortable, you may have to be transferred to another case.

## GOALS TO KEEP IN MIND AS YOU CARE FOR YOUR CLIENT

All clients, whether they are ill, are disabled, have a chronic condition, or are having an acute attack, will have a plan of care.

As the homemaker/home health aide, you will be asked to follow this plan of care. A plan is carefully made up by the professional nurse, supervisor, and therapists who care for the client. Your maintenance of this routine is most important. Your careful observation and reporting to your supervisor is also important.

The goal of the client's care plan will be established by the professionals and the client. It is essential that the client and his caregivers share the same goals. Then they are all working toward the same end. Although each client has his own individual care plan, certain broad goals are present in all care plans:

- Promote self-care
- Promote self-respect
- Promote behavior appropriate to the client's condition and age
- Promote a safe, clean environment

# Section 4 Mental Health and Mental Disability

<table>
<tr><td>

## Objectives: What You Will Learn to Do

</td><td>

- Identify some characteristics of good mental health.
- Identify some misconceptions about mental disabilities.
- Describe your role as a homemaker/home health aide when caring for a client who is mentally disabled.

</td></tr>
</table>

## Introduction: Mental Health/Mental Disability

**mental health** the ability to function satisfactorily in a society; a sense of well being

**Mental health** is the ability to function effectively and satisfactorily in a certain society. Mental health is a condition of the whole person. It reflects how a person deals with daily life and crisis. Our mental health is the basis for our behavior and relationships with others.

Mental health is also a matter of degree. At times everyone shows behavior that may be judged unusual. The difference between a mentally healthy person and one with a mental disability is that the person who is mentally disabled adopts characteristics or behaviors that no longer enable him to function within society.

Mentally healthy people can:

- Adapt to change
- Give and receive affection and love
- Tolerate stress to varying degrees
- Accept responsibility for their own feelings and actions
- Distinguish between reality and unreality
- Form and keep relationships with people

### MENTAL DISABILITY

**mental disability** the temporary or permanent disruption in the ability of a person to function satisfactorily in a society

**contagious** readily transmitted by direct or indirect contact

Not long ago **mental disability** was thought to be a punishment or a curse. Many people thought mental disabilities were **contagious,** that is, that they could be spread. People who were mentally disabled were put in institutions so that the rest of society would not catch their disease. We now know that mental illnesses are not contagious and that there are many different causes for mental disabilities and socially unacceptable behavior. Not all mental disability is permanent. With treatment many people recover and go on to lead productive lives.

Mental disabilities often start slowly, and people are unable to tell you when the problem started. They can, however, say when the behavior became such that it was no longer acceptable. There are many levels of mental dysfunction. Do not try to label a client. Just treat him with respect, support him and his family, see to his safety, and follow the plan of care.

Some of the causes of mental disability are:

- Isolation
- Medication
- Drugs
- Environment
- Chronic stress
- Alcohol

- High fevers
- Family and interpersonal relationships
- Venereal disease
- Heredity
- Circulatory diseases

Besides reacting to illness and disability in physical ways, people also have mental reactions. Some people even become mentally disabled as a result of a physical ailment. In these cases caring for the client's mental disability will be an added component to caring for his physical condition.

Different people show their disability in different ways. One of the classic symptoms is a marked change in behavior patterns. If you notice any change in your client's behavior or his family tells you that his behavior is changed, report it to your supervisor immediately. After a careful assessment, your supervisor will be able to change the patient's plan of care to reflect his mental needs.

Other symptoms of mental disability are:

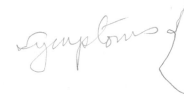

- Hallucinations
- Sleeplessness
- Fears
- Decreased memory
- Disorientation *(what day it is)*
- Forgetfulness
- Mood swings
- Withdrawal

### Defense Mechanisms

**defense mechanism** a thought used unconsciously to protect oneself against painful or unpleasant feelings

When a person is subjected to stress, he reacts with certain defenses. This is normal. When **defense mechanisms** are used so often that a person is not in touch with reality, he is said to be mentally disabled. The most common defense mechanisms are:

- **Denial**—"It's not possible."
- **Depression**—"It's no use. It's hopeless."
- **Regression**—acting like a child or becoming very dependent.
- **Repression**—forgetting about the situation, putting it out of mind.
- **Projection**—"It's not my fault but the fault of the medical people."
- **Rationalization**—explaining how one's behavior is acceptable even though it isn't.
- **Aggression**—behavior that attacks everyone regardless of cause.

You will be asked to care for clients with many combinations of mental disabilities. Two of the most common ones you will see are depression and overdependence.

### Depression

**depression** low spirits that may or may not cause a change of activity

**Depression** may be an illness or depression may be another way in which a person deals with illness. Depression can also be the result of an illness or a side effect of medication. The primary sign of depression is lack of any interest in the present situation and the present environment. Some other signs of depression are:

- Poor appetite
- Disinterest in people and things that were previously of interest
- Statements like "I'm not up to that" and "What does it matter anyway?"
- Being overappreciative of help
- Lack of activity or social interaction
- Lack of expression in face or voice

Some depression is to be expected when a person realizes he does not have as much control over his life as he once had. You should allow him to take part in as much of his care as he wants and is able to. Point out that there are still decisions he can make. Consult the client whenever you can. Encourage his decisions and opinions. Try to establish routines that are both good for the client and have a high rate of success. For example, it may be more convenient for you to help the client exercise before his bath. But the client may want to do his exercises after his bath, and he does them better at that time. It would then be appropriate for you to alter your schedule and do the exercises when the client feels they are most helpful. You must remember that some clients will remain depressed no matter what you do. Do not become discouraged. Continue to try to interest them in meaningful activities.

### Overdependence

Some people adopt this type of behavior because they have learned it brings them rewards. Some people cannot function any other way.

When some people realize they are no longer in total charge of their situation, as with the new diagnosis of a chronic disease, they are unable to adjust to this change. Instead, they become totally dependent on others and take no responsibility for their care. When a client does not assume the responsibility he is able to take, he is said to be overdependent. It is important to assist the client in assuming, at his own pace, the role of being somewhat dependent, while continuing to be responsible for himself when possible. No matter how ill he is, a client still may be able to take some part in his care. You must point out this responsibility to the client and his family. Remember, though: clients will assume their independence when they are ready to meet their own needs. Until then, it is your responsibility to assume the care.

## Your Role as a Homemaker/Home Health Aide

As society recognizes the causes of and develops better treatments for mental disability, more and more people are being returned to the community after hospitalization. Communities have set up clinics, foster homes, day care programs, and halfway houses to help these former institutionalized patients adjust to community life.

You may be assigned to a client with a mental disability or you may be in a home where a family member is disabled. Be sure you understand your responsibility to the person. Your plan of care will be your guide to both the physical and emotional care of the person. Care of the client who is disabled mentally is very similar to the care of any other client. One of the important parts of your care will be to support the client's family. Encourage them to discuss their feelings and concerns with their doctor. For the client to reach his maximum ability it is necessary that his environment be an accepting one. Remember:

- Your observations of the client and family are very important.
- Report your observations objectively.
- Your friendly, understanding manner will show how you feel about the client. It will encourage others to feel positively about the client.
- Be aware of your body language.
- Encourage the client to take part in his own care as is appropriate.
- Speak to the client in simple sentences. Do not shout or talk baby talk to him.
- Should you find out information about the client's care when you are away from the home, be sure to tell this to your supervisor.

# Section 5  Substance Abuse

## Objectives: What You Will Learn to Do

▪ Understand what is meant by *substance abuse*.
▪ Identify some misconceptions about substance abuse.
▪ Describe your role as a homemaker/home health aide when a substance abuser is in the home where you work.
▪ Describe your role as a homemaker/home health aide when you are caring for a client who is a recovering substance abuser.

## Introduction: Substance Abuse

**substance abuse** the use of anything, usually alcohol or drugs, to an excess and to the detriment of the person

There are many types of **substance abuse**. A person can abuse drugs, alcohol, or a combination. There are many reasons people use drugs and/or alcohol to excess. Some people think it is a way of escaping their problems; some people do it because their friends do it; some people start out using drugs to help them with an illness and then discover they are unable to stop; still others start out using alcohol slowly and do not realize they are in trouble until it is too late. The term *substance abuse* means that a person uses a drug or alcohol to excess and that his behavior is altered due to the abuse. There was a time when society felt that there was no help for substance abusers. We know now that is not the case. Many of them can receive treatment and return to living useful and productive lives. The treatment is usually not easy and it takes a long time, but for those who are able to continue in the treatment, the result may well be a complete cure.

### GENERAL MISCONCEPTIONS ABOUT SUBSTANCE ABUSE

#### *"Everyone does it."*

This is not true. Everybody does not do it. We read a great many stories in the newspapers about famous people who use drugs and we read about everyday people who try them. This leads some readers to believe that *everyone* is doing it. Actually, nobody knows how many people really use drugs and abuse alcohol, and although the number certainly seems to be growing, "everyone" does not do it!

#### *"I can control it."*

Wrong! The body gets used to drugs and alcohol and then no longer reacts to the usual amount that is taken. Therefore, the person must now increase the "dose" to get the same feeling. As the dose increases, so does the price. There has never been an addicted person who could control it. Sooner or later, the habit controls the person.

#### *"No one will know."*

Wrong! It is entirely possible that when the user starts, no one will know. But as the body accustoms itself to the foreign substance, there are definite changes in behavior. Soon employers know. Families can no longer deny the problem. Finally, somebody must confront the user.

*"It makes me feel good."*

When someone starts to use drugs or alcohol, they may do so to get "high." But this is not a state in which a person can remain for long periods of time. Some people may enjoy this feeling because they feel they are avoiding their real problems. When they are no longer high, however, they do not feel good and their problems are still present.

## GENERAL SIGNALS OF SUBSTANCE ABUSE

There are many signs associated with abuse of specific substances (Fig. 3.7). The most important sign is a change in the person's behavior. Some general signals that there should be further investigation into the person's behavior are:

1. Personality changes, such as mood swings, bizarre activities, or change of friends; disinterest in familiar activities
2. Change in the way money is spent
3. Change in employment or in relationship with present employer
4. Change in school habits
5. Alteration in physical appearance, such as weight gain or loss, reddened eyes, dilated pupils, nausea/vomiting
6. Change in eating habits or the consumption of fluids
7. Change in sleep habits
8. Liquor missing

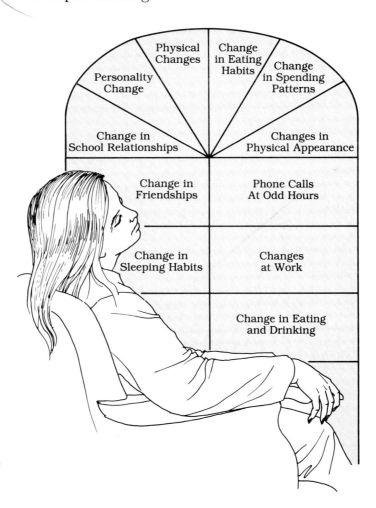

*FIGURE 3.7* Be alert to subtle changes in behavior of both clients and family members.

9. Unusual breath odor, unusual smell on clothing
10. Change in gait; change in sense of smell, vision, or hearing
11. Change in breathing pattern
12. Continued discussion about drugs or alcohol
13. Phone calls at odd hours

## Your Role as a Homemaker/Home Health Aide

You may be assigned to care for a client who is in a house with a drug user or an alcoholic. First you must be sure your client is in no danger and that the abuser is not able to harm your client—or harm you. Discuss the situation with your supervisor so that a plan can be made to offer help to the abuser. Do not try to obtain help on your own. Offering help to a long-time abuser can be a complicated affair and must be carefully planned. It is important that the correct help be offered and that the most appropriate community resource be used. Your supervisor will know how to plan this.

Do not tell the abuser he must stop. The chances are he would if he could but is unable to do so without help.

Do not make the family members feel guilty that they have permitted the situation to continue. They may not know what to do. But with your help and support and that of your supervisor, a plan can be made. Families of abusers need a great deal of support. Your understanding and demonstration of nonjudgmental behavior will be very important in this household.

If you are assigned to a client who is presently under treatment for having been an abuser, you will act in the manner we have already discussed. In addition, you will have to be observant to detect if the client has reverted back to his previous habits of abuse. Report to your supervisor any actions that suggest to you that the client is not drug or alcohol free. Follow the care plan carefully, and support the client. Recovery from drug abuse or alcoholism is not easy. With your presence and support, it can be made easier.

## Topics for Discussion

1. Review the needs of different clients. List those that are the same and those that are different. Then list how you would meet these needs.
2. Think about how you and your family react to illness, to death, to the aging process.
3. Discuss your feelings about mental illness.
4. Discuss how you would feel if you worked in a house where a family member was an alcoholic or abused drugs.

# Chapter 4

# Caring for a Geriatric Client

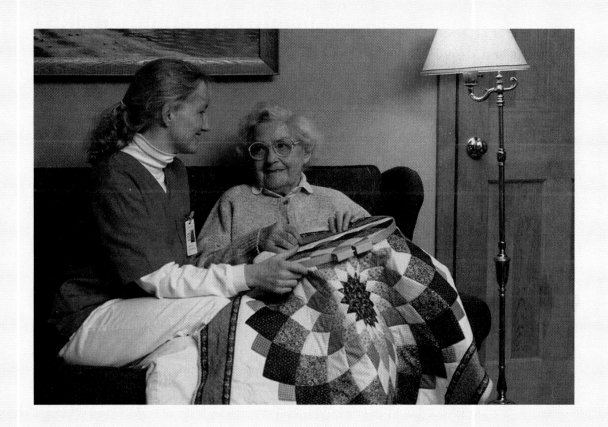

# Section 1  Aging

**Objectives: What You Will Learn to Do**

- Describe the general aging process.
- List some of the common problems facing the aged.
- Discuss your feelings about aging.
- Become familiar with your role as a homemaker/home health aide caring for an elderly client.

## Introduction: The Aged

The elderly population is growing faster than any other segment of our population. Here are some interesting facts:

- There are about 50 million people over 65 years old in America.
- The fastest growing segment of the elderly population is the over-85 age group.
- The largest source of income for the elderly is Social Security.
- Over 7 million elderly live at the poverty level.
- Women live longer than men and outnumber them 3 to 2.
- Half of the people over 65 work part-time although they have at least one chronic disease.
- Eighty percent of the elderly have more than one chronic disease that requires medical attention.

Although about 5 percent of the elderly live in nursing homes, the rest live in the community. It is expected that as medicine, nutrition, and the general standard of life improve, the number of aged will increase. As this happens, more and more people who remain at home will need some assistance. The home health care system is changing to meet the needs of these people. Many of your clients who are aged will require some assistance so they can remain in their own homes and have some measure of independence and self-respect. Some of your clients will need minimal assistance; some will need maximal assistance. It is important that clients receive the type of help that is most appropriate for their individual needs.

There are many different types of living arrangements for the elderly. Some live in their own homes; some live in supervised homes with several other clients; some live in communities with various levels of assistance, such as meals, medical supervision or homemaker services, provided by professional caregivers.

The world has changed so much in the last 50 years that the aged are often unfamiliar with what now exists. It is not that they cannot learn about the new machines or the new systems, but rather that no one has ever taken the time to teach them. They often find themselves in a strange world. The adjustment to all the changes is often difficult for clients and their families. Although many clients have a well-tested and strong system of coping, enabling them to adjust to changes and new roles, many elderly are unable to cope with all the changes.

**geriatric** refers to persons over 65

The term **geriatrics** refers to the knowledge and care of the elderly. You will be using this specialized knowledge as you care for your elderly clients.

# AGING

aging to get older

Aging is universal and starts the moment we are born. The way in which society views the aging citizen varies. In some cultures, the aged are of no value and are often neglected because they are unable to contribute to the society. In some cultures and some professions, the aged are well respected and cared for and are given a place of honor. American society often appears to value youth for its beauty and not to value the contributions of its elderly citizens. At this time, however, it seems that society is also gaining a greater understanding of the aged. There are many signs that our American society is coming to see all ages of man as valuable. More advertisements for products that are of interest to the elderly are appearing. Community programs designed for the elderly are gaining popularity. We are also seeing laws passed that meet the concerns of our older citizens and that protect them. American society is coming to the conclusion that, although youth has its value, age has its also.

There are some facts that are important for you to remember as you care for older people:

- They want to remain independent.
- They enjoy sexual relationships.
- They can maintain good health.
- Senility is not the same as old age.
- They want to be contributing members of society.
- They can learn although they often take longer than younger people to do so.

## HOW YOU FEEL ABOUT THE AGED

Everyone has feelings about the aged. Some people are afraid of them, some people feel sorry for them, and some people avoid them because they are a reminder of what may happen when they age. Think about the following statements about the aged. Get to know what your feelings are. Which of these statements are true? Are they true about all older people?

1. Old people are untidy and messy.
2. Old people tend to worry about financial matters.
3. It is normal for the elderly to withdraw from society.
4. Old people prefer to be with people their own age.
5. Old people have no friends.
6. Old people live in the past, and that is boring.
7. Old people only talk about death and are afraid of dying.
8. Old age is not a problem for rich people, only for poor people.
9. Old people prefer to be waited on hand and foot.
10. Old people remind us of what is in store for us when we age.

aging process changes in the body caused by growing older

The aging process has many phases (Fig. 4.1). The exact combinations of physical, mental, and social changes vary from person to person. Some changes are obvious, and some are not. Some changes are more easily acceptable, and some are not. There are several theories about how we age, but the results of aging are the same.

As people age, they have the same needs as they did when they were younger. The main difference is that the needs of an older person are often met in a different way than the needs of a younger person.

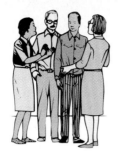
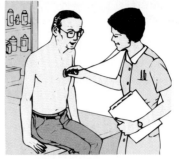
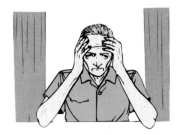

Social Changes      Physical Changes      Mental Changes

**FIGURE 4.1** Putting the many phases of the aging process into perspective is the best way to ensure a well balanced life.

## PHYSICAL CHANGES

As we age, there are visible changes in our body and the way it functions. It takes longer to walk, longer to make decisions, and longer to execute a task. In addition, there are many other visible changes. The physical changes of aging are the most obvious and, for some, the most difficult to accept. These changes occur at different rates and at different ages. Everyone is an individual whose body has its own unique schedule. Some physical changes that occur in everyone are:

- Reflexes slow.
- Circulation becomes less efficient.
- Hair turns gray and may change in texture.
- All bodily processes slow.
- Skin loses elasticity and underlying fat and becomes thin and more fragile.
- Senses become less acute and aids are needed, such as glasses or hearing aids.
- Posture becomes more stooped, and walking becomes more difficult.
- Muscles lose strength, and familiar tasks become more difficult.
- Sensing of temperature of water and air becomes less accurate.
- Healing takes longer.
- Short-term memory often decreases so directions have to be repeated often.

| Body System or Organ | "Normal" Aging Change | Possible Problems Consequence |
| --- | --- | --- |
| Skin | Decreased response to pain sensation, temperature changes, and vibration | Accidents; inability to feel hot and/or cold objects, weather changes, injury and/or pain |
| | Loss of fat under skin (subcutaneous fat) and fatty padding over bony prominences (i.e., hips); change in number of blood vessels | Veins appear more prominent; wrinkles, especially facial, and folds in skin appear; occurrence of pressure sores (bedsores); slower healing; loss of hair; fluid balance of skin is difficult to maintain |
| | Decrease in number of sweat glands | Difficulty in regulating body temperature |
| | Decrease in oil production | Dry skin, itching, easily injured |
| | Formation of pigment cell clusters | Moles and "old age spots" (liver spots), graying of hair |

| Body System or Organ | "Normal" Aging Change | Possible Problems Consequence |
|---|---|---|
| Eyes | Clouding of lens | Development of cataracts |
| | Decrease in ability to focus | Difficulty seeing at night or in fluorescent lighting |
| | Decrease in production of tears | Dry eyes |
| | Inability to blink as quickly | Easier to get a foreign body in the eye |
| | Muscle degeneration in 50 percent of people over 70 | Central vision loss |
| | Less light reaching retina | Need for adequate lighting |
| | Eyelids tend to evert or invert | Irritation |
| Ear | Decrease in ability to hear high-frequency sounds (presbycusis) | Hearing loss |
| | Stiffness and inflexibility of ear structure | Distortion of sound and pain if volume is too high |
| Sense of taste | Decrease in number of taste buds | Food may become tasteless |
| | Salty taste decreases the most, sweet next | Use of salt and sugar |
| Sense of smell | Generally declines | Difficulty smelling smoke, gas, etc., or enjoying pleasant odors |
| Mouth and teeth | Loss of gum and bone structure around teeth | Periodontal disease, loss of teeth |
| Brain | Change in reaction time, in verbal and vocabulary skills | Slowed reactions and reflexes; inability to learn quickly |
| | Memory loss may occur after age 50 | Recall, recognition may be slightly slowed (i.e., "Where are my keys?") |
| | Decrease in deep sleep | Periods of wakefulness during sleep hours |
| | Decrease in need for sleep | Hours of sleep may change |
| Lungs and chest | Stiffness of respiratory muscles | Expansion of the lungs |
| | Decrease in elasticity of rib cage | Mild barrel chest due to structural changes |
| | Decrease in area for oxygen and carbon dioxide exchange | Less oxygen available during physical exercise and activity |
| | Diminished activity of cilia (help to clean lung) and diminished cough reflex | Difficulty coughing and eliminating foreign particles from lung; incidence of bronchitis and pneumonia |
| Heart and circulatory system | Decrease in cardiac muscle strength | Cardiac output is decreased |
| | Narrowing of arteries and veins | Blood pressure is increased |
| Musculoskeletal system | Decrease in absorption of calcium | Osteoporosis (thinning of bone) |
| | Decrease in bone replacement | Incidence of fractures is increased |
| | Loss of muscle mass and tone | Fatigue and weakness |
| Balance | Less efficient balancing mechanisms and reactions | Incidence of falls is increased; standing position tends to be with flexed hips and knees |
| Gastrointestinal system | Decrease in esophageal muscle action | Indigestion is more frequent, slower transport of food to stomach; slower digestion |

| Body System or Organ | "Normal" Aging Change | Possible Problems Consequence |
|---|---|---|
| | Decrease in large bowel mobility, nervous stimulation | Constipation, diminished frequency of BMs, incomplete emptying of the bowel |
| | Decreased sensitivity to thirst | Dehydration |
| Renal system | Decrease in size of urinary bladder | Frequency of urination |
| | Decrease in kidney size | Sensitivity to medications |
| | Slowing of filtration, blood flow to kidney | Decreased ability to eliminate toxic wastes |
| Genitalia | *Men* Enlarged prostate gland | Urinary system obstruction |
| | Increased time to urinate | Increased urinary retention, frequency, and infections |
| | Penis may be less hard | Decreased ability to delay ejaculation |
| | *Women* Decreased vaginal and cervical secretions, thinning of vaginal walls | Uncomfortable intercourse, longer time to experience orgasm |
| | Changes in estrogen after menopause | Changes in secondary sexual characteristics |
| Hormones | Decreased insulin response | Blood sugar elevation |

## MENTAL CHANGES

It was once thought that all older people became senile. This is now known to be a myth. All older people do not get confused, forgetful, and dependent. Those who do must be treated carefully just as you would treat any other impaired client, not as an object of pity or as a child.

Decreased circulation to the brain can cause mental changes. Medications can cause mental changes. Some changes are temporary, and some are permanent. Obvious changes in brain function are forgetfulness, disorientation, and irritability. A physical reason may cause some mental changes. Other mental changes are brought about as a reaction to social changes.

**dementia** loss of mental powers

**Dementia** is the gradual decrease in a person's ability to make judgments. This is not a normal part of the aging process. The presence of dementia and the type of dementia can only be diagnosed by a physician. Dementia is the condition that used to be called senility.

There are two main types of dementia: those that are reversible and those that are not. Reversible dementia is often caused by a physical, social, or chemical stimulus. When that stimulus is removed, the person reverts to his predementia status. Irreversible dementia can be caused by small portions of the brain losing function due to small strokes. This condition leads to confusion, decreased mental acuity, decreased physical abilities, and decreased ability to make judgments. The client may not have the same problems all the time; he may have "good days" and "bad days." Irreversible dementia can also be caused by Alzheimer's disease (see Chapter 19, Section 8).

It is important for you to discuss with your supervisor the reason for your client's behavior. Knowing why people act in a certain way will help you in caring for them. For aged clients who are confused and forgetful, special precautions are necessary. It may be necessary to

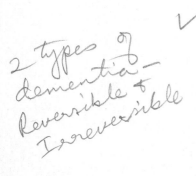
2 types of dementia — Reversible & Irreversible

remind them where they are, who they are, and who you are. Safety is the key to the care of these clients because they are unable to make judgments on their own.

Caring for these clients takes time, understanding, and patience. It can be very tiring for you to be continually with a mentally impaired client. When you feel you are no longer able to handle your feelings, talk with your supervisor. It may be time for a change of assignment. After all, to care for a client at the expense of a homemaker/home health aide is not good home health care.

Families of elderly clients are often very stressed. Caring for an elderly relative brings with it several responsibilities. Caring for a mentally disabled elderly client is an additional set of responsibilities. Encourage your client's family to discuss their feelings with professionals. It would not be helpful for the caregivers to suffer family problems.

## SOCIAL CHANGES

There are many social changes that affect the elderly. Some are brought about as a result of physical changes, some are brought about by society, and some just happen:

- Retirement
- Change in income
- Change in level of activity
- Fear of illness
- Isolation from friends and family
- Death of a spouse
- Change in housing
- Increased dependence on others

One or two of these changes may not cause any change in your client's behavior. However, several of these changes can cause a person to change his usual behavior patterns because he will no longer be able to cope with the situation. Your client's reaction to change will depend on his usual coping ability and the result of the changes. He may become anxious, depressed, or withdrawn, or he may increase his activity. His eating habits, sleeping habits, or memory may change. He may no longer show interest in those things he used to enjoy. He may suddenly develop an interest in activities he always disliked. If you notice any of these changes in your client's behavior, report them to your supervisor immediately.

## REALITY ORIENTATION

**reality orientation** a technique to orient people to their surroundings

**Reality orientation** is a technique utilizing the remaining brain cells to reduce the confusion often seen in clients with dementia. This program must be carefully individualized by your supervisor and requires the continued backup of the client's family and caretakers. Usually, the reality orientation board, which is visible to the client, contains simple information useful to him so that he can function at home (Fig. 4.2).

The homemaker/home health aide must continually reinforce the use of this program. Your supervisor will want to know how the program is progressing, so report at least the following:

- Does the client understand the subjects on the board?
- Does the client remember the information? For how long?

■ Is the family supportive of the reality orientation program?

■ List your other observations.

**REALITY ORIENTATION BOARD**

| | |
|---|---|
| Day: | Monday |
| Date: | Feb 3 |
| Year: | 1988 |
| Weather: | Sunny ☼ |
| Address: | 154 Tulip Street |
| City: | Millville |
| State: | Rhode Island |
| Activities: | • Watch T.V. |
| | • Clean linen drawer |

**FIGURE 4.2** Orienting a client to his surroundings assists him in feeling secure.

## Your Role as a Homemaker/Home Health Aide

The needs of the aged are the same as the needs of all other people. It will be your responsibility to help meet these needs. By giving the necessary assistance in a safe, warm, understanding manner, you enable the client to remain at home in familiar surroundings and to be an independent person.

■ Assist with all phases of personal care. A complete bath may not be necessary every day. Remember that many clients have dry, flaky, fragile skin. Lubricate the skin with lotion or oil as the client wishes. Expensive lotions are not necessary, but lubrication is.

■ Observe the client for irritation, redness, bruises or for areas on the body that do not heal.

■ Teach the client how to maintain his own personal hygiene when you are not in the home. A squeeze bottle filled with warm soapy water can be used after urination and bowel movements while the client is seated on the toilet. Remind him to rinse the area thoroughly.

■ Provide an environment for safe, simple exercise, such as walking up stairs or getting from room to room.

■ Plan your care around the client's usual household schedule and ethnic customs.

■ Provide for warmth and ventilation in the home. Aged clients often react to temperature differently than do younger people. They often wear sweaters in the summer. Dress and groom them in what makes them comfortable and is appropriate for their age.

■ Protect them from extreme heat or cold.

■ Do not disturb personal belongings, letters, pictures, and so on. You may suggest moving them, however, to another obvious place where the client can still enjoy them so that you can give better care.

■ Do not use baby talk with the client.

■ Do not speak about the client to others as though he were not there.

■ Have patience!

# Section 2   Special Considerations in Caring for the Elderly

## Objectives: What You Will Learn to Do

- List the important safety measures to remember while caring for an elderly client.
- Discuss how exercise benefits the elderly client.
- List some considerations to remember while assisting elderly clients with medications.
- Become familiar with the role sexuality plays in the life of your elderly client.
- List the signs of elderly abuse and your responsibility for reporting this.

### Introduction: Areas of Special Concern as You Care for the Elderly

Although caring for an elderly client is much the same as caring for a younger client, you must be aware that the elderly often need special attention in certain aspects of their care (Fig. 4.3). You will have to be extra alert in the areas of safety and exercise and in assisting them with medication. In addition, because elderly people often are unable to report abuse or to find someone to talk to outside of their home, you will have to be their voice. This is a very important role. Because you may be the only person who sees the client regularly, you will develop a special relationship with him and will be able to notice changes in mood and activity. Report every change to your supervisor no matter how slight so that your client's status can be assessed and monitored. Remember, your overall goal as you care for your client is to preserve his independence, self-worth, and safety.

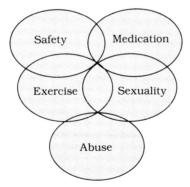

FIGURE 4.3  Clients may need help in meeting these needs. Be sure your client is safe and basic needs are met when you assist him.

### SAFETY

Safety for the elderly is always a prime concern. As their activity level changes, so do those things that are considered safe (Fig. 4.4). A situation that at one time was considered safe may, as a person ages, become a hazard. Poor eyesight, decreased reflexes, and poor hearing all contribute to accidents. In addition, many elderly attempt tasks they cannot execute and, thus, cause themselves harm. In an effort to be independent, a client may take unnecessary risks.

As people age, the ability to sense and then react to hot water is decreased. Many elderly are severely burned each year because they cannot feel that water is too hot. Teach your client to test his washing and bathing water *before* he uses it. If hot water has been run through a faucet, the faucet itself may be hot enough to cause burns should someone touch it. Briefly running cold water through the faucet after the hot will cool the metal and prevent such burns.

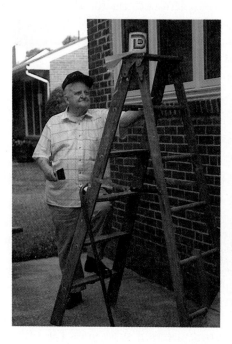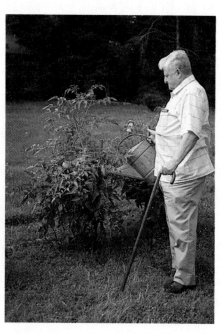

**FIGURE 4.4** Assist your client in accepting his limitations and making the right choice for safety's sake.

It is easier to prevent accidents than it is to heal. People who fall and break bones take months to heal and then may never regain full use of the limb again. The elderly heal slower than younger clients, so the prevention of falls for your elderly clients is even more important than for younger patients. Safety remains one of your primary responsibilities as a homemaker/home health aide. Help your clients maintain a safe environment:

- Encourage your clients to discuss their capabilities realistically.
- Help provide good lighting with switches that are easy to operate.
- Encourage the use of banisters and properly installed grab bars.
- Encourage safe practices in the kitchen. Never let clients wear long, flowing sleeves while cooking.
- Set the thermostat on the water heater so that hot water is at a safe level.
- Plan emergency exits.
- Help provide for smoke detectors.
- Encourage patients to discuss their driving capabilities with their physician.

It is important to discuss your activities with your supervisor. If you find yourself in an unsafe situation, both you and your supervisor may have to confront the patient. Although we can never forget that the client has the right to act in any way he wants in his own house, it is not part of your job to remain anywhere that is unsafe. It is also important to determine if the patient is acting in such a way as to cause harm to others. For example, does he smoke in bed? In this case, your supervisor will have to report the situation to the appropriate source. Should your client want and need structural changes in the house, your supervisor will be able to arrange for a reputable person to perform this work. There are often community groups that do such work for minimal pay.

## EXERCISE

Health professionals now feel that planned exercise is important for everyone (Fig. 4.5). Planned exercise is also important to older clients. The benefits are many:

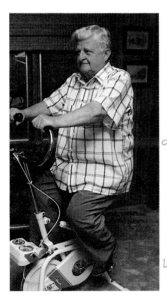

FIGURE 4.5 Always consult your physician before starting an exercise regime.

- A feeling of well-being
- Increased strength of bones
- Increased cardiac and respiratory capacity
- Increased strength and tone of muscles
- Decrease of weight
- Decrease of blood pressure
- Decrease of anxiety
- Better sleep habits

All clients should consult their physician before they start an exercise regime. There are many considerations before the proper regime is chosen, and only a physician is able to make the most informed decision. Be sure to report any change in the client's level of exercise or if you notice him having difficulty.

## MEDICATIONS

Elderly patients react to medications differently than do younger patients. Often elderly patients have several diseases and disabilities and take several medications for each one. The interaction of these medications often results in unexpected side effects (Fig. 4.6).

- The older body retains medications at a different rate than a younger body.
- Clients may stop taking medications due to financial reasons, forgetfulness, or because they read or hear some news about the drug.
- The kidneys and liver of older clients remove waste products more slowly than do those of younger clients.

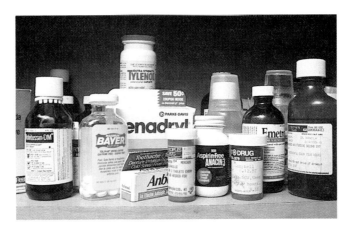

FIGURE 4.6 Keeping medication in a cluttered manner fosters medication errors.

- Older clients often forget they have taken medications and repeat them.
- Some clients may save medications that become outdated and then start taking them again.
- Older clients tend to have several physicians, each of whom may not be aware of all the medications that have been prescribed by other physicians.
- Clients may not discuss their reactions to medications with the physician because they feel the physician will be disappointed in their inability to take the drug.

Your role as a homemaker/home health aide is to assist your client with maintaining a safe medication schedule. Help your client maintain a foolproof organized method of taking his medications. This method should be established by your supervisor with input from you and the client. Be sure all your client's medications are prescribed for him. Borrowing medications can be dangerous! Report all, no matter how slight, side effects to your supervisor. Be sure your client knows why he is taking his medication and the possible side effects. Talk to your supervisor if you think your client is unaware of the reasons he is taking his medications.

When your client visits his physicians, encourage him to take all his medications with him. In that way, the physician will have a clear picture of the medications your client is taking and can prescribe new ones accordingly. Encourage your client to throw out old, outdated medications and to return medications that are not his.

Many medications are now packaged in childproof bottles. These bottles are difficult for the older client to open. Help your client get his medications packaged in containers that are easy for him to open and close. Often clients will not take their medication because they cannot open the bottle.

## SEXUALITY

The need for intimacy does not disappear with age, although there is a gradual slowing of response in sexual activity and a decreasing frequency of activity. Sex and the need for closeness and companionship and touching are not the same. Sexual performance may decrease, but the need for human companionship does not. Sexual desire, response, and activity is also often affected by medications. Therefore, any change in sexual activity or any concern expressed by your client should be referred to your supervisor immediately.

You may have preconceived notions about sex. You may have feelings about sexual activity between older people. It is important for you to prevent these ideas from interfering with your relationship with your client. Clients may have sexual practices that are unfamiliar to you. If you have concerns or questions, talk to your supervisor.

Your role as a homemaker/home health aide is to encourage your client to continue his sexual activities. If you are caring for a couple, respect their privacy and confidentiality. If your clients or their family have questions or concerns, report them to your supervisor so that counseling can be arranged.

## ABUSE

**abuse** any act that causes another harm; using a substance to excess

**Abuse** is any act that causes another harm. Abuse of anybody is a disturbing situation. Abuse of the elderly is especially disturbing because the abused are helpless to fight back and are often unable to call for help. Today, the health professions are seeing more and more cases of the elderly being physically and emotionally abused and neglected. There may be many reasons for abuse, but the result is always the same—an elderly person is hurt or in danger.

As you work in your client's home, you will be privileged to see and hear activities that no one else sees. Be alert for signs of abuse or neglect. Some of the signs are:

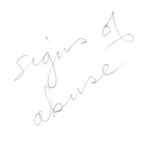

- Bruises on a patient that are hard to explain
- Fear of one particular person
- A request from a patient not to be left alone with a particular person
- Conflicting stories from family members
- A "feeling" that things are not right
- Lack of nourishment and care for the client
- Lack of family concern for the safety of the client
- Exchange of abusive words between family members
- Unexpected deterioration of the client's health

The accusation that a person is abusing an elderly client is a very serious one. Do not make it lightly. But do report immediately all activities you see that indicate the possibility of abuse. Most states require that any case of suspected elder abuse be reported. It is your responsibility to become familiar with the laws of your state and the proper reporting agency in your area. Remember, most abuse is inflicted by a family member. Be alert!

## Topics for Discussion

1. Discuss the way in which you would care for a client by taking into account all the considerations in this chapter.
2. Discuss your feelings about elderly abuse. How would you report any suspicions about abuse?
3. Discuss how you would feel taking care of an elderly person twenty-four hours every day.
4. Discuss some of the effects that the responsibility of an elderly relative would have on you, on your family.

# Chapter 5

# Working with Children

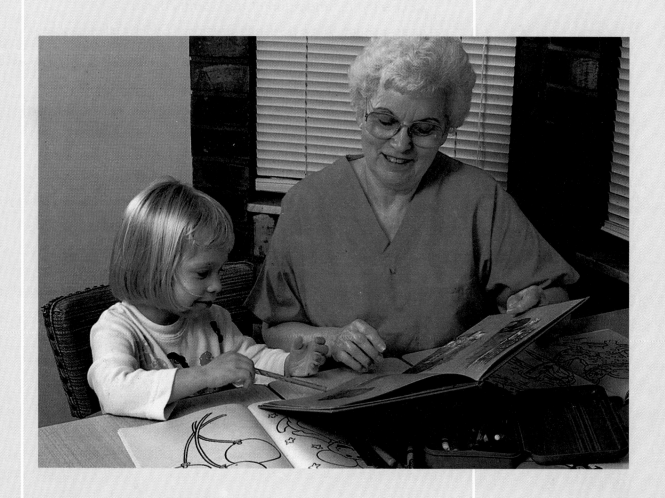

# Section 1 Basic Needs of Children

## Objectives: What You Will Learn to Do

- List the basic physical and emotional needs of children.
- List some common ways in which children react to the stress of illness.
- Know the difference between discipline and punishment.
- Describe ways in which a homemaker/home health aide would care for a child as a client.
- Describe ways in which a homemaker/home health aide would relate to a child who is not a client.

### Introduction: Caring for a Child

As a homemaker/home health aide, you will relate to children as clients. That means a child will be assigned to your care. In addition, there may be a time when you will teach a parent or family member how to care for a child.

You will also relate to children when they are in the house of your assigned adult client. They may live there or just be visiting. This interaction calls for a different relationship than when the child is your assigned client. It is important for you to know what your relationship is with the child and his parents or guardian.

When meeting a child, bend down so you are at eye level. Spend a few minutes alone with the child. This will signal the child's importance and allow both of you to get to know each other. You will also be able to learn about any special concerns or questions the child may have.

#### REASONS WHY A HOMEMAKER/HOME HEALTH AIDE MAY CARE FOR A CHILD

- The main caregiver becomes ill or suffers a disability.
- The main caregiver needs a rest from or assistance with the care of a child with an illness or disability.
- The main caregiver must be taught, by your example, how to care for the child.
- The main caregiver must leave the house to work.
- Child abuse or neglect has been reported or suspected.

#### BASIC NEEDS OF CHILDREN

Children have the same physical and emotional needs as adults (Fig. 5.1). However, they often depend on adults for the fulfillment of these needs.

Just as adult needs change in importance and fulfillment, so do those of children. Depending on the age of the child, certain needs may take on more importance. Children are not little adults. Their reactions and needs are based on their experiences as children. Researchers feel that a child must successfully meet specific needs at a certain age before he can mature. Often when the child is ill or a family member is ill, meeting the needs completely is difficult. That is your most important role—to meet the needs of the child.

## BASIC NEEDS OF CHILDREN

| Physical Needs |  | Emotional Needs |
|---|---|---|
| • Shelter | | • Recognition |
| • Activity, Rest, Exercise | | • Independence |
| | | • Socialization |
| • Avoidance of Pain | | • Acceptance |
| • Safety | | • Affection |
| • Clothing | | • Security |
| • Food | | • Trust |
| | | • Love |

*FIGURE 5.1* Children are often unable to meet their own needs and may not be able to ask to have them fulfilled. Be alert to signals that your help is needed.

## Stages of Childhood from Birth to Adolescence

| Stage of Development | Age | Key Characteristics or Tasks of the Age | Guidelines for Activities |
|---|---|---|---|
| Infancy | Birth–1 yr. | Rapid growth; totally dependent on adults; experiences first relationship; starts to distinguish the world through his senses | Provide calm routine, taking into account infant's schedule; encourage family to participate in care; stimulation includes brightly-colored objects held high or tied to crib, music, different shapes and textures; swings, carriages, rockers; toys he can put into larger containers; smooth objects that do not injure |
| Training period | 1–3 yrs. | Begins independence and exploration; learns to say "no"; puts everything in mouth; shows food likes and dislikes; frightened of loud noises and absence of primary caregiver; can understand simple honest explanation; may or may not share; usually starts to toilet train by age three | Attachment to mother and regular caregivers is strong; tell familiar stories again and again; do not lie, as the child does not know fact from fiction; help child become familiar with those objects that are part of his care; help toilet train as the family wishes without punishment but with positive reinforcement; likes pull toys, balls, stackable objects, mirrors, threads, large beads, windup toys |
| Love triangle | 3–5 yrs. | Girls mature more quickly; discovers sharing of friends and parents; affection and jealously apparent imitation; attempts to please; assumes some of his own personal care; assists with simple household chores; vivid imagination leads to stories | Approval of family important; older children like to take active part in care; enjoy activities with hands and crayons, simple puzzles; like to use familiar objects over and over; simple ball games and tag; always give simple reasons for activities |
| Middle childhood | 6–12 yrs. | Peer acceptance important; easily embarrassed; asserts independence and makes his friendships; secretive and argues with adults; growth spurts 10–12 yrs.; sexual curiosity | Reasons for actions important; explain; give time frame for schedule; enjoy scientific play, jigsaw puzzles, table games, board games, electronic and video games, music, puppets, sewing and crafts, model building |

| Stage of Development | Age | Key Characteristics or Tasks of the Age | Guidelines for Activities |
|---|---|---|---|
| Adolescence | 13–18 yrs. | Rapid change physically and emotionally; sexual development; mood changes; relationship very sensitive; need for privacy; peer relationships important; independence very important | Respect need for privacy; sexual concerns; explain all actions logically, honestly; reading, use of telephone, music; may reject familiar objects or foods; exerts his opinions, may reject suggestions from parents or caregivers but accept them from strangers; idol worship is common; concern for appearance and virility; encourage child to express his desires and interests |

## CONGENITAL ANOMALIES—BIRTH DEFECTS

**congenital anomaly** a deviation from the normal present at birth

**Congenital anomalies** is another term to describe birth defects. The definition of this condition is: "any abnormal organ or part of an organ present at birth, even though it may not be noted at that time." Such defects may result from a genetic disorder or from external factors, such as exposure to toxic substances, drug use, or alcohol abuse during pregnancy. Some congenital anomalies are visible, such as a child born with a shorter arm or one born with no fingers. Some anomalies are not visible, such as a child with a mental deficiency or with only one kidney.

When you work in a home with a child who has a congenital anomaly you will be called upon to assist the family as they learn to cope with the situation and the way it will affect the whole family. It is not unusual for the family to experience anger, guilt, denial, and emotional difficulties as they learn to care for this child. You must show an accepting behavior and encourage the family to seek help and support.

Discuss your feelings with your supervisor so that your actions will complement the plan of care for the whole family. Do not be disturbed if you need support during this assignment. This situation may cause you to have feelings that you will need help to understand. As you work in this house, however, be alert to separating your feelings from those of the family.

## CHILDREN UNDER STRESS

Everyone reacts to stress and change differently. Children are especially sensitive to threats to their security and familiar routines. This is true both of children who are ill and those who are in homes where there is illness. You may notice a child behave in a manner that is unusual, offensive, and difficult to explain.

You may notice:

■ Refusal to follow familiar household routines
■ Shyness, fear, withdrawal
■ Aggressive behavior
■ Jealousy
■ Nightmares and fears
■ Denial of the condition

- Overdependence
- Bed-wetting
- Regression

When illness is present in a home, many things affect the child indirectly. Some of these are:

- Noise restrictions
- Attention restrictions
- Financial conditions
- Family fears
- Activity restrictions

## DISCIPLINE AND PUNISHMENT

**discipline** a system of rules

You may be faced with the subject of discipline or punishment. There is a difference. Remember we are discussing a subject from the point of view of a homemaker/home health aide in a work setting. **Discipline** is a set of rules that govern conduct and actions, resulting in orderly behavior. Discipline can be strict or loose. The rules can be well known or not well known. Discipline can be accepted or just followed for fear of punishment. **Punishment** is a harsh act given as a result of an offense or wrongdoing, as when a rule or discipline is broken.

**punishment** action performed as the result of wrongdoing

The goal of directing children is to teach them behavior that will be accepted by society and will foster self-reliance and independence. Children must feel good about themselves and their actions. They should not act because it will prevent punishment. Self-esteem is developed early in a child's life and is directly related to the way in which behavior is taught and reinforced.

Your role is usually to maintain the discipline already in the home. If you are going to set up new rules in the house, your supervisor will plan this carefully with you. Remember, you will be leaving this house but the other people will stay. You must set up rules *they* can live with when you are gone. Should you be unable to follow the discipline already in the household, report this to your supervisor. If discipline seems unusually harsh or punishment seems severe, report this with objective data. Punishment is not within your role as a homemaker/home health aide. If you feel that a child deserves punishment, discuss this with your supervisor. As you work with children, remember:

- Treat each child as an individual.
- Discuss with the child the expectations related to his behavior or a particular task. "I expect . . . . Do you understand?"
- Encourage and praise children whenever possible.
- Use positive suggestions—avoid saying "Don't." Rather say, "Please make your bed," or "Please lower the television because it is disturbing your grandfather and he cannot sleep now. Thank you."
- Explain the limits that are set upon the behavior before the child makes a mistake. "You may play outside until it is dark. Then you are to come in. Do you understand?"
- Make mealtime a pleasure.
- Prepare food the child enjoys.
- Encourage parents to take an active part in making decisions.
- Do not take sides in arguments.
- Suggest that people separate during an argument before harsh words are said or physical punishment has taken place.

- Do not be judgmental.
- Report changes in family members.
- Report changes in family activities.
- Report feelings or suggestions and the objective happenings that lead you to your suspicions.
- Report child abuse or neglect.

## Your Role as a Homemaker/Home Health Aide

Your role in each family will be different. Be sure you discuss your role with your supervisor so you understand exactly what is expected of you. Usually, you will be expected to assume one or more of the following roles:

- Teacher
- Primary caregiver
- Observer
- Stabilizer
- Assistant caregiver

Try to maintain the routine familiar to the family. The fewer the changes, the better. Familiarity maintains a feeling of security. If a child has always been involved in household tasks, it would be best to continue this. However, if the child has never taken an active part in the house or its care, this time of illness might not be the best time to start. On the other hand, it might. Use your judgment. Discuss your opinions and plans with your supervisor. It is most important that your plan reflects the best possible plan for that house and that child.

Report all your observations of behavior changes of the child and the adults in the house. You may notice many changes, or very few. When caring for children, remember that they are part of a unit and depend on that unit. Therefore, the behavior of other family members is important.

Be alert for observations concerning behavior in the home when you are not there! What does the child say? Do your observations agree with the child's report or the adult's report? Your personal opinions as to the responsibilities children should or should not have are not important at this time. The most important point is what works in this house!

# Section 2   Child Abuse

## Objectives: What You Will Learn to Do

- Define the various kinds of abuse.
- Become familiar with some of the reasons for child abuse and why children do not report it.
- Discuss your role as a homemaker/home health aide when working in a home where child abuse has taken place.

## Introduction: Child Abuse

**abuse** any act that causes another harm; using a substance to excess

**Abuse** is any act that is considered to be improper and that usually causes harm or pain to another. No one knows exactly how many children are harmed, and no one knows exactly why some people abuse children. Many possible reasons for abuse have been explored. None of these reasons have been proven. Abuse may be linked to increased stress in a house and may only happen once in a while. Even if it occurs only once or even occasionally, it must be reported to protect the child and help the family as a whole.

No matter what the reasons for the abuse of children, all of them result in children being either physically or emotionally traumatized. Sometimes the children report these events; but most often they do not (Fig. 5.2).

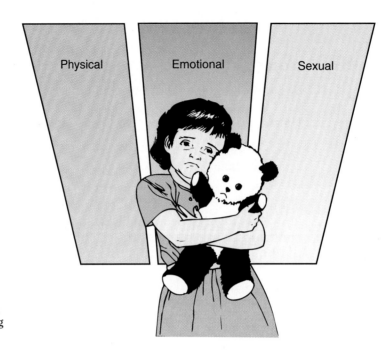

Physical    Emotional    Sexual

**FIGURE 5.2** Abuse comes in many forms. Be alert and report any concerns you have regarding abuse or neglect.

## SOME REASONS FOR ABUSE

- The abuser was also abused and learned this type of behavior.
- The abuser cannot cope with the stress of having children.
- The abuser is not the parent, but the parent is unable to stop the event.

## REASONS CHILDREN DO NOT REPORT ABUSE

- They are ashamed.
- They do not know who to tell.
- They do not know any other type of behavior.
- They are afraid the abuse will increase.
- They feel they deserve it.

## KINDS OF ABUSE

There are three main kinds of child abuse:

1. *Physical:* This abuse is seen when a child is beaten, tied up, burned. The evidence of this abuse is visible, except in the case of broken bones when the evidence must be verified by X-ray.
2. *Emotional:* This abuse is seen when a child is scared, neglected, screamed at, not permitted to feel safe.
3. *Sexual:* This abuse exists when a child is forced to submit to sexual acts because of fear of either physical or emotional harm.

Many people have definite feelings about child abuse and the punishments they feel are just for abusers. Some people think children should be removed from the house where they were abused. Some people feel the abusers should be put in jail. It is important to think about your feelings on this subject. It is also important to be able to work in a home where there has been abuse without judging the people. Your responsibility will be to care for the child in the family without punishing the parent or family member who is the abuser. If at any time you feel you are unable to work in a home where abuse has occurred, report your feeling to your supervisor.

## Your Role as a Homemaker/Home Health Aide

It is possible that you will have different roles in different cases. It is important for you to understand what is expected of you in each house. Keep in close contact with your supervisor so she can reinforce your actions and alter the plan of care as is necessary.

Your role will be determined by the situation. Sometimes the courts will insist that a homemaker/home health aide be in the home. In this case, the parents may feel you are acting as a "policeman." In a sense you are. But your main role is to provide a safe environment for the child and to support the parent in learning to cope with the problem. Learning new behavior is difficult, and your support is crucial in this situation. You will be calm and nonjudgmental and will demonstrate the proper way to interact with the child.

In some cases, the parent will be removed from the house and you will be placed there instead. In this case, you will act in a supportive way to the child and provide a safe, calm environment for him.

It is possible you will be assigned a client who is a member of a family where abuse is taking place. In this case, you will come by this information by accident. Report it immediately! In some states, it is a crime *not* to report such information.

No matter what the case, if you are in a home where child abuse has taken place, here are some general guidelines:

- Be supportive to the parents. Do not be judgmental. Do not compare one case with another. Do not compare their life with yours.
- Be observant! Observe the family dynamics. How do the people in the family interact? Do they scream? Do they tease? Do they talk nicely to one member and in a hostile tone to another?
- Are there any signs of further abuse? Do the children have marks on them? Are they fed? Is there food in the house? Do they have a place to sleep? Are they clean? Do they laugh? Do they play? Do they seem afraid?
- Have you noticed any unusual behavior?

Your feelings are important in these cases. If you suspect that something is wrong in the family dynamics, report your feelings and the objective observations to your supervisor immediately! Do not wait! Children cannot always protect themselves. They need adults to do it for them.

- Do the parents have activities that can be considered "adult"? Do they have friends? Do they go out?

- Is the family keeping its counseling appointments?
- Listen to what the children say. If you do not understand what they are saying, report the entire conversation to your supervisor.

# Section 3   Developmental Disabilities

## Objectives: What You Will Learn to Do

- Discuss the concept of developmental disabilities.
- Discuss the role of a homemaker/home health aide when caring for a child with developmental disabilities.

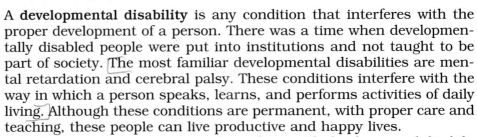

### Introduction: What Is a Developmental Disability?

**developmental disability**
any condition that interferes with the normal development of a person

A **developmental disability** is any condition that interferes with the proper development of a person. There was a time when developmentally disabled people were put into institutions and not taught to be part of society. The most familiar developmental disabilities are mental retardation and cerebral palsy. These conditions interfere with the way in which a person speaks, learns, and performs activities of daily living. Although these conditions are permanent, with proper care and teaching, these people can live productive and happy lives.

The exact reason some people are born with developmental disabilities is not known. However, we do know that these conditions are not contagious. Four reasons some people have developmental disabilities are:

1. Deficiency in the development of the fetus
2. Infection or injury during birth
3. Accident during developmental stages of a child
4. Heredity

### Your Role as a Homemaker/Home Health Aide

As you care for children who have developmental disabilities, remember that they have the same needs as other children. As they become adults, they are expected to be able to meet more and more needs themselves. Your client, however, may never be able to do that. Therefore, you, or another adult, will have to continue to help him meet his needs throughout his life.

Your feelings as you care for your client are important. Do you feel as though you are doing a worthwhile activity? Do you feel as though you are contributing to the family life of your client? Do you feel that your activities are a waste of time? Discuss your feelings with your supervisor so that the two of you can put your activities into perspective.

As you work with your client, the plan of care will be determined by what your client can do when you receive the assignment and by what is expected of him in the future. Follow the plan carefully. You will be instructed in the ways to specially feed, carry, and ambulate your client. It is important that each step be carefully planned so that the client does not get discouraged or attempt an activity that is dangerous for him. In addition, it is necessary to establish a plan the family can follow when you are not in the home and they must assume the care of the client. Stimulation of the client is an important activity of the caregiver. You may be asked to "play" with the client. Do not neglect this activity, as it is necessary for proper development of the senses. However, there are different activities that are appropriate for different ages; so, do not assume one activity is correct until you discuss it with your supervisor. All of your activities will fall into one of these categories:

- Supporting the family in the form of demonstration, respite, or discussion
- Encouraging independence up to the ability of the client
- Providing physical and emotional care
- Providing a safe general environment, in particular with feeding and ambulation

Each family reacts differently to having a disabled member. Do not compare one family with another, but accept the family as they are. If you have concerns, discuss them with your supervisor.

As you work in the home, observe the family dynamics. How do the members of the family interact with each other? with the client? Do they consider him a part of the family or merely an imposition? Are the family members following the care plan when you are not in the home? The care of a developmentally disabled child can be a draining experience on all family members. Each one is affected in a different way. It is your role to observe and report family interactions that may affect the care and safety of your client. With prompt reporting, your supervisor can intervene and provide support, counseling, or other aid to the family.

# Section 4 Newborn and Infant Care

## Objectives: What You Will Learn to Do

- Assist the mother in breast-feeding the baby.
- Prepare infant formula.
- Sterilize water, bottles, nipples, and caps.
- Carry, feed, and burp a baby.
- Provide care for an infant's umbilical cord.
- Provide care for a male after circumcision.
- Give a baby a bath.

### *Introduction: Care of the Infant in the Home*

You may be assigned to care directly for the child or you may be caring for the mother and other family members may care for the child. Or you may be assigned to care for both mother and child.
Some of the reasons you may care for an infant are:

- The mother is recovering from surgery.
- The mother is unable emotionally to assume the care of the child alone.

- There are many other children in the house.
- The child is ill.
- The child has been abused.

The most important part of your role in this house is to teach by example. You will not be in this house forever, and it is important that someone can take over when you leave. One of the tasks you will teach is how to hold the baby comfortably and safely.

Most infants are fed six times a day or about every three to four hours. Nursing babies, however, may be fed as often as every two hours. It is important to remember that some will eat more often and some less. Stick to the schedule already in place in the house. If the mother is breast-feeding her baby, it may be your responsibility to bring the baby to her when it is time for feeding. If the baby is being bottle-fed, you may need to prepare the formula. You will be given detailed instructions by your supervisor about your responsibilities. If you have a question, ask.

## CARRYING AN INFANT

Carrying an infant is a big responsibility. It is important to pay close attention to many details and safety factors.

- Always support the child's head (Fig. 5.3).
- Hold the infant close to you.
- Do not carry other objects while you are carrying a baby.
- Do not hold an infant while you are talking on the phone or cooking at the stove.

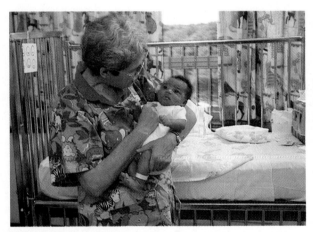
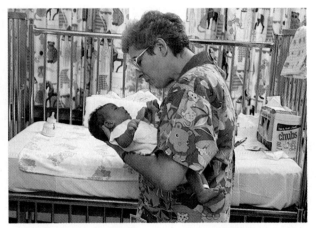

**FIGURE 5.3** Support the baby in a comfortable, safe, and secure manner so that you can see where you are going and can quickly reach the baby if needed.

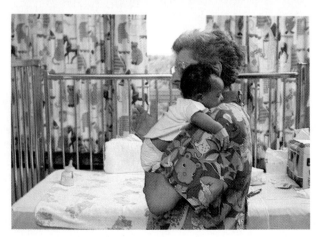

- Do not carry a baby into a dark room. Turn on the light before you enter.
- Be alert to basic household hazards, such as liquid spills, shoes, clothing on the floor, and loose rugs.
- Be alert while carrying a baby up and down stairs.
- Wear good supporting shoes with nonskid soles while you are carrying a baby.

## DIET

Children's diets vary. Different pediatricians add cereal to diets at different ages. Some pediatricians insist on breast-feeding; some do not. It is important to support the family as they learn to follow the diet their physician has prescribed. Although you may have definite feelings about the manner in which the child's diet has been ordered, do not change it. Do not change a diet or routine without discussing it with your supervisor.

Observe the pediatric client for his acceptance of the diet. If you notice the child has a great deal of gas following a meal, cries a great deal, has diarrhea or is constipated, or refuses food on a regular basis, report this to your supervisor immediately. Remember, the child is unable to get help himself. He needs you to report his distress.

## ASSISTING WITH FEEDING INFANTS

### Breast-Feeding

You will be asked to assist in the feeding of infants. In some homes, the mothers will breast-feed the babies. Breast-feeding is a natural act. Most babies and mothers learn how to do this while the mother is still in the hospital. By the time they come home the mother will probably have had an opportunity to learn some of the basic skills of breast-feeding. She will have some pamphlets with pictures. If they are not enough information, ask your supervisor for some additional literature.

The body makes milk about two to four days after the birth. The clear yellow fluid in the breast before that time is called colostrum. This is a nourishing substance and contains antibodies the baby needs. When the milk starts to fill the breasts, they become hard and full and may be uncomfortable. As the baby nurses, the body regulates the amount of milk needed to satisfy the baby, the discomfort disappears, and the breasts become soft. As the baby grows and needs more milk, the body will adjust the supply.

During the first few days after birth, nursing may stimulate the client's uterus to contract. Sometimes this is very uncomfortable, and sometimes it is not. Encourage the client to discuss any discomfort with her physician before she takes medication to relieve the pain.

Most experts recommend feeding the baby from both breasts at each feeding—usually six to eight minutes at each breast. The nutrition of the mother greatly influences the quality of the milk the body produces. The mother should eat a balanced diet, take vitamins if the physician recommends them, and increase the calorie intake slightly. The client should drink six to eight glasses of fluid each day. If the baby sleeps well and nurses seven to ten times a day during the first months of life, the milk is sufficient and the baby is nursing well.

Some families feel comfortable with having a mother feed her baby while other family members are present. Some women prefer privacy. Support the mother and the family in their decision.

You may be asked to help the mother ready herself to breast-feed. This may involve assisting the mother in getting comfortable, removing distractions, or bringing the baby, after you have changed the diaper, to the mother. Some women nurse sitting up and some lying on their side.

The mother may have questions about the timing of the feeding, ways in which to interest the baby in feeding, her diet, or the care of her breasts. Assist the mother in reading the material given to her by her physician and the hospital. This material will include advice on whether to feed from both breasts on one feeding, how long to nurse, and how to supplement feedings if necessary. If this material does not answer her questions or if you have questions, call your supervisor.

## Guidelines: Assisting with Breast-Feeding

- Remind the mother to wash her hands before each feeding. Hands should be washed with a mild soap. Nipples are usually washed with soapy water and rinsed thoroughly during daily bathing. Washing the nipples before each feeding is not usually necessary. The mother should use circular motions, from the nipple outward, when she washes.

- Assist the mother with nursing aids such as breast shields or pumps.

- The decision to stop nursing is a personal one and will affect both mother and child. Suggest the mother discuss this with her physician before any decision is made.

- If the baby does not take the breast, have the mother stroke the cheek closest to the breast with her nipple. This will cause the child to turn toward the breast (Fig. 5.4).

- Support the mother as she learns the skill of breast-feeding. Provide quiet time between feedings so the mother can rest.

- While the breast is in the baby's mouth, remind the mother to keep the breast tissue away from the baby's nose with one or two fingers (Fig. 5.5).

- If milk drips from the breast not being sucked, clean the breast. This is normal.

- To remove the breast from the baby's mouth, the mother should break the suction by either inserting her little finger in the cor-

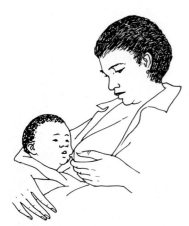

**FIGURE 5.4** Stimulate the baby to turn towards the breast.

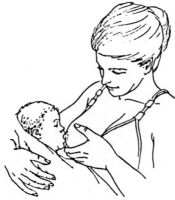

**FIGURE 5.5** Keep breast tissue away from the baby's nose so he can breathe more easily.

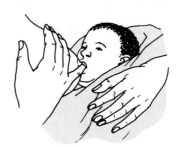

**FIGURE 5.6** Break the suction before removing the nipple from the baby's mouth.

ner of the baby's mouth or pushing on her breast tissue near the baby's mouth (Fig. 5.6).

■ The routine of feeding and the length of nursing is varied and should be decided by the mother and baby.

### Bottle-Feeding

The decision to bottle-feed an infant, or to supplement breast-feedings with formula, is made by the mother and her physician. Choosing the type of formula is also made with medical advice. Your role is to support the mother and the family with their decision. In some cases, the mother will use a special pump to remove her breast milk and put it in a bottle for use later.

## Guidelines: Assisting With Bottle-Feeding

■ Make sure that the formula is fresh and the bottles have been properly stored.

■ Follow the mother's wishes as to the temperature of the bottles when the baby is fed. If you do not agree with her wishes, discuss this with your supervisor. Check the temperature of the formula before you feed the baby (Fig. 5.7).

■ Babies should be held while they are given bottles. Do not prop bottles. Do not leave babies unattended while they are drinking bottles (Fig. 5.8).

■ Hold the bottle so that the nipple is full of formula and the baby does not suck air (Fig. 5.9).

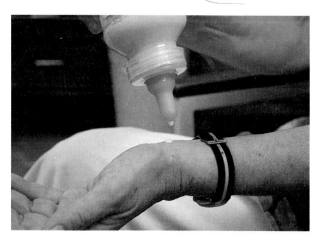

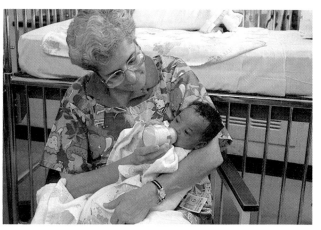

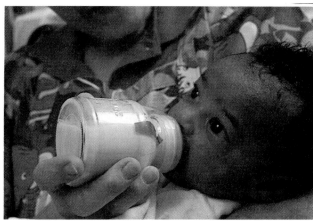

FIGURE 5.7 Always check the temperature of the liquid in the bottle before giving it to the baby.

FIGURE 5.8 Infants should be held during bottle feeding.

FIGURE 5.9 The nipple should be full of liquid to prevent the baby from sucking and swallowing air.

## STERILIZING BOTTLES AND NIPPLES

Bottles and nipples are sterilized to destroy bacteria that might cause illness. There are many opinions as to the age when sterilizing bottles is no longer necessary. Some physicians do not require sterilizing bottles for newborns. You will be asked to follow the instructions of your supervisor. If you do not agree or have questions, ask for an explanation. Do not alter the procedure without being given permission to do so.

Some people sterilize bottles and nipples in the dishwasher. Some people have found microwave ovens to be acceptable. The most common method of sterilizing bottles and nipples, however, is on the top of the stove.

## Procedure 1: To Sterilize Bottles

1. Assemble your equipment:
   Bottles
   Nipples, caps, and jar
   Bottle brush
   Dish detergent
   Hot water from the tap
   Large pot with cover or a special sterilizing pot for baby bottles
   Small towel
   Tap water
   Stove or cooking source of heat
   Timer, watch, or clock
   Tongs
2. Wash your hands.
3. Scrub bottles, nipples, and caps with hot soapy water. Use the bottle brush to clean inside the bottles. Always squirt hot soapy water through the holes in the nipples to clean out any dried-on formula.
4. Rinse thoroughly with hot water.
5. Fold the small towel to fit in the bottom of the pot, and lay it there. This will prevent the bottles from breaking. (This is done when you do not have a bottle rack.)
6. Stand the washed bottles on the towel in a circle around the inside of the pot.
7. Place the caps and nipples into the clean, empty jar. Place into the pot at the center of the bottles.
8. Pour water into and around the bottles and into the jar with the nipples until two-thirds of each bottle is under water (Fig. 5.10).
9. Cover the pot.
10. Place the pot on the stove burner, and turn on the burner to the high or full setting.
11. When the water comes to a full boil, begin timing. Allow the water to remain at a full boil for 25 minutes.
12. Remove the jar with the nipple and caps 10 to 15 minutes after the full boil begins. With the nipples still inside the jar, stand the jar on the table to cool.
13. Turn off the burner.

- Ask your supervisor if you may use alcohol. Follow her instructions.
- At every diaper change, wash the cord with plain rubbing alcohol on a cotton ball. The alcohol will help speed up the drying process and will keep the cord clean.
- Never pull on the cord. Let it fall off by itself. Laying the infant on his abdomen will not hurt the cord. Binders or belly bands are not advised.
- Never give the infant a tub bath until the cord has fallen off.

### CIRCUMCISION

**circumcision** removal of the foreskin of the penis by a surgical procedure

**prepuce** foreskin of the penis, often removed in an operation called a circumcision

**Circumcision** is the surgical removal of the loose piece of skin, **prepuce** (foreskin), from the end of the penis (Fig. 5.15). It is usually done to increase the cleanliness of the penis. Sometimes, if the foreskin is not removed at birth, it shrinks and constricts the penis. This is both dangerous and painful. Circumcision can be done in the operating room before the baby comes home. It is done on a voluntary basis. That means that the mother of the baby must give her permission to have it done. In the Jewish faith, there is a ritual circumcision on the seventh day after birth. This is done either in the hospital or at home.

The physician will give the mother special instructions as to the care of the penis. Be sure and follow these instructions carefully to prevent complications.

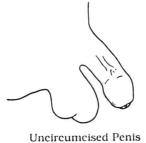

Uncircumcised Penis          Circumcised Penis

*FIGURE 5.15* The choice of whether or not to circumcise a son is a personal one. Support the family with their decision.

## *Guidelines: After Circumcision*

- Keep the penis protected from rubbing on a diaper. The pediatrician will leave instructions.
- Ask about bathing the child.
- Keep the penis clean and free of fecal matter.
- Observe for bleeding or drainage. Report these to your supervisor.

### BATHING THE INFANT

#### *Sponge Baths*

While the umbilical cord is still attached to the baby, a sponge bath with warm water or baby lotion can be given daily. More frequent bathing is usually not necessary. A tub bath is not permitted until the cord has fallen off.

Sponge bathing an infant means gently washing each part of the baby's body with mild soap and warm water, but not submerging the infant in water. Safety of the infant is very important. Whenever in doubt about anything, call your supervisor. A safe table or counter is a convenient place to give a sponge bath. Clear off the counter and wash it well. Spread a towel on the counter to make a soft warm place on which to place the baby. Prepare warm water, mild soap, washcloth, blankets, and towels before bringing the baby to the counter. Only one part of the body is washed at a time. Wash, rinse, and dry each body part or area very well. Then cover the body part right away with a towel or blanket.

### Tub Baths

After the cord has fallen off, the infant can be given a tub bath. You can use a large sink or a baby bath tub. If you are using a sink, be sure to clean the sink and counter. Scrub the sink with a cleanser and rinse it thoroughly. Assemble your equipment before you begin so you will not need to leave the room to get something that you may have forgotten. Lock the front door so no one can come in and distract you or the infant's mother. Taking the phone off the hook, if the mother agrees, will prevent it from ringing during the bath. You cannot leave the infant in the tub or on the counter while you answer the phone or the doorbell.

Bath time should be a pleasant and enjoyable time for the mother and baby. Try to involve the mother as much as she is able, and take the opportunity to teach her how to care for the baby. The infant's safety is your first responsibility. Keep your hands and eyes on the baby throughout the bath.

## Procedure 2: Giving the Infant a Tub Bath

1. Assemble your equipment:
   Infant tub or sink
   Two bath towels (soft)
   Cotton balls
   Washcloth
   Warm water (warm to the touch of the elbow)
   Baby soap
   Baby shampoo (optional)
   Baby powder, lotion, or cream
   Diaper
   Clean clothes
2. Wash your hands.
3. Wash the sink or tub with a disinfectant cleanser and rinse thoroughly.
4. Line the sink or tub with a bath towel.
5. Place a towel on the counter next to the sink or tub, as you may want to lay the infant down to dry him.
6. Fill the tub or sink with 1 to 2 inches of warm water (warm to the touch of the elbow).
7. Undress the infant, wrap him in a towel or blanket, and bring him to the tub or sink (Fig. 5.16).
8. Using a cotton ball moistened with warm water and squeezed out, gently wipe the infant's eyes from the nose toward the ears. Use a clean cotton ball for each eye (Fig. 5.17).

FIGURE 5.16

wrapping the baby

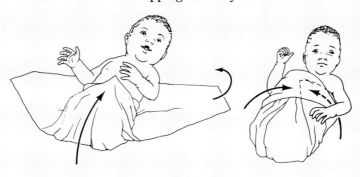

Fold Lower
Corner of Blanket
Over the Legs
and Feet. . .

Fold the Two Side
Corners Under the Arms
and Over the Chest

FIGURE 5.17

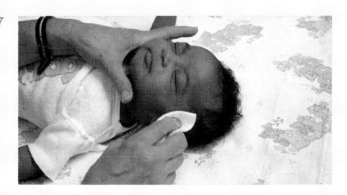

9. To wash the hair, hold the infant in the football hold, with the baby's head over the sink or tub. This will free your other arm to wet the hair, apply a small amount of shampoo, and rinse the hair.

10. Dry the infant's head with a towel.

11. Unwrap the infant, and gently place him on the towel in the sink or tub. One of your hands should always be holding the baby. Never let go, not even for a second.

12. Wash the infant's body with the soap and the washcloth, being careful to wash between the folds (creases) of the skin (Fig. 5.18).

FIGURE 5.18

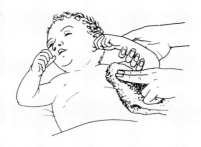

FIGURE 5.19

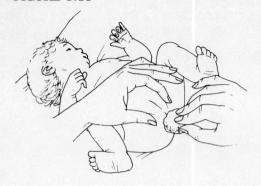

FIGURE 5.20

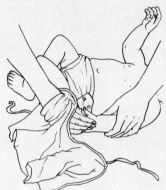

- Slip the fingers of one hand inside the sleeve of the shirt.
- With that hand, take the baby's hand. With your other hand, pull the sleeve up over the baby's arm.
- Turn the baby gently on his side.
- Slip the shirt down over his back.
- Turn him gently back, and draw the shirt to the other side.
- Put the baby's other arm into its sleeve in the same way.
- Fasten the ties or snaps.

13. If the infant is female, always wash the perineal area from front to back (Fig. 5.19).

14. If the infant is male, clean the foreskin by gently retracting it. If the child has been circumcised, this is not necessary.

15. Rinse the infant thoroughly with warm water.

16. Lift the infant out of the water and onto the towel you laid out on the counter.

17. Dry the infant well, being careful to dry between the folds of the skin.

18. Now you can apply powder, lotion, or cream to the infant, whichever the mother prefers, or as instructed by your supervisor.

19. Diaper and dress the infant (Fig. 5.20).

20. Place the infant in his crib, or allow the mother to hold him. Show the mother how to hold the infant in either the upright or the cradle position.

21. Clean and return the equipment and supplies to their proper place.

22. Clean the area where the bath was given.

23. Wash your hands.

## INFANT SAFETY

When you are caring for an infant, you must take special precautions to protect the baby from preventable accidents. Even if an infant has not yet learned to roll over, he can wiggle and kick until he falls off beds, chairs, tables, or counters. Never leave an infant unattended on any of these surfaces. If you are far from the infant's crib and you must leave him unattended for a few seconds, put him on the floor. The safest place for an infant is in his crib with the side rails up. Some people keep babies in a carriage or a drawer because they do not have a crib. Here are other things you can do to prevent accidents when caring for an infant:

- Wash your hands before handling the infant or his supplies.
- Place the infant on his side or belly after feeding to prevent aspiration.

- Keep the crib rails in the up position when the infant is sleeping or playing.
- Use only 1 to 2 inches of bath water, and never leave the infant alone in the water.
- Never place an infant in an infant seat on tables, chairs, beds, or counters.
- Keep all medications and cleaning solutions out of the reach of all children.

## ASSISTING WITH MEDICATION

Sometimes the child you are caring for will require medication. In that case the family will take the responsibility for giving the medication. Although you may assist, you may not be the person who assumes the responsibility of giving the medication.

Your role is to observe the child after he has received the medication. If you notice any of the behaviors shown in Figure 5.21, call your supervisor immediately.

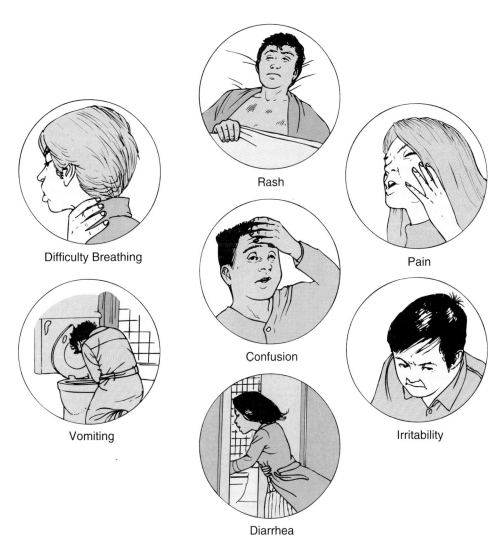

Difficulty Breathing

Rash

Pain

Confusion

Vomiting

Diarrhea

Irritability

**FIGURE 5.21**  Changes in usual patterns of behavior may indicate a medication reaction. Report any change you notice or are told about.

## Topics for Discussion

1. Discuss the way you would assist a new mother in organizing her day so that she could properly care for the baby and herself.
2. What would you do if you returned to your client's house and found it dirty and disorderly and found the whole routine changed?
3. If there were no clean place to bathe the baby such as sink or tub, what would you do? Share your thought process and how you would make the decision as to what to do first.

# Chapter 6

# Care of the Dying in the Home

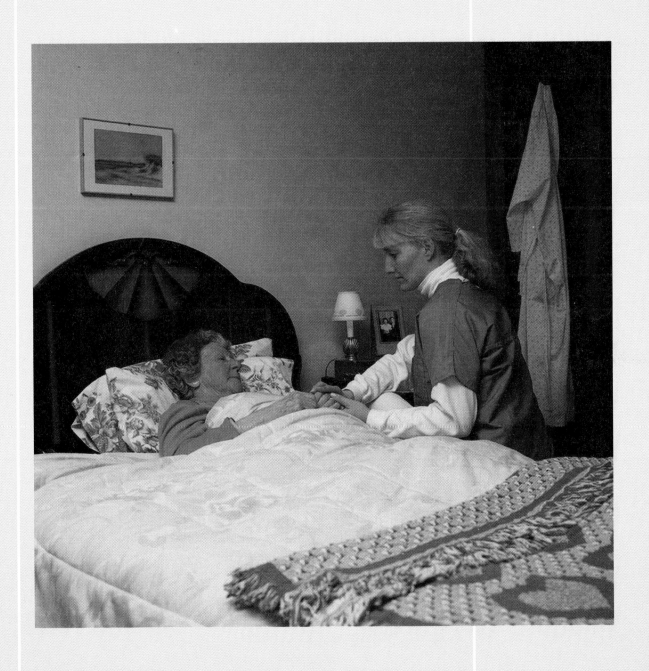

# Section 1  Dying

**Objectives: What You Will Learn to Do**

- Understand the steps that occur when a person is dying.
- Understand the client and family's special emotional needs.
- Be a good listener to the client and family.
- Examine your first experience with death, and understand how it has affected you.
- Become familiar with the hospice concept, and use part of it when working with the client.

## Introduction: Working with the Client Who Is Dying

Many of us feel uncomfortable when we are around a person who is dying. We may not know how to act or what to say to them. We may feel sad or helpless or angry. These feelings may be extra strong if the person is the same age we are or a member of our family. Sometimes, to deal with our feelings, we try to avoid working with the person who is dying, or we rush through our tasks as quickly as possible so that we can leave the room. This often leaves the dying person feeling isolated, lonely, or deserted.

To avoid this happening, as a homemaker/home health aide, it will be your responsibility to help meet the very special needs of the dying person and his family. Do not be frightened by the thought of helping the client who is dying. By using the same caring, consideration, and understanding you use with clients who will recover, you will be able to work with clients who are dying. After all, we all will die one day, and we must remind ourselves to treat these people as we would like to be treated if we were dying.

Many clients are told they are dying. This must be done by a family member or physician. If a family decides not to let your client know he is dying, you are obligated to carry out their wishes even though at times, keeping up this charade is most difficult. Discuss your feelings and activities with your supervisor.

### STEPS IN THE DYING PROCESS

Doctor Elisabeth Kübler-Ross spent many years talking with the dying and studying how people die (Fig. 6.1). She found there are certain stages or steps involved. It is most important to remember that:

- All clients are different.
- The family of the person who is dying will go through all of these steps.
- Everyone will not experience every step.
- Clients and families will go from step to step at any time.
- Clients do not go through these steps in any given order.
  Step 1: *Denial*—"Not me!"
  Step 2: *Anger*—"Why me?"
  Step 3: *Bargaining*—"Me, but . . ."
  Step 4: *Depression*—"Ah, me."
  Step 5: *Acceptance*—"Yes, me."

**STAGES OF DYING**

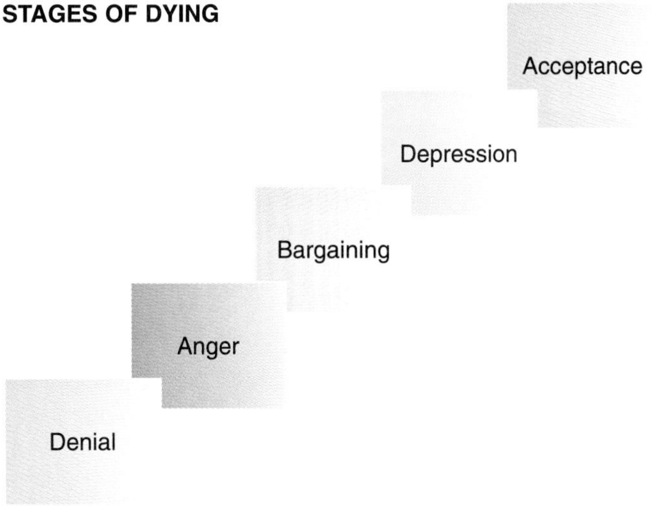

Acceptance

Depression

Bargaining

Anger

Denial

*FIGURE 6.1* Everyone passes through these stages at different rates and sometimes in a different order.

## SPECIAL EMOTIONAL NEEDS OF THE DYING

Clients who are dying are still living people and have the same needs as you (Fig. 6.2). Some of these are:

- The *need to be normal:* to know that the thoughts and feelings they are having are like those of others in their situation.
- The *need for meaningful relations:* a chance to talk to friends and family members on a meaningful level.
- The *need for love:* to feel that they are the object of someone's love. (Couples may have sexual exchanges.)
- The *need for recreation:* some way to pass the time. It may be knitting, playing cards, watching TV, reading books, or talking to loved ones.
- The *need for safety and security:* to know that they will be cared for carefully up until the moment of death.

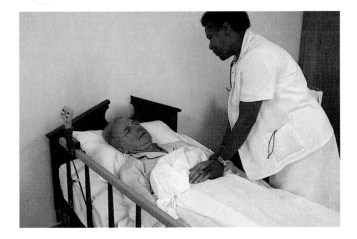

*FIGURE 6.2* The dying have the same basic human needs as everyone else. Plan your care to meet these needs.

## BE A GOOD LISTENER

When a client suspects that he is going to die, he may react in various ways:

- He may ask everyone about his chances for recovery.
- He may be afraid to be alone and want a lot of attention from you.

- He may ask a lot of questions.
- He may seem to complain constantly.
- He may make requests that seem unreasonable.

Usually, when a client asks questions of his caregivers, he is sending a signal that he wants information. Many times you may not have all the information needed to answer the questions. Assure the client that you will either get the information or provide someone who will.

Here are some guidelines you may wish to use when talking with a client who is dying:

1. *Honesty.* If you don't know, be honest and say so. The client probably does not expect you to know everything about his condition anyway.

2. *Do not offer false hope or reassurance.* By telling a dying person that he will be better soon, the homemaker/home health aide is proving she cannot be trusted. Offer realistic short-term goals, or say nothing.

3. *Do not say too much.* A caring look, an unhurried manner, a nod or word at the right time tells the client that you care. Example: "I understand how you feel. I think I would feel the same way."

4. *Let the client take the lead.* Often a question represents a fear or concern of the client. He may feel relieved if you allow him to express the concern. Example: "I don't know when you'll die. Why do you ask?"

5. *Do not destroy hope.* If the client really feels that he will recover, even if we know he won't, do not destroy this hope. Hope is an important part of life. The client who has hope usually lives longer than the client who does not. Example: "I'm happy to hear of your plans to go on a trip next year."

**hospice** program of care that allows a dying client to remain at home and die at home while receiving professionally supervised care

Many areas of the country have **hospice** programs. These are organized systems of professional care that help families care for dying clients at home up to and including the time of death. The hospice concept is not appropriate for everyone because not everyone is able to die at home without any heroic methods. You can now even apply many principles of hospice care to your work with clients without actually having a hospice program.

Most hospice clients do not wish any treatment except to remain comfortable and pain-free. This is often difficult for families to accept. These programs provide the support and help to the dying client and his family without the use of curative methods and include:

- Treating the client/family as a unit of care
- Allowing the client/family as much choice as possible in determining care in the home
- Making use of team professionals who are experienced in home health care
- Helping the family through the dying process
- Helping the family after the death of their loved one

In addition, hospice programs use trained volunteers to help with transportation, shopping, and assisting the client with hobbies and other important things that paid employees seldom have time to do. Volunteer training sessions are run by hospice programs to prepare community members to work with the dying and their families.

You may find yourself caring for a client in a family where you feel hospice-type care is most appropriate. In that case, talk to your supervisor. She will discuss the client's situation with the physician. Do not take it upon yourself to recommend hospice care.

You may also find yourself caring for a client who has refused aggressive treatment and has decided to die. This may be hard for you to accept. Remember, this is the client's decision and you must accept it. If you have difficulty working in this house, discuss it with your supervisor.

## Understanding Your Feelings About Death

A person's first exposure to death (usually as a child) affects how the person will react to death for the rest of his life. The time, place, and manner of death we experience may be different, but the feelings are the same. To help you deal with your feelings, it is often helpful to think about death and your feelings. You may want to think about the different feelings you experience when you discuss the death of a baby, a young person, an older person, or a terminally ill person. Some people feel differently about the death of a person when it occurs suddenly. You may want to share these feelings with a close friend, member of the clergy, or someone you trust.

There is no right or wrong way to feel about death or to react to death. It is a very individual experience.

Some families treat death as a very solemn religious experience; some do not. You will be asked to support the family as they deal with this experience within their culture, their coping mechanisms, and their family dynamics.

# Section 2 Physical Care of the Dying

## Objectives: What You Will Learn to Do

■ Make the client who is dying as comfortable as possible.
■ Help meet the physical needs of the client and family.

## Introduction: Physical Needs

The client who is dying usually needs careful attention to physical needs. You will have to attend to many needs that the person used to attend to himself. Allow the client to do as much as possible for himself. This permits him to be independent for as long as he is able. Discuss with your supervisor your activities and what the family will do. Here are some guidelines for care:

■ *Skin care.* Bathe daily, with partial bathing as necessary. The skin may be fragile, so wash gently with mild soap. Apply lotion to bony prominences.

■ *Positioning.* Do not allow tight clothing, stockings, garters, or tight bed linens. Use pillows and rolled blankets for careful positioning. Change the client's position often, at least every one and one-half to two hours. Change soiled linens and protective pads. Change nonsterile dressings when soiled. Reinforce sterile dressings.

■ *Mouth care.* Cleanse teeth and mouth at least twice daily. Remove dentures, or brush teeth. Cleanse mucous membranes with glycerine swabs, as needed.

■ *Bowel care.* Keep a careful record of bowel movements, and notify the nurse if the client has not had a bowel movement in several days.

■ *Circulation.* The circulation slows as death approaches, and the arms and legs may feel cold and look ashen. Elevate the limbs as needed to aid blood return and do not allow the limbs to be in a "dependent position."

■ *Food/water.* Assist the client to a comfortable position, cleanse the mouth. Wash his hands, refresh the linen. Air the room of any odors. Do not try to mask odors with perfume or spray, but remove the source of the odors. Ask the client and his family about food choices, and try to get as much variety as possible. Offer small portions of food and frequent sips of water so as not to tire the client with long meals. Arrange portions in a neat, appetizing manner.

■ *Breathing.* Remove secretions from the mouth as necessary. Urge the client to cough up mucous for as long as possible. Elevate the head of the bed, or prop the client on pillows if this makes breathing easier.

## THE MOMENT OF DEATH

Many clients are now choosing to die at home rather than returning to the hospital. Usually, the nurse has prepared the family for the moment of death and the other events that will occur.

Many clients die as they have lived. The fearful die in fear, the angry die in anger, and the peaceful die in peace. Some simply slip into a coma for days before the death, and others will cling constantly to a loved one's hand.

Dying is a spiritual process for some people. Many clients and families will ask to see a priest, minister, rabbi, or person who shares the same concept of spirituality. As the time of death nears, services or prayer rituals may be held at the bedside, and privacy will be requested.

**Cheyne-Stokes** a type of noisy breathing alternating with periods of no breathing; usually precedes death

Breathing may become very irregular and stop for periods of up to thirty seconds or more. This breathing is called **Cheyne-Stokes** breathing, and although it may be upsetting to the family, it is a very usual occurrence. As death approaches, the gurgling breathing called the death rattle may begin. At this time, the client is usually unconscious, so it does not bother him, but it may be distressing to the family. Notify the supervisor when it begins.

Talk openly and in a concerned way to the client, even when he is seemingly unconscious. Hearing is the last sense to be lost, and loving words from a family member, up until the moment of death, are comforting. Plan with your supervisor exactly what you will be expected to do when the death occurs. Whom should you call? What should you do?

Your reaction to the actual death depends on your experience with death, your culture, your religion, and how open you are in expressing and voicing your feelings. Usually, homemakers/home health aides feel sadness and loss when a client dies. This is normal. The agency you work for may hold special "support sessions" for those aides and nurses who have had a client die, so that they can discuss their feelings and help each other. Check with your agency regarding the availability of support services.

# Section 3   Postmortem Care

## Objectives: What You Will Learn to Do

■ Describe postmortem care.

### Introduction: Postmortem Care in the Home

postmortem after death

Care of the body after death is called **postmortem** care. Most of the time when death occurs at home, the family has been prepared for what to do by the doctor and nurse who care for the client. Usually, the client's doctor, the nurse from the home health agency, and the funeral director are notified. If the client's doctor is not available to make a home visit, an ambulance may have to be called to take the client to the emergency room so a physician can pronounce him dead. Check with your agency for the policies and procedures to be followed at the time of death.

The body must be prepared for removal in any case. After death occurs, the family may sit at the bedside and say their final goodbyes. Families handle grief in many ways, and they should have time and privacy as they need it. Be sure to inquire as to specific religious practices that should be observed at this time.

When appropriate, prepare the body in the following manner:

■ Remove all pillows except one under the head.
■ Bathe the body, removing secretions, reinforce dressings.
■ Place dentures in the mouth if possible.
■ Close the eyes, but do not press on the eyeballs.
■ Keep the body flat on its back, straightening the arms and legs.
■ Move the body gently to avoid bruising.
■ Check with the family regarding any jewelry the client may be wearing.
■ Fold the arms over the abdomen.
■ Check your agency's policy about the removal of catheters. Usually, you will not be asked to remove a tube after death if you did not care for it when the client was alive.

After the body is removed from the home, strip the bed and air the room. Remove any equipment. Check with the family regarding the proper disposal of these items. Place personal items carefully at the bedside so family members can remove them at the appropriate time.

In addition, the aide may help the family by answering phone calls from friends and neighbors, making coffee, or sitting with grieving family members. Ask the family how you can help, and try to do whatever is necessary to help them through this difficult time.

Some caregivers wish to attend the funeral of the client. It gives them a formal chance to say goodbye and shows the family how much they cared for the client. You must examine your own feelings on the subject and do as you feel best.

## Topics for Discussion

1. How do you feel about working with a dying client? How do you think you will feel when he dies?
2. Discuss how you feel about the hospice concept.

# Chapter 7

# Anatomy and Physiology

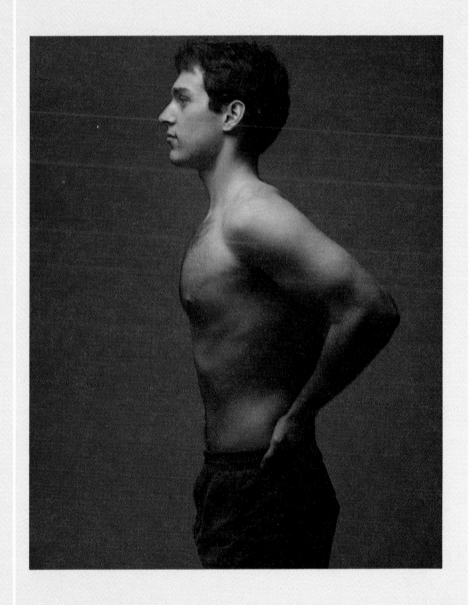

# Section 1  An Introduction to Anatomy and Physiology

## Objectives: What You Will Learn to Do

- Describe the structures and functions of cells, tissues, organs, and systems.
- Explain how body systems work together.
- Discuss ways your knowledge of body systems will help you to give better client care.

## Introduction: An Introduction to Anatomy and Physiology

**anatomy** the study of the structure of the body

**physiology** study of the functions of body tissues and organs

**Anatomy** is the study of the structure of the body. **Physiology** is the study of how the body functions. It is difficult to discuss one without the other. Knowledge of how the human body is constructed and how it works will help you give better care to your clients. The vocabulary of these subjects will help you understand your supervisor's instructions.

### THE CELL

**cell** basic unit of living matter

The **cell** is the fundamental microscopic building block of all living matter. The human body is made up of millions of cells. Each has a special task within the body, but they all have certain things in common:

- They come from preexisting cells.
- They use oxygen to break down food into energy.
- They need water to live.
- They grow and repair themselves.
- They reproduce.
- They die.

### TISSUES

**tissue** group of cells of the same type

Cells usually do not work alone. Groups of cells of the same type that do a particular kind of work are organized into **tissues**.

## Tissues to Systems

**organ** several types of tissues grouped together to perform a certain function

**system** group of organs acting together to carry out one or more body functions

Tissues, each having a special function, are grouped together to form **organs,** such as the heart and lungs. Each organ, in turn, has a specific function that cannot be carried out without its various tissues. Organs that work together to perform one or more body functions make up **systems:** for example, the digestive system, respiratory system, and circulatory system. Always remember that a system cannot work by itself. Systems are dependent on each other. What happens to one system affects all the others (Fig. 7.1).

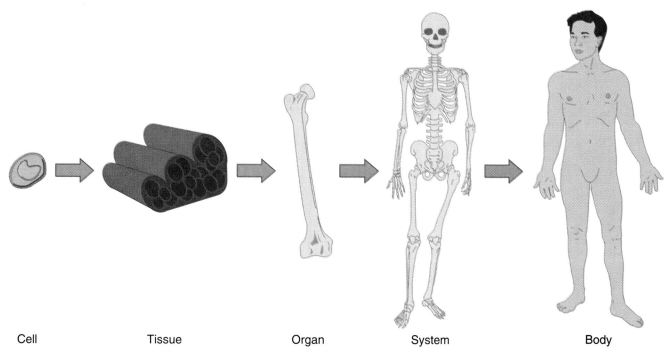

| Cell | Tissue | Organ | System | Body |

FIGURE 7.1 Cells combine to form tissues, tissues combine to form organs, and organs combine to form systems.

## Primary Kinds of Tissues

| Type of Tissue | Function | Location in the Body |
| --- | --- | --- |
| Epithelial | Protect, secrete, absorb, receive sensations | Lining of mouth and nose, skin, lining of stomach |
| Connective tissue | Connect, support, cover | Tendons, bones, layer of fatty tissue under skin |
| Muscle tissue<br>  a. Striated<br>  b. Smooth<br>  c. Cardiac | Movement—stretch, contract | Muscle groups in arms, legs, abdomen, back, and internal organs |
| Nerve tissue | Transmit impulses to and from the central nervous system and to the body systems | Throughout the body |
| Blood and lymph tissue | Circulate nutrients, oxygen, and antibodies throughout the body: remove waste products | Circulatory system |

## THE SKIN

**skin** the largest organ in the body whose functions include protection from infection, temperature regulation, and removal of waste products

**dilate** expand; get bigger

The **skin,** which is our largest system, has many functions. It covers and protects internal organs from injury, bacteria, and environmental changes. The skin also contains nerve endings from the nervous system that aid the body in awareness of its environment. The skin helps regulate the body temperature by controlling the loss of heat from the body. To increase heat loss, the blood vessels near the skin **dilate** or enlarge and the increased blood flow brings more heat to the skin. Then the skin temperature rises, and more heat is lost from the hot skin to the cooler environment. Even more important in heat loss is the **evaporation** of fluid **perspiration** from the sweat glands found in the skin. These glands open by **ducts** or **pores** to the outside skin.

When the body is conserving heat, perspiration stops and blood vessels constrict (contract). This prevents the blood from carrying heat to the skin. The skin temperature falls, decreasing heat loss. We know this as goose bumps. When illness is present and the body cannot release heat as quickly as it is produced, a person is said to have a fever. The body also rids itself of certain waste products through perspiration.

Skin secretes an oily substance through ducts that lead from oil glands. In this way the skin is kept lubricated, soft, and flexible. The oil provides a protective film for the skin. In elderly persons, these oil glands sometimes fail to function properly and the skin becomes quite dry, scaly, and delicate. In addition, as we age, our skin loses its elasticity and fatty padding, and the skin becomes thin, wrinkly, and saggy.

Other parts of the skin include the hair and the nails. Each hair has a root under the skin into which the oil glands of the skin open. Fingernails and toenails grow from the nailbed at the base underneath the skin. If the nailbed is destroyed, the nail stops growing.

The outer layer of the skin that you can see is called the **epidermis** (Fig. 7.2). Cells are constantly flaking off or being rubbed off this layer of the skin as they naturally die. Beneath the epidermis is the **dermis.** These cells replace the cells that are lost from the epidermis. **Pigment**, which is responsible for the color of the skin, is found in the epidermis.

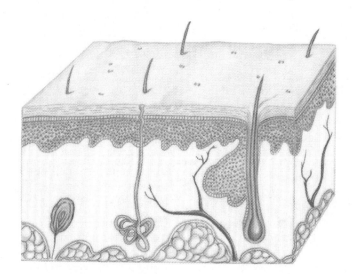

*FIGURE 7.2* Magnified cross section of skin.

Keeping the skin clean removes waste products, those naturally secreted through the skin and those from the environment that are on the skin. Waste products that remain on the skin can cause irritation, disease, and odor. This is the main reason for keeping the skin clean.

Watch for changes in your client's skin. Be aware of changes in color; temperature; bruises; breaks in skin, such as scratches or cuts; dryness or oiliness; and thinness or thickness of skin. Be particularly aware of whether both limbs are the same temperature and color. If you should notice any changes or areas on the client's body about which you have a question, report it to your supervisor.

## THE SKELETAL SYSTEM

**skeletal system** bones of the
body which give the body
shape and protection

The **skeletal system** is made up of more than 206 bones. The bones act as a framework for the body, giving it structure and support. Bones also protect several internal organs. The bones of the skull, joined together during the first year of life, totally surround the brain. The **vertebral column,** or spinal column, protects the spinal cord. The rib cage guards the heart, lungs, and major blood vessels. Bones are the passive organs of motion. They do not move by themselves. They must be moved by muscles, which shorten or contract. This is an example of how systems work together.

**vertebral column** backbone

Bones also store minerals that are necessary for many other body activities and are involved in the constant reproduction of blood cells. There are four types of bones:

1. *Long bones,* like the bones in your arm, provide support (Fig. 7.3).
2. *Short bones,* like the bones in your fingers, provide flexibility (Fig. 7.3).
3. *Flat bones,* like the bones of the rib cage, provide protection (Fig. 7.4).
4. *Irregular bones* include the vertebrae that make up the spinal column (Fig. 7.5).

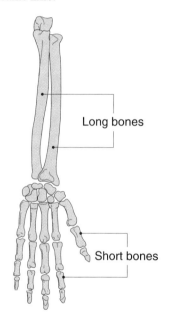

*FIGURE 7.3* Long bones and short bones may be found in the same limb.

Long bones

Short bones

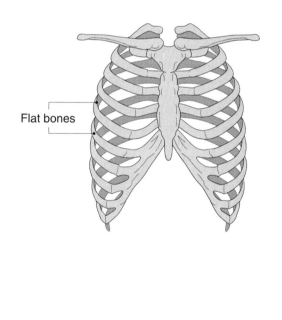

*FIGURE 7.4* Flat bones.

Flat bones

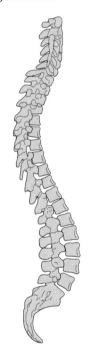

*FIGURE 7.5* Irregular bones are held together to form one working structure.

Irregular bones

**fracture** break

Broken or **fractured** bones usually mend solidly, but the process is slow and gradual. Bone cells grow and reproduce slowly compared to other types of cells. The hardening of the new bone is a gradual process of depositing calcium. As we age, our bones become more brittle. The blood supply is often decreased, calcium is not as readily stored, and the body's powers of general resistance to infection and healing are decreased. For this reason an elderly person who breaks a bone will require a longer time to heal than a younger person. In addition, when an elderly person falls, because his bones are so brittle, he is more subject to fractures than a younger person. Protect your clients from falls!

**Joints** are areas in which one bone connects with one or more other bones. The tough white fibrous cord that connects a bone to a bone is called a **ligament**. The fibrous material that connects muscle to bone is called a **tendon**. The joints in the shoulder, hip, and knee are each enclosed in a strong capsule lined by a membrane that secretes a lubricating fluid. This is called a **bursa**. Movable joints are constructed so that two ends of the bones do not rub against each other. A pad of **cartilage** at the end of the bone absorbs jolts and cushions the bone ends. Injury to joints may cause a ligament or tendon to be strained in what is called a **sprain.**

There are several kinds of joints in the human body. The hinge joint, such as in the knee, is freely movable. There are also less movable joints, such as those between the vertebrae. Some joints do not move at all, such as joints between the bones of the head that protect the brain.

## THE MUSCULAR SYSTEM

The **muscular system** makes all motion possible. Groups of muscles work together to perform a body motion (Fig. 7.6). Two groups of muscles that work together are called **antagonistic groups.** For example, **flex** your forearm, bending it toward your shoulder. Your biceps **contract** or shorten, and the triceps relax. **Extend** your forearm. The biceps muscle relaxes while the triceps contracts. **Flexion** and **extension** are two terms you should know (Fig. 7.7). Two others are **abduction** (Fig. 7.8), which means moving a part away from the body, and **adduction,** (Fig. 7.9), which means moving it toward the body.

Muscles can also be classified as **voluntary** (those muscles we move consciously, such as an arm) or **involuntary** (those that move without conscious control, such as the heart) or **smooth** or **striated,** depending on what they look like under a microscope.

**joint** part of the body where two bones come together and there is movement

**ligament** a tough band of tissue connecting bone to bone

**tendon** tough cord of connective tissue that binds muscles to bony parts

**bursa** sac of fluid within a joint capsule that provides lubrication for joint movement

**cartilage** tough connective tissue that holds bones together

**sprain** to twist a ligament or muscle without dislocating the bones

**muscular system** group of organs that allow the body to move

**flex** to bend

**contract** get smaller

**extend** to straighten an arm or leg

**flexion** to bend a joint

**abduction** to move an arm or leg away from the center of the body

**adduction** to move an arm or leg toward the center of the body

**involuntary** action taken with out conscious input

**smooth muscle** appears smooth under a microscope; usually associated with involuntary actions

**striated muscle** appears to be lined under a microscope; usually associated with voluntary action

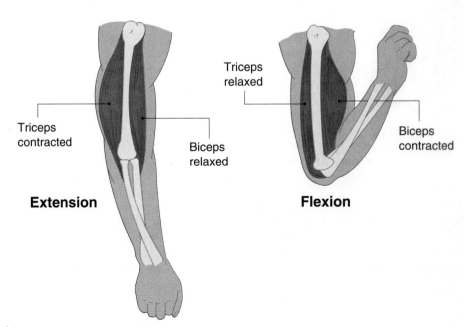

Extension

Triceps contracted

Biceps relaxed

Triceps relaxed

Biceps contracted

Flexion

**FIGURE 7.6** Adduction of a limb moves out toward the body.

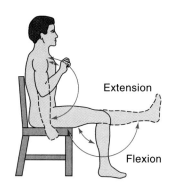

Extension

Flexion

*FIGURE 7.7* Abduction of a limb moves it away from the body.

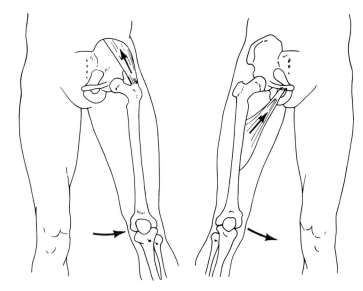

*FIGURE 7.8* Muscles work in coordination with each other to move bones and provide movement.

*FIGURE 7.9* Every muscle has two activities: flexion—bending the limb, and extension—straightening out the limb.

Atrophy — muscle inactive that shrinks and wastes away.

Muscle is the most infection free of all the body's basic tissues. This is largely because of its rich blood supply. Muscles not only move the body but also help to keep the body warm, especially during activity. If a muscle is kept inactive for too long, it tends to shrink and waste away. This is called atrophy. **Contracture** is a permanent muscle shortening or loss of function and a permanent flexed position of the limb. Range-of-motion exercises are often given to inactive clients to prevent these problems.

### THE CENTRAL NERVOUS SYSTEM

The central **nervous system** controls and organizes all body activity, both voluntary and involuntary (autonomic nervous system). The nervous system is made up of the **brain,** the **spinal cord,** and the **nerves.** The nerves are spread throughout all areas of the body. Nerve tissue is made up of specialized cells called **neurons.** All body organs receive messages from the brain by way of the nervous system (Fig. 7.10). Any change in our external or internal environment that is strong enough will set up a nervous impulse in these receptor organs. This impulse is carried through the spinal cord to the brain. The impulse is then interpreted by the brain, which sends other impulses back to a part of the body that must respond to the first impulse.

When part of the brain is damaged, as in a stroke or accident, either the path along which impulses travel or the brain itself is dam-

**spinal cord** one of the main organs of the nervous system. The spinal cord carries messages from the brain to other parts of the body and from parts of the body back to the brain. The spinal cord is inside the spine (backbone)

**nerves** bundles of neurons held together with connective tissue. They go to all parts of the body from the central nervous system, that is, from the brain and spinal cord

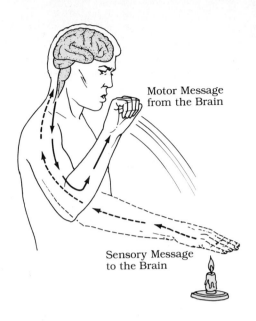

**FIGURE 7.10** All messages travel to the brain, which directs appropriate activity in response to the message.

Motor Message from the Brain

Sensory Message to the Brain

aged. Remember that nerve cells do not grow back once they die. If possible, another part of the brain or impulse pathway can be trained to take over the function of the part that has been damaged. You will work with the rehabilitation therapists in your agency, helping clients learn to do things again after such damage has occurred.

The right half of the brain controls most of the activity on the left side of the body. And the left half of the brain controls the activity on the right side of the body. Specific parts of the brain are responsible for movement, all emotional thoughts, learning, and memory.

The nerves that serve your entire body as pathways to and from your brain branch off the spinal cord as it is housed inside the spinal column (Fig. 7.11). The small cushion of cartilage that separates the **vertebrae** or backbones is called a **disc**. It prevents the two bones from rubbing each other and squeezing the nerve. When the disc is damaged and there is increased pressure on the nerve, pain is often the result.

**vertebra** one of the bones of the spinal column

**disc** round piece of cartilage between the vertebrae

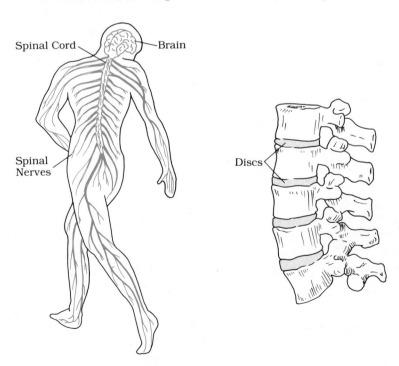

Spinal Cord

Brain

Spinal Nerves

Discs

**FIGURE 7.11** The nervous system provides the pathways for messages to and from the brain.

Chapter 7 ■ Anatomy and Physiology

**autonomic nervous system** part of the nervous system that carries messages without conscious thought

**sense organs** groups of tissue that make it possible for us to be aware of the outside world through sight, hearing, smell, taste, and touch

Much of the activity of the organs of the body is involuntary. In other words, we are unable to regulate it. The part of the nervous system that controls such things is called the **autonomic nervous system.**

**Sense organs** contain specialized endings of the sensory neurons. These are activated by sudden changes in the outside environment called **stimuli.**

- Eyes respond to visual stimuli.
- Ears respond mainly to sound stimuli.
- Membranes of the nose respond to odors.
- Taste buds, located mostly on the tongue, respond to sweet, sour, and other sensations.
- Skin responds to touch, pressure, heat, cold, and pain.

**nerve impulse** regular wave of negative electrical impulses that transmit information along a neuron from one part of the body to another

Remember, these sense organs must send their messages to the brain and receive directions as to how to respond to the stimuli. This message is called a **nerve impulse.** If this pathway is broken, the sense organ cannot function and the client loses the use of it. For example, if the nerve pathways to the eye are damaged, the client will not be able to see.

## HORMONES AND THE ENDOCRINE SYSTEM

**hormone** protein substance secreted by an endocrine gland directly into the blood

The endocrine glands secrete liquids called **hormones** into the bloodstream (Fig. 7.12). These chemicals are secreted in one place, but work

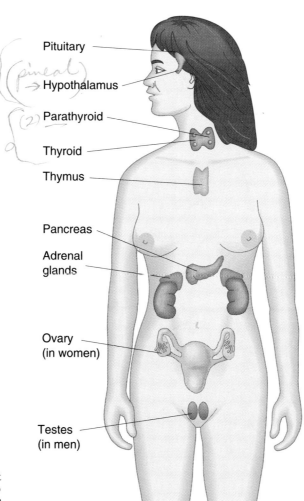

Pituitary

Hypothalamus

Parathyroid

Thyroid

Thymus

Pancreas

Adrenal glands

Ovary (in women)

Testes (in men)

**FIGURE 7.12** Endocrine glands secrete hormones that travel throughout the body to regulate proper body function.

**endocrine glands** ductless glands in the body that secrete hormones into the blood

**feedback mechanism** process whereby the output of a system is fed back into the system (input) to change the way the system works or what it produces

in another. The organs that manufacture the chemicals are called **endocrine glands.**

The endocrine gland works by a **"feedback mechanism."** When the body requires more of a specific hormone, the gland supplies it. When the level is high enough, production stops (Fig. 7.13). This is a very sensitive balance. If it is not perfect, the body produces too much or too little of a hormone. This results in some body misfunctions. Through the feedback mechanism, the endocrine glands regulate bodily functions and interact with other systems to keep our bodies working at their best.

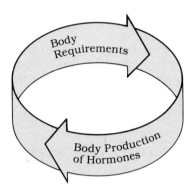

**FIGURE 7.13** Hormones are produced as the body needs them. Any imbalance in this system results in illness, disease, or body changes.

**Endocrine Glands and Their Functions**

| Gland | Function |
|---|---|
| Pituitary<br>Direct (hormones into bloodstream) | Regulates growth and sexual development, salt and water in body, milk production in women after birth |
| Indirect (acts on other glands) | Metabolism of food; reaction of body to stress; sexual development; regulation of circulation, respiration, and urinary output |
| Thyroid | Regulates growth and general metabolism; stores iodine |
| Parathyroid | Works with thyroid to regulate levels of calcium and phosphorus; affects muscle and nerve function |
| Pancreas | Produces insulin |
| Adrenal | Produces adrenalin; helps regulate body fluid and electrolyte balance; influences metabolism; influences sexual organs; helps body cope with stress |
| Ovaries (female) | Produce estrogen and progesterone, which regulate menstruation and female characteristics |
| Testes (male) | Produce testosterone, which causes the production of sperm and is necessary for male characteristics |

**circulatory system** organs of the body concerned with circulation

**heart** four-chambered, hollow, muscular organ in the chest cavity, pointing slightly to the left, that pumps blood throughout the body

**lymph** clear colorless fluid carried by an independent system of vessels which returns the fluid to the heart

**blood vessels** the tubes that carry the blood throughout the body

**artery** blood vessel that carries blood away from the heart

**vein** blood vessel that carries blood to the heart

**capillaries** minute blood vessels that connect arteries to the veins

**nutrients** food substances that are required by the body to repair, maintain, and grow new cells

## THE CIRCULATORY SYSTEM

The **circulatory system** is made up of the **blood,** the **heart,** the **lymph system,** and the **blood vessels—arteries, veins,** and **capillaries.** The heart actually acts as a pump for the blood, a liquid that carries the **nutrients** (food) and oxygen to the cells of the body and removes waste products.

## Important Facts to Know About Blood

- The blood carries oxygen from the lungs to the cells.
- Carbon dioxide is a waste product carried by the blood from the cells to the lungs.
- Nutrients are absorbed by the blood from the duodenum (small intestine) and brought to the cells.
- The hormones from the endocrine glands are transported by the blood.
- Dilation and contraction of the blood vessels help regulate body temperature.
- The blood helps maintain the fluid balance of the body.
- The white cells of the blood help defend the body against disease.
- Blood is continually recirculated through a closed system in our bodies.
- Red blood cells exchange oxygen, iron, and other nutrients for waste products from all body tissues.

The blood vessels leading away from the heart are called arteries. Usually, these vessels carry blood rich in oxygen. (This is true of all arteries except the pulmonary artery.) Arteries have thick elastic walls. These walls can absorb the pressure of the heart's constant pumping of blood (Fig. 7.14).

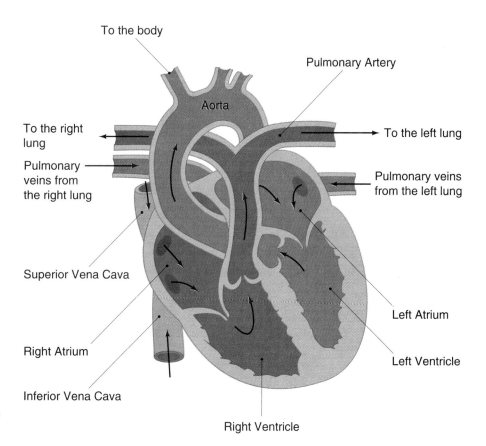

**FIGURE 7.14** The heart acts as the pump that moves the blood and nutrients through the circulatory system.

Arteries branch into a vast network throughout the body. As they branch, the blood vessels become smaller and smaller until they are so small that they become capillaries. The walls of the capillaries are only one cell layer thick. Through these walls, gases, nutrients, waste products, and other substances are exchanged between the red blood cells in the capillaries, the tissue fluid, and the tissue cells.

After the blood has given up its oxygen, which is carried on the surface of the red blood cells, it returns to the heart through the veins. The veins, which carry blood to the heart, have valves in them. These function as trapdoors so that the blood flowing against gravity will not fall backward. When these valves do not work well and blood pools in veins, they stretch. This condition is known as **varicose veins.** People who have too few red blood cells have anemia: people with too many red blood cells have too much iron and oxygen in their circulatory system.

The heart is made up of four chambers—the two **atria** and the two larger and more powerful **ventricles.** The right atrium receives the blood from the body that is high in carbon dioxide and other waste products. This blood flows into the right ventricle. Then it is pumped through the **pulmonary** artery to the lungs. Here, in the lungs, the blood exchanges the carbon dioxide for oxygen and returns to the heart through the pulmonary veins. It reenters the heart in the left atrium, flows to the left ventricle, and is pumped out to the body through the aorta. The **aorta** is the largest blood vessel in our body. This cycle is then repeated.

It is necessary that heart muscle be supplied with blood carrying oxygen. The **coronary** arteries, which surround the heart, carry the needed oxygen and nutrients to the cardiac muscle tissue. When one of the branches of the coronary artery is blocked, as by a blood clot, the client suffers a heart attack. This can result in death of some heart tissue. This event is called a **myocardial infarction** (MI).

The liquid portion of the blood, called **plasma,** transports both the red blood cells (carrying oxygen and iron) and white blood cells (that fight infection). When a person has an **inflammation** or injury, white blood cells rush to the infected area to help fight the foreign material. The waste product of this battle is **pus.**

The **liver** is the place where **toxins** or poisonous substances are removed from the blood. Damage to the liver can be caused by drinking alcoholic substances or taking drugs that are harmful to its tissue. The liver is also responsible for the production and storage of some elements necessary for proper circulation of the blood and for blood-clotting. Blood clots are not always bad. When a blood vessel has been injured, a clot may form that holds the blood within the closed vessel until healing occurs. Sometimes, however, a blood clot can be dangerous because it may prevent new blood from passing through the vessel. This means that part of the body will not receive its nutrients or get rid of its waste.

A person's circulation tends to slow down when he is in bed. Therefore, when you have orders to help a client out of bed, remember that his circulation is not at its peak. Make sure that he moves carefully and slowly. Allow him to sit at the edge of the bed until his circulation **stabilizes,** that is, comes back to normal. Then assist him to a standing position. If the client becomes dizzy or feels faint, have him sit down again.

The **lymphatic system** is considered part of the circulatory system. The function of this system is to assist the circulatory system in draining fluid from the body tissues. Lymph channels are located in the body near veins. The channels get bigger as they get closer to the heart. Two large lymph vessels empty into the venous blood system in

**varicose veins** abnormal swelling of veins

**atria** the two upper chambers of the heart

**ventricles** lower two chambers of the heart

**pulmonary** refers to the lungs

**aorta** major artery that carries blood away from the heart

**coronary** pertaining to the heart

**myocardial infarction** death of a part of the heart due to blockage in a blood vessel

**plasma** liquid portion of blood

**inflammation** reaction of the tissues to disease or injury. There is usually pain, heat, redness, and swelling of the body part

**pus** a waste product of inflammation

**liver** body's largest gland located in the upper left quadrant of the abdominal cavity, which helps process some waste products

**toxin** substance that is toxic

the neck area. Lymph fluid is always moving toward the heart. Lymph contains fluid plasma, white blood cells, carbon dioxide, and other chemicals, depending on what the body must flush out.

Lymph **nodes** are lymph tissues. They help the body fight infection. While doing this, they often enlarge and become tender. This is called enlarged nodes or swollen glands.

Two glands, the **spleen** and the **thymus,** are also part of the lymphatic system. The spleen produces, stores, and destroys blood cells. The thymus gland is one that we do not know much about. We do know, however, that it is used by the body to fight infection.

### THE RESPIRATORY SYSTEM

The respiratory system provides a pathway for oxygen to get from the air into the lungs and for the blood to exchange carbon dioxide for this oxygen. Breathing is regulated in part of our brain. It is an **involuntary** act.

The organs that make up the respiratory system include the nose, mouth, **pharynx** (throat), **trachea** (windpipe), **larynx** (voicebox), **diaphragm, bronchi,** and **lungs** (Fig. 7.15). Because this exchange must take place all the time, it is necessary that this pathway always be kept open. The structures themselves help do this. The trachea and bronchi are kept open by their anatomical structure. The tiny hairs in the nose trap dust so that it does not reach the lungs. On the

**spleen** abdominal organ

**thymus** ductless gland, part of the lymphatic system, located in the chest cavity just above the heart

**involuntary** action taken without conscious input

**pharynx** area behind the nasal cavities, mouth, and larynx that opens into them and the esophagus

**trachea** organ of the respiratory system. It is located in the throat area. The trachea is commonly called the windpipe

**larynx** area of the throat containing the vocal cords

**diaphragm** muscular partition between the chest cavity and the abdominal cavity

**bronchi** two main branches of the bronchial tree that lead to the lungs

**lungs** primary organs of breathing

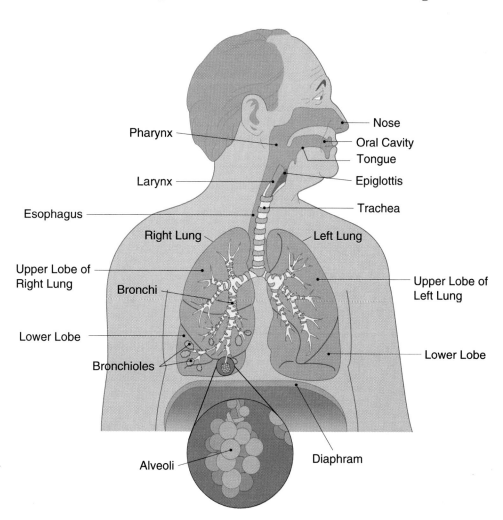

*FIGURE 7.15* The respiratory system exchanges waste products for oxygen through a filtering system in the lungs.

top of the trachea, opening from the pharynx, is a structure known as the larynx. It is not only the opening to the trachea; it also contains vocal cords that make it possible for us to have a voice. An important piece of cartilage, the **epiglottis,** covers the opening to the trachea. When food is swallowed, the epiglottis prevents the food from going into the lungs.

A very weak client or one who is having trouble breathing must be watched carefully while eating so that food does not get into the trachea. This is known as **aspiration** of food. An unconscious client who vomits may also be in danger of aspirating that material. Turn the client's head to the side at once.

The exchange of oxygen and carbon dioxide occurs in the small air sacs (**alveoli**), which are the last branches of the bronchi. As you **inhale** and the diaphragm moves toward the abdominal cavity, oxygen fills these sacs and is exchanged for the carbon dioxide that the blood brings to the sacs from the heart. As you **exhale,** the diaphragm compresses the lungs and forces the carbon dioxide out of the lungs into the air. The oxygen-rich blood then returns to the heart to be sent around the body. If your client has difficulty breathing, that means he has difficulty exchanging the carbon dioxide in his blood for fresh oxygen in his lungs. As a result, all the cells in his body have less oxygen.

If the weather is very humid or pollution is thick, people with heart or lung disease may have difficulty breathing. Always be alert for a sign of distress from the client. This may signal to you that his airway is blocked. If you are assigned to a client who may have difficulty swallowing or breathing, be sure to discuss with your supervisor any emergency procedures of which you should be aware.

## THE DIGESTIVE (GASTROINTESTINAL) SYSTEM

The **digestive system** is responsible for breaking down food into a form that can be used by the body cells. This action is both chemical and mechanical. The digestive tract is about 30 feet long. Its entire length is important in reducing food to the form of body needs (Fig. 7.16).

**Digestion** begins in the mouth, where food is chewed and mixed with **saliva.** This is the first step of digestion. During swallowing, the food moves in a moistened ball down the **esophagus** to the **stomach.** The stomach churns and mixes the food at the same time it is being broken down chemically. The most important part of digestion and absorption of nutrients occurs in the **duodenum.** This is the first part of the **small intestine.** It is here that digestive juices from the duodenum and the **pancreas** and **bile** from the **gallbladder** finish the job of breaking down the food. Bile is stored in the gallbladder, but manufactured in the liver.

The lining of the duodenum is composed of thousands of tiny fingerlike projections called **villi.** Each villus is capable of absorbing the end products of digestion. The products are then moved into the bloodstream, where they are carried to individual cells (Fig. 7.17).

A lot of water is necessary for the chemical reduction of food into its end products. Food is moved along the length of the intestines by the rhythmic contraction of the muscle walls. This is called **peristalsis.** What is left of the food, after some has been absorbed by the small intestines, moves through the **large intestines,** where water is reabsorbed into the body. The material that cannot be used by

**alveoli** microscopic air sacs in the lung where oxygen passes into the blood in exchange for waste products

**inhale** to breathe in air in respiration

**exhale** to breathe out air in respiration

**saliva** secretion of the salivary glands into the mouth. Saliva moistens food and is necessary for digestion

**esophagus** muscular tube for the passage of food, which extends from the back of the throat (pharynx), down through the chest and diaphragm into the stomach

**stomach** part of the digestive tract between the esophagus (food pipe) and the duodenum

**duodenum** first part of the small intestine

**bile** substance needed for digestion that is secreted by the liver and stored in the gallbladder

**villi** tiny fingerlike projections in the lining of the small intestines into which the end products of digestion are absorbed and distributed through the bloodstream

**peristalsis** movement of the intestines that pushes food along to the next part of the digestive system

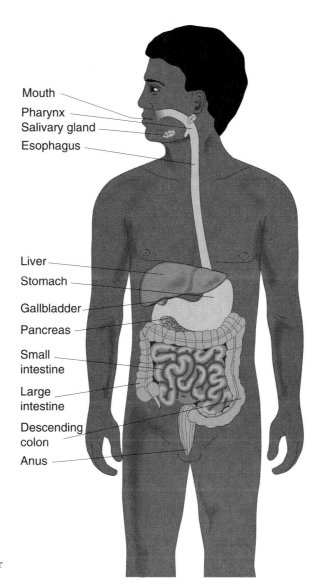

Mouth
Pharynx
Salivary gland
Esophagus

Liver
Stomach
Gallbladder
Pancreas
Small intestine
Large intestine
Descending colon
Anus

**FIGURE 7.16** The digestive system changes food into chemical nutrients the body can use or store for future use.

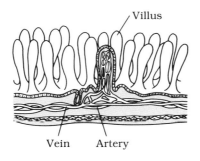

Villus

Vein    Artery

**FIGURE 7.17** The finger-like lining of the small intestine increases the area for absorption of nutrients.

**anus** opening of the rectum onto the body surface

**glucose** sugar

**colon** large bowel

**appendix** slender growth attached to the large intestine

the body is excreted from the rectum through the **anus** as **feces** or waste.

The liver is part of the digestive system. Besides manufacturing bile, the liver is a storage area for **glucose**. This form of sugar is released in large amounts when the cells need it for energy.

On the right side of the **colon,** or large intestine, at the junction between the small intestine and the large intestine, there is a pouch with a projection called the **appendix.** Because there is little peristalsis in this area, the appendix may have material trapped in it and become infected. This is known as appendicitis. Surgery is usually performed to remove the appendix and correct this condition.

The lowest portion of the large intestine curves in an S shape into the **rectum.** The rectum is made up of delicate tissue. It has an internal and an external **sphincter** muscle. When the rectum has fecal matter in it, a message is received by the brain. The brain returns a message to the muscles of the rectum, allowing them to relax. This is called a bowel movement. Sometimes blood vessels that supply the rectal area become enlarged and filled with blood clots, resulting in **hemorrhoids.**

**rectum** lower eight to ten inches of the colon

**sphincter** ringlike muscle that controls the opening and closing of a body opening

**hemorrhoid** swelling of a vein near the anus

## THE URINARY SYSTEM

One of the systems that rids the body of waste products is the **urinary system.** This system filters out waste products and toxins from the blood and disposes of them in the liquid called **urine.** The organs that make up the urinary system include the **kidneys,** the **ureters,** the **urinary bladder,** and the **urethra** (Fig. 7.18).

As all blood passes through the kidneys, an exchange of substances takes place between the capillaries and the filtering units of the kidney, which are tiny **tubules.** There are hundreds of these tubules in each kidney. As the filtered material flows through these tubules, the blood vessels surrounding them reabsorb those materials still needed by the body, particularly the water. Near the end of the winding tubules, substances from the blood, such as toxins and some drugs, pass into the urine. The material that is left is collected in a larger tube, the ureter. From here it drips steadily through the ureter, helped by a peristaltic motion very similar to that of the gastrointestinal tract, to the urinary bladder. The urinary bladder is capable of expanding and storing about 500 cc of urine. There are **stretch receptors** in the muscular wall of the bladder. When these receptors are stimulated by a full bladder, messages are sent to the brain, causing urinary tract muscles to release the urine from the bladder. This is called **urinating** or **voiding.**

**urine** liquid waste manufactured in the kidneys and discharged from the urinary bladder

**kidney** organ lying in the upper posterior portion of the abdomen that removes wastes from the bloodstream and discharges them in the form of urine

**ureter** tube leading from the kidneys to the urinary bladder

**bladder** membranous sac that serves as a container within the body such as the urinary bladder, which holds urine

**stretch receptors** nerve cells that relay messages to the brain as the organ enlarges

**void** to urinate, pass water

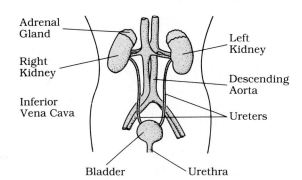

*FIGURE 7.18* All blood passes through the kidneys so that chemicals can be filtered out in the form of urine.

Because the urethra is open to the outside of the body, it may also provide a passageway for disease-causing microorganisms to enter the bladder. A bladder infection is known as **cystitis.** The infection may also spread through the ureters to the kidneys, causing kidney damage. Cystitis is most commonly found in women because of the shortness of the urethra.

You may have a client who has a urinary **catheter** in the urethra. This is a tube from the bladder to a bag that collects the urine. (This

**cystitis** inflammation of the bladder

**catheter** a tube used to remove body fluids from a cavity

does not have to hamper women's sexual activity. If your client has questions about this, tell your supervisor.)

Remember, the urinary system determines the water content of the blood, and the blood content, in turn, determines the content of the tissue fluid. The urinary system also determines the content of other nutrients in the blood, such as salt and potassium.

When ill, a client is sometimes unable to void. This condition must be reported to your supervisor immediately. You will notice the color, odor, and amount of urine your client voids as you care for him. Discuss usual color, odor, and amount for your client so you will be alert to changes and report them. Many changes in client kidney functions can be detected from changes in urine.

## THE REPRODUCTIVE SYSTEM

### Female Reproduction

**ovary** one of a pair of organs in the female that produce mature eggs and the primary female sex hormones, estrogen and progesterone

**fallopian tubes** also called the oviducts, through which an egg travels from the ovary to the uterus

**uterus** expandable female reproductive organ in which an embryo grows and is nourished until gestation is complete

**vagina** the birth canal leading from the cervix to the outside

In the female, the reproductive organs are two **ovaries,** two **fallopian tubes,** the **uterus,** and the **vagina** (Fig. 7.19). The main task of the ovary is the production of eggs or ova. These are specialized cells that may unite with a sperm cell (released from the male during sexual intercourse) and then grow over a period of forty weeks into a new human being.

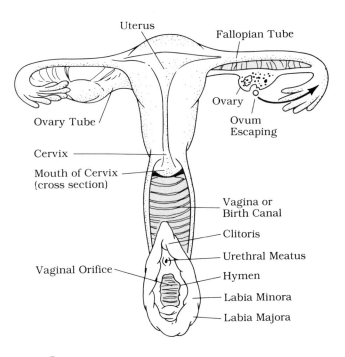

*FIGURE 7.19* Internal female genitalia.

Ovulation is the process whereby an **ovum** is released from one ovary into the opening of a fallopian tube and moves through this tube to the uterus. This occurs approximately once each month, usually fourteen days before the onset of the next menstrual period. During this time a woman is **fertile** (able to become pregnant). During ovulation, the hormone estrogen is released into the bloodstream. This causes a buildup of the **endometrium** (lining of the uterus), preparing it for a possible pregnancy. If the ovum is fertilized, the mouth of the uterus closes to protect the developing embryo.

The uterus lining now helps to nourish the embryo. If the ovum is not fertilized, the lining of the uterus is not necessary and is shed.

This process is called **menstruation.** Menstruation is the periodic loss of blood and a small part of the lining of the uterus. The discharge flows out of the vagina for four to seven days.

The process of ovulation is controlled by hormones from the pituitary gland and the ovaries. These hormones from the pituitary gland are involved in the development of the ovum and in maintaining pregnancy.

Ovulation and menstruation usually begin between the ages of ten and thirteen. At this time a girl develops breasts, body hair, and starts to look more and more like a woman. Once a female starts to menstruate, she can become pregnant, no matter how young she is. Menstruation usually continues uninterrupted, except for pregnancy, until a woman enters menopause.

**menopause** period of life in the female usually between 45 and 50 when menstruation stops; change of life

When a woman is about forty-five, her menstrual cycles change. They become farther apart and finally stop. In addition, she may have emotional changes and changes in her skin and hair. This process is called **menopause** or "the change of life." Some women may feel depressed, get hot flashes, or have difficulty sexually. If one of your clients, or a member of her family, mentions to you that she finds this time of life difficult, suggest she discuss this with her physician. Of course, you will report this conversation to your supervisor. Many cultures have customs or superstitions connected with menstruation. As a homemaker/home health aide, you will have to show tolerance and understanding for customs that may be different from your own.

**meatus** opening of the urethra to the outside of the body

In the human female there are three openings from the body to the outside area: (1) the external urinary **meatus,** the end of the urethra; (2) the vagina, which is not only the organ for intercourse, but also the birth canal; and (3) the anus, the last portion of the gastrointestinal tract (Fig. 7.20). These three systems are not connected and function independently of each other.

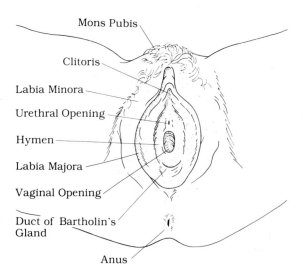

*FIGURE 7.20* External female genitalia.

Mons Pubis

Clitoris

Labia Minora

Urethral Opening

Hymen

Labia Majora

Vaginal Opening

Duct of Bartholin's Gland

Anus

**hysterectomy** removal of the uterus

You may have a client who has had a **hysterectomy.** At the time of surgery the physician removes the uterus and/or ovaries. This procedure is done for many reasons. Women who have had this operation are often concerned about their sex lives. This operation will usually have no effect on your client's sex life. If a client voices concerns to you, communicate them to your supervisor and discuss with the nurse the most appropriate plan of care. Do not pass on old wives' tales or stories you may have heard about other women.

## Male Reproduction

The male internal reproductive system has two **testes,** two **epididymides,** two **seminal ducts** and **vesicles,** two **ejaculatory ducts,** two **spermatic ducts,** the urethra, and the **prostate gland.** The **penis** and **scrotum** are considered external reproductive organs (Fig. 7.21).

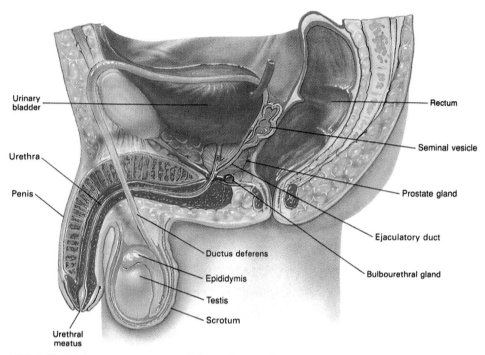

*FIGURE 7.21* A cross section of the male genitalia.

**Testicles,** or testes, are paired glands that lie outside the body in a sac called the scrotum. The function of the testes is to produce **sperm,** the male cell of reproduction. During intercourse, sperm travel up the **vas deferens,** or sperm duct, to a point where they enter the urethra. They enter along with secretions from other glands in the male reproductive system. These glands—the seminal vesicle, the prostate gland, and **Cowper's glands**—contribute water, nutrients, and vitamins, which, added to the sperm, make up the **semen,** a fluid that is **ejaculated** (expelled) at the same time the male has an orgasm. There is only one duct in the penis. It is used for the flow of urine and for the ejaculation of sperm in its carrying medium, the semen. During intercourse the internal sphincter of the male's urinary bladder closes tightly, so there is no chance for the urine to become mixed with the semen. The penis has three columns of spongy tissue. During sexual excitement, blood rushes in through the penile artery and the veins constrict, trapping the blood so it fills these spaces. Then the penis becomes erect and hard. All of this activity occurs under the influence of **testosterone,** the primary male sex hormone, which is also manufactured in the testes. It is secreted into the blood through the influence of hormones from the pituitary gland.

Sometimes during the aging process the prostate gland, which encircles the urethra like a doughnut, becomes enlarged. When the prostate expands, it squeezes the urethra, causing painful urination. Many men fear surgery on their prostate glands, because they believe it will end their sex life. The amount of semen ejaculated will be less, but otherwise, men who have had prostate surgery are almost always capable of having normal sexual relations.

**The Body Systems**

| System | Function | Organs |
|---|---|---|
| Skeletal | Supports, protects the body; provides a place for muscles to attach | Bones, joints |
| Muscular | Gives movement to the body; protects | Muscles, tendons, ligaments |
| Gastrointestinal (digestive, GI) | Processes nutrients into usable units of absorption for the body; eliminates waste | Mouth, teeth, tongue, esophagus, salivary glands, stomach, intestines, liver, gallbladder, pancreas |
| Nervous | Controls movements and activities of the body | Brain, spinal cord, nerves |
| Urinary (excretory) | Removes waste from the blood, produces urine, and eliminates urine | Kidneys, ureters, bladder, urethra |
| Reproductive | Reproduces the species | Male: testes, scrotum, penis Female: ovaries, uterus, fallopian tubes, vagina |
| Respiratory | Eliminates carbon dioxide; supplies oxygen | Nose, pharynx, larynx, trachea, bronchi, lungs |
| Circulatory | Carries nutrients, oxygen, and water to the body cells and removes wastes | Heart, blood, arteries, veins, capillaries, spleen, lymph nodes, lymph vessels |
| Endocrine | Secretes hormones directly into the blood, regulating body function | Thyroid and parathyroid glands, adrenal glands, testes, ovaries, pancreatic islands of Langerhans, pituitary gland |
| Skin | Provides first line of defense against infection; maintains body temperature, regulates fluids, and rids body of waste | Skin, hair, nails, sweat and oil glands |

## Topics for Discussion

1. Discuss how the circulatory and respiratory systems work together.
2. Pick any two systems and see if you can think of ways they work together to keep a person healthy.
3. Can you remember any superstitions or old wives' tales you have heard about the way the human body functions?

# Chapter 8

# Infection Control in the Home

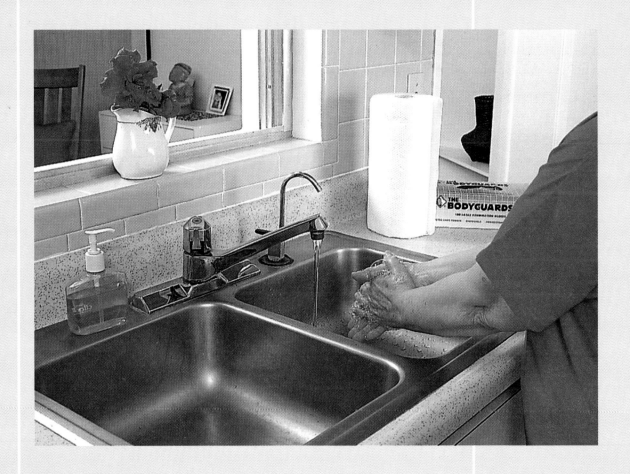

# Section 1  Medical Asepsis in the Home

## Objectives: What You Will Learn to Do

- Explain the relationship between microorganism and infection control.
- List the conditions necessary for microorganisms to grow.
- List the ways microorganisms are spread.
- Define *medical asepsis*.
- Define *clean* and *dirty*.
- Demonstrate the procedures for sterilization of equipment in the home.

## *Introduction: The Nature of Microorganisms*

**microorganism** living thing so small it can be seen only through a microscope

**organism** living thing

People once believed that sickness was caused by evil spirits. About 500 years ago scientists began to suspect that some diseases were caused by very small living things called **microorganisms.** *Micro* means very small. *Organism* means a living thing. Microorganisms can be seen only under a microscope.

Some microorganisms are helpful to people. Microorganisms in the human digestive system break down foods not used by the body and turn them into waste products (feces).

**pathogen** disease-causing microorganism

**toxin** substance that is toxic

**bacteria** microorganisms that may or may not be pathogens

There are some microorganisms, however, that are harmful. They cause disease and infection. Disease-producing microorganisms are called **pathogens.** Pathogens destroy human tissue by using it as their food and give off waste products called **toxins.** Toxins are poisonous to the human body. Every living organism has its own natural environment where it can exist without causing disease. When an organism moves out of its normal environment and into a foreign one, it can become a pathogen. For example, the **bacterium** *Escherichia coli* belongs in the colon where it helps to digest our food. When it gets into the bladder or into the bloodstream, it can cause a urinary infection or a blood infection. Pathogens may enter the body through any opening, such as the mouth, nose, or a cut in the skin.

### CONDITIONS NECESSARY FOR BACTERIA GROWTH

Just as human beings need proper conditions to live, so do microorganisms. Microorganisms need five conditions to grow (Fig. 8.1).

### MEDICAL ASEPSIS

**asepsis** free of disease-causing organisms

Medical **asepsis** means preventing the conditions that allow pathogens to live, multiply, and spread. As a homemaker/home health aide, you will share the responsibility for preventing the spread of disease and infection by using aseptic techniques. The main purposes for medical asepsis are:

**reinfection** to become ill again with the same microorganism

**cross-infection** infection by a new or different microorganism from a visitor or health team member

- Helping the client overcome a current infection or preventing the spread of that infection
- Protecting the client against a second infection by the same microorganism. This is called **reinfection.**
- Protecting the client against infection by a new or different type of microorganism from a visitor or member of the health care team. This is called **cross-infection.**

## CONDITIONS NECESSARY FOR BACTERIA GROWTH

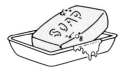

1. *Moisture.* Microorganisms grow well in damp places.

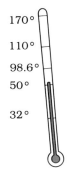

2. *Temperature.* Microorganisms need the correct temperature to live. Most cannot survive at high temperatures, but live well at body temperature.

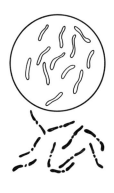

3. *Oxygen.* Microorganisms require a specific oxygen content.

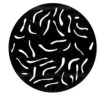

4. *Darkness.* Microorganisms grow best in darkness.

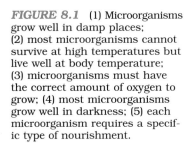

Nourishment
Living or Dead Matter

5. *Nourishment.* Microorganisms need food. Each one requires a different type of food specific to its needs.

*FIGURE 8.1* (1) Microorganisms grow well in damp places; (2) most microorganisms cannot survive at high temperatures but live well at body temperature; (3) microorganisms must have the correct amount of oxygen to grow; (4) most microorganisms grow well in darkness; (5) each microorganism requires a specific type of nourishment.

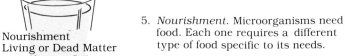

- Protecting the family and health care team against infection by microorganisms passed from caregiver to client, client to caregiver. Diseases that can be passed from person to person are called **communicable** diseases.
- Protecting the client from infection from his own organisms. This is called **self-inoculation.**

### Clean and Dirty Areas in the House

One way to control the spread of disease is to have a **clean** area in the house and a **dirty** one. The kitchen is considered clean, and the toilet is considered dirty; or the area of dishwashing is considered clean, and the area of toileting is considered dirty (Fig 8.2).

**communicable** spread from one person to another

**self-inoculation** infecting oneself with one's own organisms

**clean** uncontaminated by harmful microorganisms

**dirty** contaminated by harmful microorganisms

| MICROORGANISMS ARE IN MANY PLACES | MICROORGANISMS ARE SPREAD IN MANY WAYS |
|---|---|
| • In the air we breathe<br>• On our bodies<br>• In our bodies<br>• On our clothing<br>• In liquids<br>• In food<br>• On animals<br>• In animals<br>• In human waste<br>• In animal waste | • Touching secretions, urine, feces<br>• Touching objects: dishes, bed linen, clothing, instruments, belongings<br>• Sneezing, coughing, talking<br>• Contaminated food, drugs, water, blood<br>• Dust particles and moisture in the air |

**FIGURE 8.2** Microorganisms are in many places and spread in various ways during the day.

**Clean:** This means uncontaminated. It refers to those articles and places from which disease cannot be spread. Clean areas contain food, dishes, and clean equipment. No waste material is ever brought into this area.

**Dirty:** This refers to those areas that have come in contact with disease-causing or-carrying agents. In the home, there are differing degrees of dirty. We make a distinction between being dirty with human waste, such as wound drainage or fecal matter, and bed sheets that are only soiled. Articles that are dirty with potentially infectious material are brought into the dirty area for initial cleaning or disposal. This could be linen, bath water, or equipment. Articles that are only soiled are cleaned in the usual way.

# Section 2  Handwashing

**Objectives: What You Will Learn to Do**

▪ Discuss the importance of handwashing.
▪ Demonstrate the correct method of handwashing in the home.
▪ Discuss when you wash your hands.

### Introduction: The Importance of Handwashing

In your work you will be using your hands constantly. You will be touching clients. You will handle supplies and equipment used in the treatment and care of clients. Microorganisms will get on your hands. They will come from clients or from the things they have touched. Your hands could carry these microorganisms to other persons and places. They could also be moved to your own face and mouth. Washing your hands frequently with a lot of soap and friction is the best way to prevent this transfer of microorganisms.

## Guidelines: Handwashing

▒ Handwashing must be done before and after each task and before and after direct client contact.

▒ The water faucet is always considered dirty. This means there may be pathogens on it. This is why you use paper towels to turn the faucet on and off.

▒ If your hands accidentally touch the inside of the sink, start over. Do the whole procedure again.

▒ Take soap from a dispenser, if possible, rather than using bar soap. Bar soap leaves pools of soapy water in the soap dish, which is then considered contaminated.

## Procedure 3: Handwashing

1. Assemble your equipment:
   Soap or detergent
   Paper towels
   Warm running water (if possible)
   Wastepaper basket
   Nailbrush

2. Open a paper towel near the sink. This is considered your clean area. Put all your equipment on it. Leave it there until you are ready to leave the house.

3. Turn the faucet on with a paper towel held between your hands and the faucet. Adjust the water to a comfortable temperature.

4. Discard the paper towel in the wastepaper basket.

5. Completely wet your hands and wrists under the running water. Keep your fingertips pointed downward. Hold your hands lower than your elbows while washing. This is to prevent microorganisms from contaminating your arms. Holding your hands down prevents backflow over unwashed skin (Fig. 8.3).

6. Apply soap.

7. Work up a good lather. Spread it over the entire area of your hands and wrists. Get soap under your nails and between your fingers. Add water to the soap while washing. This keeps the soap from becoming too dry.

8. Use the nailbrush on your nails.

9. Use a rotating and rubbing (friction) motion for one full minute.
   a. Rub vigorously.
   b. Rub one hand against the other hand and wrist.
   c. Rub between your fingers by interlacing them.
   d. Rub up and down to reach all skin surfaces on your hands and between your fingers.
   e. Rub the tips of your fingers against your palms to clean with friction around the nailbeds.

10. Wash at least 2 inches above your wrists.

11. Rinse well one hand at a time. Rinse from 2 inches above your wrists to hands. Hold your hands and fingertips down under the water.

FIGURE 8.3

FIGURE 8.4

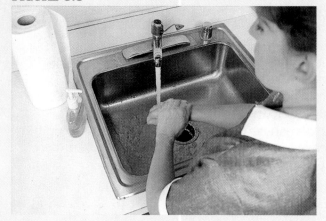

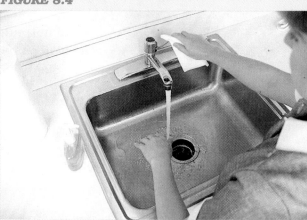

12. Dry thoroughly with paper towels.
13. Use a paper towel to turn off the faucet. Never touch the faucet with your hands after washing (Fig. 8.4).
14. Throw the paper towel into the wastepaper basket. Do not touch the basket.

# Section 3  Disinfection and Sterilization

**Objectives: What You Will Learn to Do**

- Discuss the differences between disinfection and sterilization.
- Demonstrate the procedure for wet or dry sterilization in the home.
- Discuss when wet-heat sterilization would be appropriate and when dry-heat sterilization would be appropriate.

## Introduction: Disinfection and Sterilization in the Home

While you are caring for your client, you will always try to prevent the spread of pathogens. Despite the best efforts of health care personnel, there are always some harmful microorganisms around us. They can be made harmless, however, by simple cleanliness procedures. We can keep ourselves clean by bathing and frequent handwashing. We can keep the environment and equipment clean with soap, water, and solutions that assist in keeping down bacterial growth.

Two other important methods for killing microorganisms or keeping them under control are:

**disinfection** process of destroying most disease-causing organisms

1. **Disinfection:** the process of destroying as many harmful organisms as possible. It also means slowing down the growth and activity of the organisms that cannot be destroyed.

sterilization process of destroying all microorganisms including spores

spore microorganism that has formed hard shells around themselves for protection. They can only be destroyed by sterilization

2. **Sterilization:** the process of killing all microorganisms, including spores, in a certain area.

**Spores** are bacteria that have formed hard shells around themselves as a defense. These shells are like a protective suit of armor. Spores are very difficult to kill. Some can even live in boiling water. Sterilization is necessary if the article comes in direct contact with a wound, as in the case of surgical instruments or solutions used for cleaning a wound. Sterilization is the responsibility of a specialized department within a health care institution. However, in the home, such specialized equipment does not exist. Depending on the item, it can be sterilized in one of two ways: wet heat or dry heat.

## Procedure 4: Wet-Heat Sterilization

1. Assemble your equipment:
   Items to be sterilized, cleaned, and dried
   Clean, covered pot large enough to hold items
   Cold water to cover the items in the pot
   Timer or clock
   Sterilized tongs
   Pot holder
   Source of heat (stove, Sterno, fire)
2. Wash your hands.
3. Place the equipment in the pot so that water touches all parts of it. If there are glass parts, put a clean piece of cloth in the bottom of the pot to protect them.
4. Cover the contents of the pot with cold water. Be sure there is head room left in the pot.
5. Put the pot on a source of heat that is big enough to heat it. Turn handles away from the edge of the burner.
6. Bring water to a boil. *Do not open the pot. Note the steam escaping under the cover.*
7. Boil the contents undisturbed and covered for twenty minutes.
8. Turn off the heat.
9. Allow the contents to cool undisturbed. Leave the equipment in the pot until you are ready to use it.
10. With the sterilized tongs remove the contents to a sterilized holder (Fig. 8.5).

FIGURE 8.5

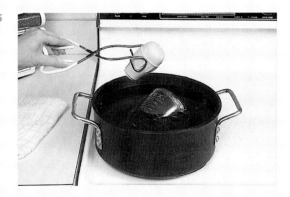

## Procedure 5: Dry-Heat Sterilization

1. Assemble your equipment:
   Pie tin
   Dressing or cloth to be sterilized
   Oven
   Pot holder
2. Wash your hands.
3. Place the clean dressings wrapped in a clean cloth in the pie tin.
4. Place the pie tin in an oven at 350°F. Allow the dressings to bake for one hour. Then allow them to cool (Fig. 8.6).
5. Unwrap carefully. Do not touch the dressings; they are considered sterile.
   *Note:* A hot iron held on dressings for several seconds also sterilizes. However, the oven method is preferred.

*FIGURE 8.6*

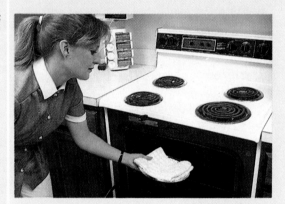

## Section 4   Special Infection Control and Isolation Precautions for Transmittable Diseases

### Objectives: What You Will Learn to Do

■ Name two diseases transmitted through exposure to blood and body fluids.
■ Discuss the need for universal precautions.
■ List the universal precautions necessary when caring for clients in their home.
■ Discuss the five types of isolation and their uses.

### Introduction: Care of Clients with Transmittable Diseases

The discovery of certain diseases within the last fifteen years has alerted health care workers to the need to lower the chance of transmission of these diseases from client to caregiver. These diseases are spread

**blood-borne pathogens** those disease-causing entities transmitted through contact with blood

through exposure to blood and body fluids and are called **blood-borne pathogens.** Two of these diseases are AIDS and hepatitis B. One of the problems with caring for clients who have AIDS is that little is known about this disease. The other problem is our personal feelings. This disease may awaken feelings because of fear or because some of the victims may have an unfamiliar lifestyle.

The U.S. Centers for Disease Control (CDC) and the Occupational Safety and Health Administration continually remind us that the chance of transmission of a disease such as AIDS or hepatitis B from a client to a caregiver is very small: however, every agency will have its own policies and procedures that should be followed when caring for clients with these diseases and that further minimize the chance of transmission.

Clients who have these diseases are entitled to caring and understanding personnel. They and their families have the same needs as other clients and their families. Do not allow your personal feelings about their lifestyle or their disease to color your care. If you have strong feelings or fear, discuss them with your supervisor.

### UNIVERSAL PRECAUTIONS

**universal precautions** those routine activities recommended to protect health care workers from contamination with blood and body fluids

Medical tests and careful medical history are often not enough to identify clients who have the HIV virus or other blood-borne pathogens. Therefore, the CDC requires health workers to decrease the risks of being exposed to blood and body fluids. These basic activities are called **universal precautions.** Remember, universal precautions are actions taken on a routine basis for all clients. It is the law that universal precautions be incorporated into the routine of all health care workers. If a definite diagnosis is made, specific types of isolation may become part of the plan of care.

Each agency has a policy discussing universal precautions and the use of protective barriers. Protective barriers are equipment to protect you. They are:

- gloves
- masks
- gowns
- goggles

Your agency will provide this equipment. If you do not have it available, ask for it! Be sure that you ask for the universal precautions policy and that you understand it.

Although AIDS, the HIV-positive virus, any blood-borne disease, and tuberculosis which is being treated cannot be transmitted from one person to another by touching, holding hands, or being in the same room, health care workers are still required to practice universal precautions.

## Guidelines: Universal Precautions

Universal precautions are commonsense guidelines. Gloves are to be worn whenever exposure to blood or body fluids may occur. Clients often feel uncomfortable when being cared for by somebody wearing gloves. Explain to the client that this is the standard of care among health care workers and that you will still touch him when blood and body fluids are not present.

If you injure yourself while caring for a client, report it. If you have any cuts or injuries on your hands or body, report them to your supervisor before you start to care for your client.

■ *Exposure to body fluids or blood.* Wear gloves if a chance exists for contamination. If splattering is possible, wear a gown or protective apron and mask. Flush waste products down the toilet. Spills should be wiped up by a person wearing disposable gloves with soap and water, then wiped with a solution of 1 part household bleach to 10 parts of water. The rag should be thrown out. Gloves should be changed frequently. When removing gloves, do not touch the outside of the gloves (Fig. 8.7).

■ Personal items, such as tampons, peripads, or razors, are not considered medical waste and should be disposed of as you would any dressing.

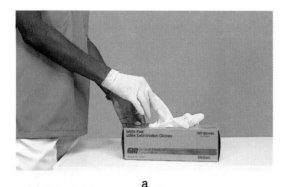

a

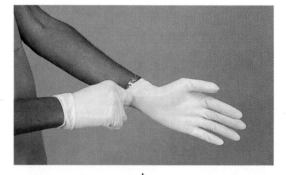

b

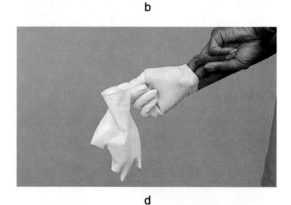

c

d

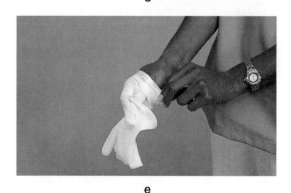

e

**FIGURE 8.7** (a) Use a clean pair of gloves for each client contact. (b) Grasp the glove just below the cuff. (c) Pull the glove over your hand while turning the glove inside out. (d) Place the ungloved index finger and middle finger inside cuff of the glove, turning the cuff downward. (e) Pull the cuff and glove inside out as you remove your hand from the glove.

■ *Sharp objects, needles, blades.* Handle carefully to prevent cutting yourself. These objects should be placed in a puncture-resistant container and disposed of according to local rules. Do not bend needles or try to recap them (Fig. 8.8).

■ *Dressings.* Wrap these items in a plastic bag, and dispose of them according to local law. You may have to double bag them if you are transporting them as medical waste. Check with your supervisor (Fig. 8.9).

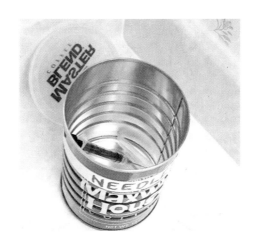

FIGURE 8.8 Carefully place sharp objects in a secure container.

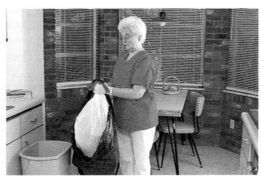

a

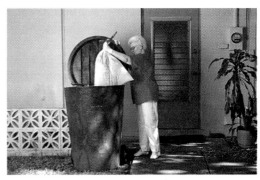

b

FIGURE 8.9 (a) Double wrapping dressings protects you, the environment, and the people who handle the bags. Double bagging may be done as part of isolation technique or as an extra precaution for all heavily soiled trash. (b) Be sure all trash goes into a covered container.

■ *Plates, glasses, dishes.* Use separate utensils—disposable, if possible. Clean reusable utensils in hot water and detergent (Fig. 8.10).

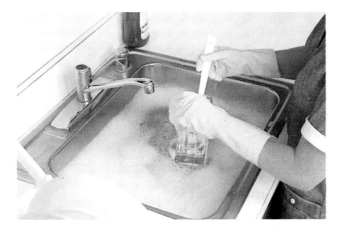

FIGURE 8.10 Use hot water, friction, and dry. Do not let dishes drip dry.

■ *Laundry.* Unsoiled laundry needs no special attention but should be washed or dry cleaned normally. Soiled linen should be separated and handled with disposable gloves. Keep soiled linen in a double plastic bag lined with a cloth bag or pillowcase. Empty the contents of the plastic bag into the washing machine without touching the items, then throw away the plastic bag. Wash soiled linen each day.

| | |
|---|---|
| *Machine washing (colorfast)* | One cup of household bleach in *hot* water and laundry detergent |
| *Hand washing (colorfast)* | Two tablespoons of household bleach in 1 gallon of *warm* water and laundry detergent; soak for ten minutes and rinse. |
| *Machine washing (noncolorfast)* | One cup of Lysol in *warm* water and laundry detergent; wash again with water only to remove Lysol. |
| *Hand washing (noncolorfast)* | Two tablespoons of Lysol in 1 gallon of *warm* water and laundry detergent; rinse at least three times to remove Lysol. |

## ISOLATION TECHNIQUES

The isolation of a client may be necessary to protect the caregiver or to protect the client. When the client has a highly contagious disease, isolation is necessary to decrease the chance of spreading the disease to others. When a client is highly susceptible to diseases caregivers may have, isolation may be necessary to protect the client until his body is able to fight an infection. The physician will determine the type of isolation and how long it must be used.

*Strict isolation* is necessary to decrease the spread of a communicable disease from a client to others.

*Respiratory isolation* is necessary to decrease the spread of air-borne pathogens.

*Drainage and secretions precautions* are used when pathogens are contained in secretions or wound drainage.

*Enteric isolation* is necessary to prevent the spread of pathogens through fecal matter.

*Blood and body isolation* is necessary when transmission of disease can be through contamination by blood or body fluids.

The use of gown, gloves, and mask should be discussed with your supervisor and individualized. A gown is put on to protect you and the client.

A mask is worn to decrease the spread of air-borne pathogens. It filters the air the wearer breathes. Sometimes a mask is worn to protect the client too. There are different types of masks, but they all filter the air and should be applied the same way and changed after every patient encounter.

Basic handwashing is necessary even though gloves are worn. Wash your hands before and after every client contact. The client may have additional restrictions placed on his activity, the washing of his linen, and the need to use disposable dishes. There will be additional laundry. Your help in arranging to get the laundry done will be important for the care of the client. Your supervisor will help you and the family incorporate the needed isolation techniques into the plan of care.

Remember, universal precautions require that you protect yourself against contact with blood and body fluids. The use of isolation status may mean some additional activities, but basic universal precautions must always be used. **Double bagging** is a technique of placing contaminated articles in a plastic bag in the isolation room and then placing the closed bag into another plastic bag as it is held outside the doorway. This can be done by either one person or two.

**double bagging** technique of putting contaminated material into two plastic bags for protection

## ▰ Guidelines: Basic Isolation

- ▰ *Dressings.* Always dispose of dressings in plastic bags and according to local regulations. If the dressings are heavily soiled, double bag them.
- ▰ *Urine/feces.* Flush down the toilet immediately. Clean urinal, bedpan, or commode thoroughly with disinfectant.
- ▰ *Dishes.* Use disposable dishes and cups, if available. Wash dishes separately in hot water and soap. Do not let dishes soak or remain in the sink.
- ▰ *Linen.* Transport to laundry area in separate plastic bags. If heavily soiled, double bag. Wash separately in hot water. Dry immediately.
- ▰ *Cleaning equipment.* Use a disinfectant. Dispose of cleaning water down the toilet. Dispose of cleaning rags in plastic bags.

## Guidelines: Using a Gown and Mask

- ▰ Gown should be long enough to cover your clothing. The outside is considered contaminated. A wet gown is contaminated also. Do not touch the outside of the gown when you remove it. A clean gown should be worn for each client contact (Fig. 8.11).

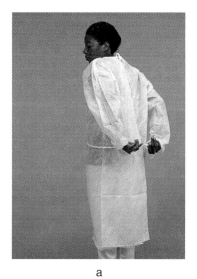

a

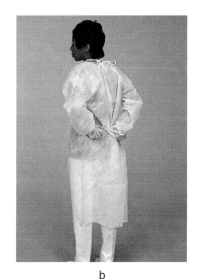

b

*FIGURE 8.11* (a) Tie the neck piece of the gown and overlap the back flaps. (b) Tie the gown securely. Put on gloves now if you need them. (c) To take off a gown, take off your gloves if you are wearing them. Untie neck & waist. Grasp shoulders. Turn gown inside out as you take it off. (d) Fold up the gown and discard. Do not reuse a gown. Wash your hands.

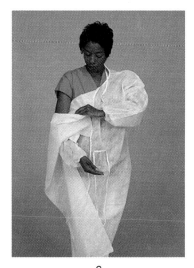

c

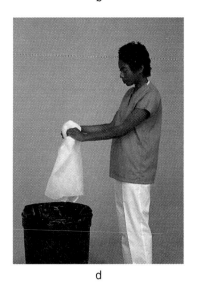

d

Masks should fit snugly over the nose and mouth. A wet mask is considered contaminated, as is the front of the mask. Do not wear a mask around your neck. A clean mask should be worn for each client contact. There are several different types of masks. Discuss with your supervisor which one is appropriate for your client (Fig. 8.12).

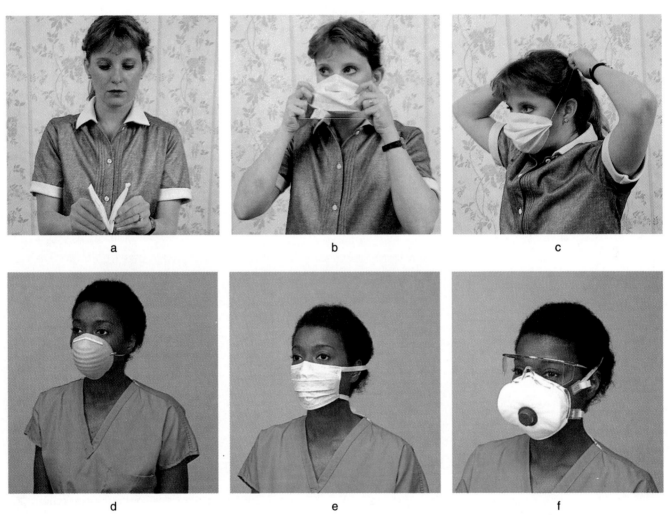

a          b          c

d          e          f

*FIGURE 8.12*   (a,b,c) Take your time to securely fasten your mask. (d) This is a rigid mask but should be molded to cover the nose. (e,f) These masks are worn when extra filtration is needed.

## Section 5   Regulated Medical Waste

**Objectives: What You Will Learn to Do**

- Define *regulated medical waste*.
- List three reasons for segregating regulated medical waste from ordinary trash.
- Demonstrate proper disposal methods for regulated medical waste.

# Introduction: Regulated Medical Waste

**regulated medical waste**
those waste products
determined by law to be in
need of special disposal

**Regulated medical waste** is defined as blood; blood products; sharp medical instruments, such as needles; and dressings contaminated with body fluids. In many communities, there are regulations that specify how the residents may dispose of regulated medical waste. It is important that you know this information so that you are able to assist the client and his family with proper disposal. In many cases, if the medical waste is not disposed of according to the local regulations, the client can be fined. Some towns make pickups, and some require residents to bring the waste to a central point.

Regulations were put into effect to protect local residents, the people who process the trash and waste, and the environment. If you or the client are not aware of the local regulations, your supervisor will be able to obtain the details.

*Human waste products:* should be flushed down the toilet immediately and not discarded in the street, backyard, or street sewers.

*Blood and bloody fluids:* should be cleaned up immediately. If the liquid can be flushed down the toilet, that is the best disposal method. Contaminated clothes should be washed separately in hot water and dried. Dressings and cleaning rags should be double bagged in plastic and disposed of according to local regulations.

*Sharps/needles:* should be kept in a metal container, such as a coffee tin. Secure the top and dispose of the can according to local regulation. Some items may be kept; some must be disposed of immediately. Discuss with your supervisor the best method of disposal.

*Medical equipment:* if contaminated, should be emptied and the equipment double bagged and disposed of according to local regulation. Discuss with your supervisor whether the used equipment can be kept or must be disposed of immediately.

## Topics for Discussion

1. Name areas in the house where bacteria could grow because of the conditions present.
2. How would you keep your hands clean if running water were not available?
3. How do you feel about taking care of a client with AIDS? with hepatitis B? with tuberculosis?
4. How would you explain the need for universal precautions to the family of your client?
5. Do you feel that the regulation of medical waste disposal is a good idea?

# Chapter 9

# Care of the Client's Environment

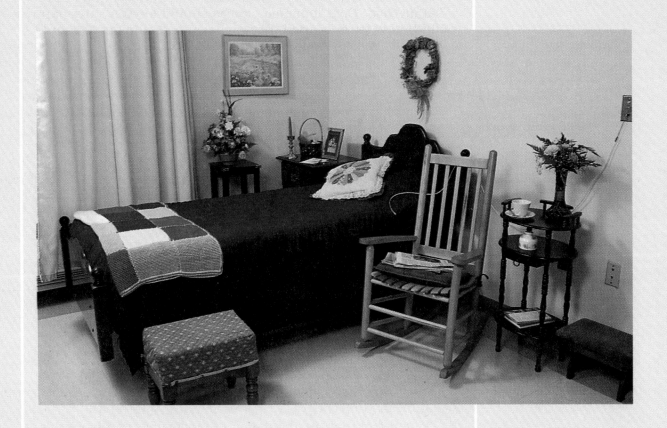

# Section 1 Homemaking

## Objectives: What You Will Learn to Do

- Understand your role as a homemaker/home health aide in maintaining a clean environment.
- Discuss ways of establishing an individual work plan with your client and his family.
- Demonstrate the correct procedures for basic household cleaning tasks.

## Introduction: Homemaking Tasks

When you receive your assignment and the client's care plan, your supervisor will tell you what housekeeping tasks you will be expected to do. They will be based on several guidelines:

- Is the task related to the personal and therapeutic care of the client?
- Can anyone else in the home or family do this task?
- Who will do this task when you are no longer in the home?

Remember, it is often difficult for families to realize what things are important in keeping a house clean and that the homemaker/home health aide is not there to perform all the housekeeping tasks. If the client and his family do not understand your assignment, discuss this with your supervisor.

Clean environments keep harmful bacteria under control. By cleaning bathrooms regularly, chances for the spread of communicable diseases are decreased. Foods stored in specific places are easy to find and can be used more often with less time and energy being spent to look for them. Accidents are prevented in areas that are kept orderly. It is especially important to keep clutter clear of stairways and areas where people walk frequently.

Clean environments also tend to make us feel better. When things are looking their best, we are more often relaxed and comfortable. It also gives us a feeling of pride when others visit. A client will tend to be healthier and happier in an environment that is clean and comfortable.

### CLEANING A CLIENT'S HOME

*Clean* usually refers to an area that is free of pathogens and clutter. To some people, a dust-free home is the only way a home may be judged clean. To others, the presence of dust may not matter.

You may find that what is clean to one person may not be considered clean by another. These differences in values are important to recognize. Try to meet the client's values. If your values and the client's needs are very different, consult your supervisor.

All housekeeping tasks that need to be done in the home should be discussed by all people concerned. You might hold a meeting with the family to decide what jobs need to be done to keep the household functioning. You might want your supervisor at this meeting, or this discussion might be very informal.

After a list of jobs has been made by the group, discuss who will do them. Remember, you will not always be in the house. It is very important to develop a routine the family can follow when you are gone.

Encourage all family members to make suggestions and offer help. Remember, the family is in a crisis situation and people who may not usually help in housekeeping may be willing to help at this difficult time. A spirit of cooperation and flexibility should be encouraged. Children are important parts of families. Do not overlook them.

If someone is willing to help but does not know how, a "teacher" (either the aide or a family member) could be found. In teaching, remember:

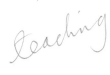

- Make the explanation of the job as simple as possible.
- Help the people, but do not do it for them.
- Let them do it their way if it gets the same results.

**Sample Work Plan**

| Day | Task | Who Will Do It |
|-----|------|----------------|
| Monday | | |
| Tuesday | | |
| Wednesday | | |
| Thursday | | |
| Friday | | |
| Saturday | | |
| Sunday | | |

## HOW TO KEEP A HOUSE CLEAN

Make a list of what you need to keep the house clean. Remember to use those products that are already in the home. Do not insist that the client purchase your brand of cleaning products. Your list might look like this:

| Necessary Supplies | Nice to Have |
|--------------------|--------------|
| Hot water | Dustpan |
| Soap or detergent | Vacuum cleaner |
| Broom | Scouring pads |
| Vinegar | Mop |
| Scrub pad, scrub brush | Wastebaskets |
| Baking soda, baking powder | |
| Bucket | |
| Trash container | |

Be sure you know how to use the appliances in the house. If you are not sure, ask!

**Basic Kinds of Cleaning Products**

| Products | Form | Uses | Cautions |
|----------|------|------|----------|
| Soaps and detergents | Liquid Powder Solid | All types of cleaning; personal cleaning | Read label; protect eyes |

## Basic Kinds of Cleaning Products

| Products | Form | Uses | Cautions |
| --- | --- | --- | --- |
| All-purpose cleaner | Liquid<br>Powder<br>Solid | All types of cleaning | Read label; protect eyes |
| Abrasives/bleach | Liquid<br>Powder | Surface soil; kills certain pathogens | Read label; protect eyes and skin |
| Specialty cleaners | Foam<br>Liquid<br>Powder<br>Spray | Specific jobs: metal, windows, etc. | Read label |

When using any cleaning product, the following care should be used:

- Read the instructions on the label. Follow the directions in the order they are given, and use the amount suggested.
- Do not mix cleaning products unless you have been instructed to do so. They may cause a chemical reaction that will hurt you and/or the surface you are cleaning.
- Do not leave cleaners on a surface for a long time. Use care in how much you scrub a surface.
- Change the cleaning water when it is only moderately dirty, and rinse if needed to avoid streaking or filming.
- Store all cleaning products safely: away from children and pets, away from heat sources, and in their original containers. Store cleaning tools and supplies safely as close as possible to where you will use them.
- Line garbage pails with plastic or paper bags. Do not put wet objects directly into paper bags. Wrap them first.

## Using Common Cleaning Products

| Task | Product | Use |
| --- | --- | --- |
| Bathtub stains | White vinegar or paste of hydrogen peroxide and baking powder | Rub stain with rag dipped in vinegar; rinse; leave paste on stain overnight; rinse |
| Tile cleaner | Sprinkle baking soda | Rub with damp rag or sponge; rinse, as this makes tile slippery |
| Windows and painted surfaces | Mix carefully:<br>5 C water<br>1 tsp detergent<br>1 pt rubbing alcohol<br>1/2 C sudsy ammonia | Wash area carefully; rinse well; dry |
| Mattress stain solution | 1/2 C water<br>1/2 C white vinegar | Dab solution on stain and let dry; rub area with water and detergent; leave on for ten minutes; blot dry; rinse; let mattress dry |

When using equipment, the following safety points should be kept in mind:

- Keep electrical equipment away from water. Never soak this equipment unless the manufacturer says that you can.
- Use equipment for the use for which it was intended.
- Do not put sharp objects such as hairpins, knives, or screwdrivers, into electrical equipment.
- When repairing an electrical object, unplug it!
- Be sure all equipment is in good condition and does not have frayed cords.

## SPECIFIC TASKS

### Dusting

Dusting is done to prevent the spread of bacteria. In homes where people are particularly sensitive to dust, you may have to dust often. Dampen the rag with a light spray of water or a commercial spray to keep the dust from spreading. Dust with motions that will gather the dust into the rag and away from you (Fig. 9.1).

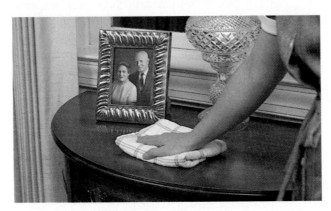

**FIGURE 9.1** Dust from top to bottom. Dust pictures, then standing objects, and finally tables and cabinets.

### Washing Dishes

Dishes should be washed properly soon after meals. If a dishwasher is used or dishes are to be washed at a later time, scrape the food off the dish (a rubber spatula is a good tool to use for this job). Then rinse or soak the dishes in a basin of water.

- Place dishes on the counter to the left of the soapy dish water in the order in which they are to be washed—least dirty first, most dirty last (glasses, silverware, plates and cups and saucers, pots, roasting pans).
- Wash dishes in the hot, soapy water and rinse in clear water in the pan to your right (Fig. 9.2).
- Drain dishes on drainboard placed to the right of the rinse water.
- Dishes are more sanitary if allowed to air dry rather than being dried with a towel.
  *Note:* If you are left-handed, reverse the placement of the soapy water pan, clear water pan, and the place where the dishes are stacked and drained.

When water is not plentiful, use water from rinsing dishes for other cleaning tasks, such as washing the floor. Wash dishes in water

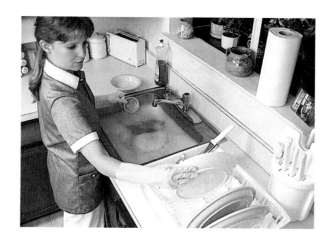

**FIGURE 9.2** Carefully place dishes in a drain that has a mat under it to catch the water.

hot enough to clean the grease from them and destroy as many microorganisms as possible.

Keeping a kitchen clean is important. Just as food keeps us alive, it is also used by bacteria. Cleaning spills and taking proper care of leftover food is very important. Trash should be disposed of regularly (before it falls out of the container). If the trash is wet, put it into a plastic bag first and then into the garbage can. Keep the garbage can clean. Wash it often!

- The stove should be wiped up regularly with soapy water to avoid spills becoming "cooked on."
- The refrigerator (or the place where food is kept cold) should be wiped out on a regular basis. Do not use sharp objects to poke at ice clumps when defrosting the refrigerator. If the refrigerator is self-defrosting, clean up spills promptly. Food tends to dry out faster in these models. If the refrigerator needs defrosting, discuss this with the family and/or your supervisor.
- Small appliances can be wiped down with soap and water or an all-purpose cleaner *after* they have been disconnected.
- Countertops should be free of food spills and grease. Counters are easier to wipe off if they are kept uncluttered. Areas around drawer handles and door pulls should be kept clean by wiping with a cloth (or sponge) and warm soap and water.

### Cleaning Bathrooms

Because of the constant moisture in the air, bathrooms need regular cleaning to keep them free of bacteria and odors. If bathroom floors are ceramic tile, any water spilled on them can make them slippery and dangerous. Keep the floors dry.

Safety in bathrooms should always be on your mind. Before a client uses a bathroom, check it:

- Are there nonskid mats in the tub?
- Are there nonskid rugs on the tile floor?
- Are there grab bars in the shower or tub?
- Is there good lighting?
- Is there ventilation?

Cleaning shower walls and bathtubs can be kept to a minimum if everyone will wipe the area out after each use. You will get people to cooperate more easily if you keep a rag or old towel handy for them to use.

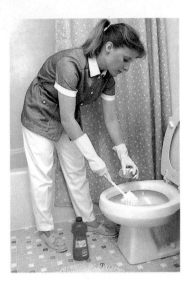

**FIGURE 9.3** The brush used to clean the toilet should be stored in a special container and used only for this purpose.

Sinks and other bathroom fixtures should be cleaned regularly with cleanser and a rag. Do not destroy the surface of enamel fixtures by using cleaners that will scratch them.

To clean the toilet bowl, you will need: soap or detergent, a toilet bowl brush, and a rag or sponge. *Note:* Do not wipe anything else with this rag or sponge. Wash it after this task (Fig. 9.3).

■ Lift up the seat and put soap or detergent into the bowl.
■ Scrub the inside of the bowl with a toilet bowl brush. Get under the rim of the bowl.
■ Let the suds stay in the bowl while you wash the outside.
■ To avoid a possible chemical reaction, do not mix toilet bowl cleaner with any other cleanser.
■ Use clean hot water to rinse off all parts of the toilet with the sponge or rag.
■ If there are water stains such as rust in the bowl, shake in 1/4 cup of toilet bowl cleaner. Let stand about thirty minutes, then scrub and flush.

### Laundry

Clean clothes are important for good health. They also make us look good and feel better about ourselves. Before washing any clothes, all tears, loose buttons, or closures should be repaired (Fig. 9.4). This will prevent the button from being lost and the repair job from becoming a much larger task. Before washing, clothes should be sorted by:

■ *Color.* Dark colors should be washed separately from light colors.
■ *Fabric.* Delicate fabrics cannot take as much scrubbing as can heavy-duty fabrics.
■ *Degree of dirt.* Heavily soiled jeans should not be washed with a silk blouse.

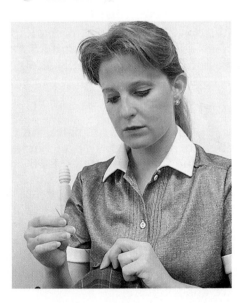

**FIGURE 9.4** Mending clothes before washing them prevents further damage.

As with any appliances that you use, either ask the client how to operate the washer correctly or read the instructions in the "use and care" booklet from the appliance manufacturer.

After sorting clothes, load the machine, being careful not to overload it. Put in the recommended amount of detergent and select the water temperature and amount of agitation. Add bleach and fabric softener (if needed) after the water has soaked all the clothes.

Clothes dried out of doors conserve energy and have a fresh, clean smell. Once dry, take clothes immediately from a dryer as they will then need less ironing and you will save energy and time.

Some homes do not have a washing machine. After you have found out how the laundry is usually done in the home, discuss with your supervisor what your responsibilities will be. Bending and lifting wet, heavy pieces of linen could cause you to injure your back. If you must do this, use good body mechanics! Protect your back!

### Care of Rugs and Carpeting

Ask your client how they usually care for their carpets and rugs. Frequent vacuuming or sweeping will preserve the rugs and decrease the lint and dust (Fig. 9.5).

If the client has a vacuum cleaner, remember:

- Treat it as you would any electrical appliance.
- Ask how to change the dirt collection bag inside.
- Use the vacuum at a convenient time for the family when it will not disturb them.

When you find stains on a carpet or rug, you may treat them as follows:

- Ask the family if the stain is new. If it is an old stain, you will probably not be able to get it out.
- You may use commercial stain removers.
- You may mix water and baking soda into a solution, and rub it into the stain. After it dries, vacuum.
- If the spot is sticky, sprinkle baking soda on it, then vacuum.

### Care of Floors

Keeping floors clean is important to the general well-being of the client and his family. Clean floors also decrease the spread of bacteria and provide a safe path in which people can walk.

- Sweep floors frequently, especially before washing them.
- Ask the family how they usually clean the floors. Wood floors often require special cleaners and are not cleaned with water.
- Use the detergent or cleanser according to directions. Do not let water remain on the floor.
- Most households will have a mop for this job. If you do not find one, discuss this with your supervisor.
- Let the floor dry before walking on it or putting furniture back in place.

### Pests and Bugs

Pests and bugs may carry diseases and be annoying to you and your client. They may bite, cause skin irritations, or even frighten people. The best way to keep an area free of bugs or rodents or other pests is to keep it clean and free of clutter.

- Put food away in closed containers; tin and glass are best.
- Clean up spills and crumbs.
- Take out garbage and trash.
- Keep garbage and trash in covered containers (Fig. 9.6).

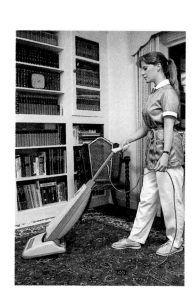

FIGURE 9.5 Be sure the noise of the vacuum cleaner does not disturb the client or the family.

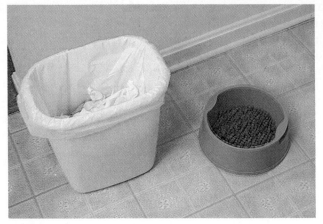

**FIGURE 9.6** Cover garbage. Do not allow moist pet food to remain out for long periods of time.

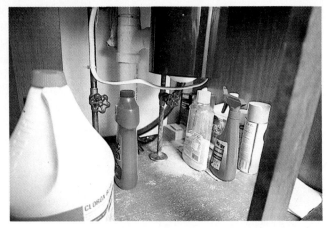

**FIGURE 9.7** Wet, damp, dark places that are undisturbed attract bugs and pests.

- Roaches and mice can pass through small cracks in walls and near pipes. Talk to your supervisor about having someone caulk up such holes (Fig. 9.7).
- Do not let water stand inside or outside.

If you or any family member wish to use a commercial product to get rid of bugs or rodents, check with your supervisor to be sure that it is safe.

## Section 2 Bed Making

**Objectives: What You Will Learn to Do**

- Make a closed bed.
- Make an open fanfolded bed.
- Make an occupied bed.
- List the reasons why a well-made bed is important.

### Introduction: Bed Making

You may have a client who spends part of the day in bed. Some of your clients, though, are unable or not permitted to get out of bed at all. As a result, many clients are fed and bathed and use a bedpan in bed.

Homemaker/home health aides should make beds with no wrinkles in the sheets. Wrinkles are not only uncomfortable, but restrict the client's circulation and can cause painful **decubitus ulcers** (bedsores). These are open wounds that often slow the client's recovery. Decubiti can form very quickly and are difficult to heal.

You may care for clients in their own beds. Your clients may decide to sleep on a couch or they may have a hospital bed in their home. Some clients may have side rails on their beds. These are used both to protect the client and to assist him as he moves in the bed by providing him with something to grab for support. If your client is in need of a side rail to prevent him from falling out of bed, you could put chairs up against the bed with their backs against the mattress. Tie the chairs together and tie them to the bed (Fig. 9.8).

**decubitus ulcer** bedsore; open wound which occurs from lack of blood supply to an area usually located on a bony prominence

The same rules and procedures apply for any type of bed.

- Keep the bed dry and clean—change linen when necessary.
- Keep the linen wrinkle-free.
- Make the bed to suit your particular client.
- Keep the bed free of food particles and crumbs.

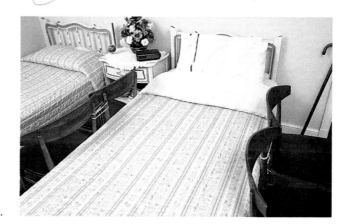

**FIGURE 9.8** This is a good way to remind a client to call for assistance. Permanent siderails have to be provided if the client uses them to frequently change position or pull himself up in bed.

## Guidelines: Bed Making

- Use the linen the client has available. If you do not have enough, report this to your supervisor.
- Try to make the bed according to the custom of the house. If you must change the custom, explain your reasons to the client and his family.
- Do not use a torn piece of linen. It may tear even more and could be dangerous.
- Never use a pin on any item of linen.
- Do not shake the bed linen. Shaking spreads harmful microorganisms to everything and everyone in the room, including you.
- Never allow any linen to touch your uniform.
- Dirty used linen should never be put on the floor.
- Put dirty linen in the place agreed upon by you and the client's family.
- Some clients use fitted bottom sheets. Others use flat sheets where the homemaker/home health aide makes the mitered corners. The mitered corner keeps the sheets firm and smooth and makes the bed neat and attractive.
- The bottom sheet must be firm, smooth, and wrinkle free. This is very important for the client's comfort.
- By fanfolding the top of the bed, you make it easy for the client to get in and out of his bed.
- The **draw sheet** is about half the size of a regular sheet. When draw sheets are not available, a large sheet can be folded in half widthwise (with small and large hems together) and used. The fold must always be placed toward the head of the bed and the hems toward the foot of the bed. You could also use a tablecloth. If you must protect the bed, a plastic tablecloth makes an excellent protective sheet. Never use plastic from a garment bag or garbage bag.
- The plastic draw sheet and disposable bed protectors protect the mattress.

**draw sheet** small sheet made of plastic, rubber, or cotton placed across the middle of the bed to cover and protect the bottom sheet and assist in moving the client

■ Plastics should never touch a client's skin. When using a plastic draw sheet, be sure to cover it entirely with a cloth draw sheet.

■ Some clients do not use a draw sheet. Instead, small disposable bed protectors are placed on the bed under the client as necessary. These are often expensive. Check with your supervisor before you suggest this to the family.

■ To save linen and washing, a used clean top sheet may be used as a draw sheet or bottom sheet.

■ Those clients who do not use their bed a great deal may not have to have the linen changed every day. Evaluate the linen, the home, the client, and the entire situation before you change the bed.

■ Always use good body mechanics, no matter what kind of bed your client is using.

■ "Bottom of the bed" refers to the mattress pad, if used, the bottom sheet, and the draw sheets.

■ "Top of the bed" refers to the top sheet, blanket, if used, and bedspread.

■ Remember that you save time and energy by first making as much of the bed as possible on one side before going to the other side.

■ Side rails are used to prevent the client from falling.

### Three Basic Beds

1. *The closed bed.* This bed is usually made when it will remain empty for a while. You can make it with a bedspread or only with a sheet and blanket (Fig. 9.9a).

2. *The open bed.* This bed is used when it will be occupied within a short period of time (Fig. 9.9b).

3. *The occupied bed.* This bed is made with the client in the bed (Fig. 9.9c).

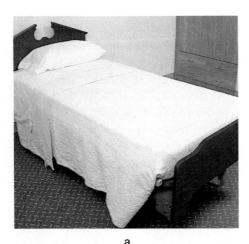
a

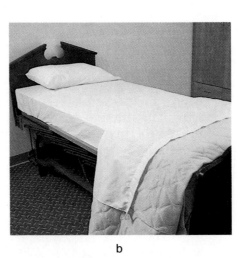
b

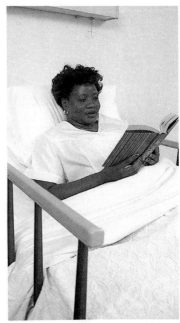
c

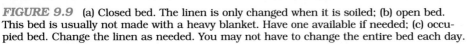
*FIGURE 9.9* (a) Closed bed. The linen is only changed when it is soiled; (b) open bed. This bed is usually not made with a heavy blanket. Have one available if needed; (c) occupied bed. Change the linen as needed. You may not have to change the entire bed each day.

## Procedure 6: Making the Closed Bed

1. Assemble your equipment:
   Mattress cover, if used
   Bottom sheet
   Cotton and plastic draw sheet (or disposable bed protector)
   Top sheet
   Blanket
   Bedspread
   Pillowcase
   Pillow
   Pillow protector, if used
   Chair
2. Wash your hands.
3. Place a chair near the bed.
4. Put the pillow on the chair.
5. Stack the bed-making items on the chair in the order in which you will use them: first things to be used on top, last things to be used on the bottom.
6. If you have a hospital bed, adjust the bed to the highest horizontal position. Lock the bed in place. If not, move the bed so you have room to practice good body mechanics.
7. Pull the mattress to the head of the bed until it touches the headboard.
8. Place the mattress pad on the mattress even with the head of the mattress.
9. Fold the bottom sheet lengthwise and place it on the bed:
   a. Place the center fold of the sheet at the center of the mattress from head to foot (Fig. 9.10).

FIGURE 9.10

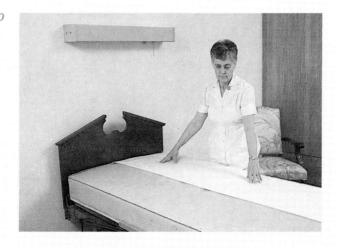

   b. Put the small hem at the foot of the bed, even with the edge of the mattress.
   c. Place the large hem at the head of the bed with about 18 inches left to tuck in.
   Always do this while practicing good body mechanics. Bend your legs, not your back.

10. Open the sheet. It should now hang evenly over each side of the bed.
11. Tuck the sheet in tightly at the head of the bed. Lift the mattress with the hand closest to the foot of the bed and tuck with the other hand. This is good body mechanics.
12. To make a **mitered corner**:
    a. Pick up the edge of the sheet at the side of the bed 12 inches from the head of the mattress (Fig. 9.11).
    b. Place the triangle (the folded corner) on top of the mattress (Fig. 9.12).
    c. Tuck the hanging portion of the sheet under the mattress (Fig. 9.13).
    d. While you hold the fold at the edge of the mattress, bring the triangle down over the side of the mattress.
    e. Tuck the sheet under the mattress from head to foot (Fig. 9.14).
13. Stand and work entirely on one side of the bed until that side is finished.
14. Place the plastic draw sheet 14 inches (two open handspans) down from the head of the bed. Tuck it in (Fig. 9.15).
15. Cover the plastic draw sheet with the cotton draw sheet, and tuck it in (Fig. 9.16).

**mitered corner** folding the bedding at the corners when making a bed so that the sheet is tightly stretched with no wrinkles

FIGURE 9.11

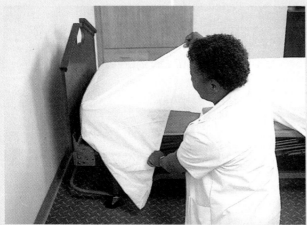

FIGURE 9.12

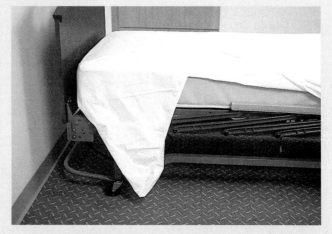

FIGURE 9.13

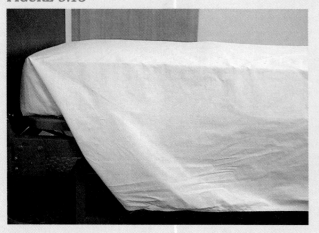

FIGURE 9.14

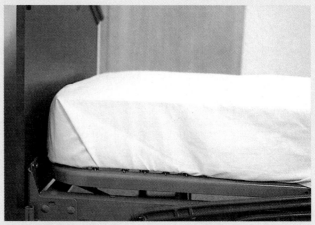

FIGURE 9.15     FIGURE 9.16

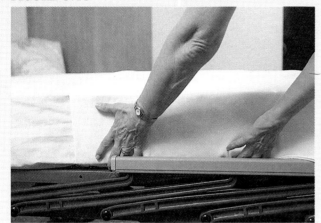
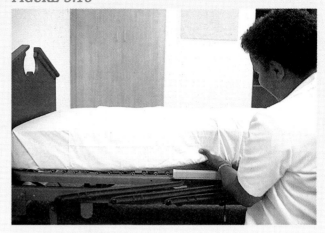

16. Fold the top sheet lengthwise and place it on the bed:
    a. Place the center fold on the center of the bed from the head to the foot.
    b. Place the large hem at the head of the bed, even with the top edge of the mattress.
    c. Open the sheet, with the rough edge of the hem up.
    d. Tightly tuck the sheet under the foot of the bed.
    e. Make a mitered corner at the foot of the bed.
    f. Do not tuck the sheet in at the side of the bed.
17. Fold the blanket lengthwise and place on the bed.
    a. Place the center fold of the blanket on the center of the bed from head to foot.
    b. Place the upper hem 6 inches from the top edge of the mattress.
    c. Open the blanket.
    d. Tuck it under the foot tightly.
    e. Make a mitered corner at the foot of the bed.
    f. Do not tuck in at the side of the bed.
18. Fold the bedspread lengthwise and place it on the bed.
19. Now move to the other side of the bed. Start with the bottom sheet.
    a. Straighten the sheet to get rid of all wrinkles. This should be done three times, first near the head, the middle, and at the foot of the bed.
    b. Miter the top corner.
    c. Pull the sheet tight so it is wrinkle free. Roll the sheet up in your hands so it is near the bed and pull slightly down and tuck in. Do this near the head of the bed, the middle, and the foot.
    d. Pull the plastic draw sheet tight and tuck it in.
    e. Pull the cotton draw sheet tight and tuck it in.
    f. Straighten out the top sheet, making the mitered corner at the foot of the bed.
    g. Miter the corner of the blanket.
    h. Miter the corner of the bedspread (Fig. 9.17).

FIGURE 9.17

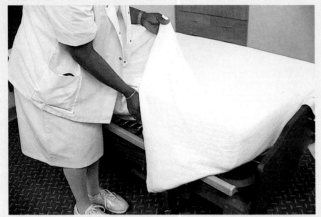

FIGURE 9.18

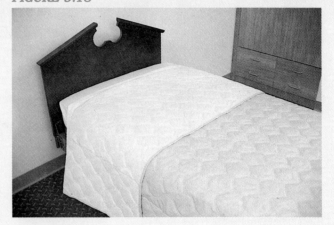

FIGURE 9.19

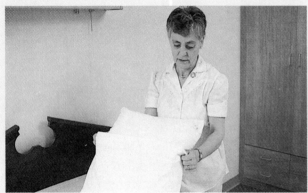

FIGURE 9.20

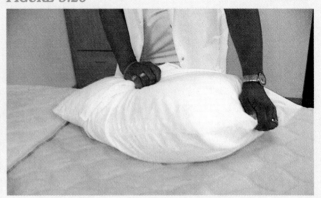

20. To make the cuff:
    a. Fold the top hem of the spread under the top hem of the blanket.
    b. Fold the top hem of the sheet back over the edge of the spread and the blanket to form a cuff. The hemmed side of the sheet must be on the underside, so that it does not come in contact with the client (Fig. 9.18).
21. To put the pillowcase on a pillow:
    a. Hold the pillowcase at the center of the end seam.
    b. With your hand outside the case, turn the case back over your hand.
    c. Grasp the pillow through the case at the center of the end of the pillow.
    d. Bring the case down over the pillow (Fig. 9.19).
    e. Fit the corner of the pillow into the seamless corner of the case (Fig. 9.20).
    f. Fold the extra material from the side seam under the pillow.
    g. Place the pillow on the bed with the open end away from the door.
22. Adjust the bed to its lowest horizontal position if you have a hospital bed.

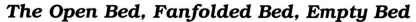

## The Open Bed, Fanfolded Bed, Empty Bed

The procedures for making the open bed, the **fanfolded** bed, and the empty bed are all the same. You will be making an open bed when the client is able to get out of bed and move around.

The open bed is made exactly like the closed bed except that the top bedding is left open so that the client can easily get back into the bed.

This is done after you finish making the cuff at the head of the bed.

## Procedure 7: Making the Open, Fanfolded Empty Bed

1. Make a closed bed.
2. Grasp the cuff of the bedding in both hands (Fig. 9.21).
3. Pull it to the foot of the bed (Fig. 9.22).
4. Fold the bedding back on itself toward the head of the bed. The edge of the cuff must meet the fold.
5. Smooth the sheets on each side neatly into the folds you have made.
6. Wash your hands.

**FIGURE 9.21**

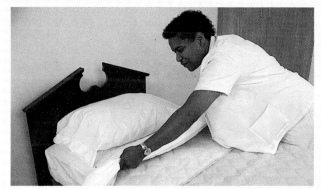

**FIGURE 9.22**

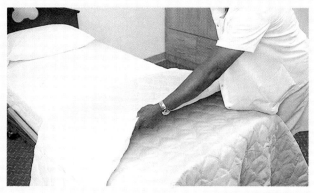

## The Occupied Bed

The occupied bed is made when the client is not able or not permitted to get out of bed. The most important part of making an occupied bed is to get the sheets smooth and tight under the client, so there will be no wrinkles to rub against the skin. When making the bottom of this bed, your job will be easier if you divide the bed in two parts—the side the client is lying on and the side you are making. By doing this, the weight of the client is never on the side where you are working. Always keep the side rail up on the client's side. Usually, the occupied bed is made after giving the client a bed bath. The client should be covered with the bath blanket while you are making the bed. The sheets must be placed on the bed so the rough seam edges are kept facing the mattress and away from the client's skin.

Some clients prefer the pillow to be moved with them from side to side as the bed is being made. Some clients will ask you to remove the pillow while making the bed. Either way is acceptable unless there is a medical **contraindication** (reason for not doing something). Your supervisor will tell you if a particular bed position must be maintained.

**contraindication** condition that forbids the use of a particular treatment or drug

Remember to talk to your client while you are making the bed. Continually notice his condition during the procedure.

## Procedure 8: Making the Occupied Bed When Side Rails Are Present

1. Assemble your equipment near the bed, in the order in which you will use them.
   A chair is useful for this purpose.
   Two large sheets
   One plastic draw sheet, if used
   One cotton draw sheet, if used
   Disposable bed protectors, if used
   One bath blanket, if available
   Pillowcase(s)
   One blanket
   One bedspread
   Container for dirty laundry
2. Wash your hands.
3. Ask any visitors to step out of the room if appropriate.
4. Tell the client you are going to make his bed.
5. If you are working on a hospital bed, lower the backrest and knee rest until the bed is flat if that is allowed. Raise the bed to its highest horizontal position and lock in place.
6. Loosen all the sheets around the entire bed.
7. Take the bedspread and blanket off the bed, and fold them over the back of the chair. Leave the client covered only with the top sheet.
8. If using a bath blanket, cover the client with this by placing it over the top sheet. Ask the client to hold the bath blanket. If he is unable to do this, tuck the top edges of the bath blanket under the client's shoulders. Without exposing him, remove the top sheet from under the bath blanket. Fold the top sheet and place over the back of a chair.
9. If the mattress has slipped out of place, move it to its proper position touching the headboard. Remember to use proper body mechanics. If you cannot move the mattress, get assistance.
10. Raise the side rail on the opposite side from where you will be working, and lock in place.
11. Ask the client to turn onto his side toward the side rail. Help the client to turn if necessary. If the client cannot turn, have him stay on his back but move as far as possible toward the side rail. Be careful as to the placing of the client's hands. Adjust the pillow to suit the client's needs. Check it for items such as dentures and eyeglasses.
12. Fold the cotton draw sheet toward the client and tuck it against his back. Protect him from any soiled matter on the bedding (Fig. 9.23).
13. Raise the plastic draw sheet (if it is clean) over the bath blanket and client.

FIGURE 9.23                FIGURE 9.24

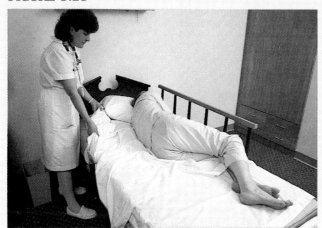
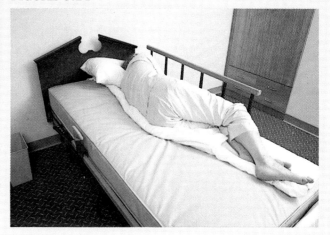

14. Roll the bottom sheet toward the client and tuck it against his back. This strips your side of the bed down to the mattress (Fig. 9.24).

15. Take the large clean sheet and fold it in half lengthwise. Do not permit the sheet to touch the floor or your uniform.

16. Place it on the bed, still folded, with the fold running along the middle of the mattress. The small hem end of the sheet should be even with the foot edge of the mattress. Fold the top half of the sheet toward the client. (This is for the other side of the bed.) Tuck the folds against his back, below the plastic draw sheet.

17. Tuck the sheet around the head of the mattress by gently raising the mattress with the hand closest to the foot of the bed and tucking with the other hand.

18. Miter the corner at the head of the mattress. Tuck in the clean bottom sheet on your side from head to foot of the mattress.

19. Pull the plastic draw sheet toward you, over the clean bottom sheet, and tuck it in.

20. Place the clean cotton draw sheet over the plastic sheet, folded in half. Keep the fold near the client. Fold the top half toward the client, tucking the folds under his back, as you did with the bottom sheet. Tuck the free edge of the draw sheet under the mattress.

21. Ask the client, or help him, to roll over the "hump" onto the clean sheets toward you.

22. Raise the side rail on your side of the bed, and lock into place.

23. Go to the opposite side of the bed and lower the side rail.

24. Remove the old bottom sheet and cotton draw sheet from the bed. Put them into the container for soiled linen. Pull the fresh bottom sheet toward the edge of the bed. Tuck it under the mattress at the head of the bed and make a mitered corner. Then pull the bottom sheet under the mattress from the head to the foot. Do this by rolling the sheet up in your hand toward the mattress and pull it as you tuck it under.

FIGURE 9.25

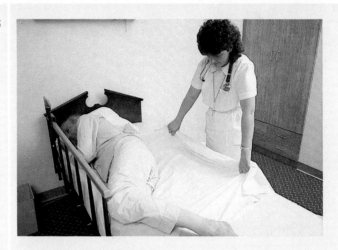

25. One at a time, pull and tuck each draw sheet under the mattress (Fig. 9.25).
26. Have the client turn on his back.
27. Change the pillowcase, and place the pillow under the client's head. If necessary, assist the client to place the pillow under his head.
28. To put the pillowcase on a pillow:
    a. Hold the pillowcase at the center of the end seam.
    b. With your hand outside the case, turn the case back over your hand.
    c. Grasp the pillow through the case at the center of the end of the pillow.
    d. Bring the case down over the pillow.
    e. Fit the corner of the pillow into the seamless corner of the case.
    f. Fold the extra material from the side seam under the pillow.
    g. Place the pillow on the bed with the open end away from the door.
29. Spread the clean top sheet over the bath blanket with the wide hem at the top. The middle of the sheet should run along the middle of the bed. The wide hem should be even with the head edge of the mattress. Ask the client to hold the hem of the clean sheet, if he can, while you remove the bath blanket, moving toward the foot of the bed. Do not expose the client.
30. Tuck the clean top sheet under the mattress at the foot of the bed. Make sure you leave enough room for the client to move his feet freely. Miter the corner of the sheet if the client likes this.
31. Spread the blanket over the top sheet. Be sure the middle of the blanket runs along the middle of the bed. The blanket should be high enough to cover the client's shoulders.
32. Tuck the blanket in at the foot of the bed if the client likes this. Make a mitered corner with the blanket.
33. Place the spread on the bed as the client prefers. Pull up the side rails.
34. Go to the other side of the bed. Put down the side rails, turn the top covers back and miter the top sheet, then

miter the blanket. Be sure the top covers are loose enough that the client is able to move his feet.

35. To make the cuff:
   a. Fold the top hem edge of the spread over and under the top hem of the blanket.
   b. Fold the top hem of the top sheet back over the edge of the spread and blanket to form a cuff. The rough edge of the hem of the sheet must be turned down so the client does not come in contact with it.
36. Raise the backrest and knee rest to suit the client if this is allowed.
37. Lower the entire bed to its lowest horizontal position.
38. Put the side rails in place.
39. Make sure the client is comfortable.
40. Put all used linen in the proper place.
41. Wash your hands.
42. Chart any observations you made during this procedure.

# Section 3   Safety and Fire Protection

## Objectives: What You Will Learn to Do

- List the general rules of home safety.
- List special safety precautions to take with yourself and with older clients.
- Explain what causes fire.
- Explain what you can do to prevent fire.
- Explain what to do in case of fire.
- Describe the special safety precautions necessary when oxygen is being used.

### *Introduction: Safety*

Safety is everyone's job. The rules that govern safety in a home must become part of every procedure and every decision you make while caring for your client. It is also important for you to remember that, by your actions, you are teaching family members. As they observe you practicing safety, they will be made aware of its importance.

It is your responsibility to protect your client and be continually aware of his safety. Make yourself aware of potential hazardous situations and their remedies in each home where you work.

It is also your responsibility to protect yourself. Be careful! Be aware! Be alert!

#### GENERAL SAFETY RULES

This section is designed to make you aware of the most common safety hazards in a home. More accidents occur in the home than in any other place. There are several reasons for this:

- We are careless.
- We do not have safety inspections in homes as we do in commercial buildings.
- We are not aware of the potential hazards that exist in homes.

### General Safety Rules You Should Follow

- Discuss emergency communication with your supervisor. If no telephone is available, what is the best route of communicating?
- Report to your supervisor any unsafe conditions where you are working.
- When you see something on the floor that does not belong there, pick it up. If you see spilled liquid, wipe it up.
- Avoid slippery floors.
- If slippery floors cannot be avoided, walk on them carefully.
- Remove scatter rugs. If you cannot remove them, tack them down.
- Be sure to set the brakes on wheelchairs when a client is getting in or out.
- Use side rails on beds if there is a chance the client will fall out.
- Do not work in poor light.
- Do not use any piece of equipment unless you are sure you know how it works.
- Keep the telephone numbers of the police, rescue squad, fire department, and poison control center near each telephone.
- Read labels. If a container does not have one, do not use the contents.
- Know how to get out of the house in case of fire.
- Be aware of what accidents are most prevalent at different ages.
- Do not attempt a task if you have any doubt that you can do it.
- Do not reach into a garbage can or trash basket. You may hurt yourself on sharp objects.

### Safety Precautions for Children

- Small children should never be left unattended when they are awake.
- Every child in a protective device should be checked frequently.
- Articles used in the child's care should be kept out of reach of a toddler when they are not being used. Watch especially for needles, water, safety pins, medications, matches, electrical equipment, syringes, or thermometers.
- Toys should never be left carelessly on the floor. Be especially alert to pick them up as they could cause someone to fall. Also, remember to clean up spills and messes such as food, urine, and feces.
- The sides of a child's crib should be up at all times except when someone is giving direct care to the child.
- Doors to stairways and the kitchen should be closed and locked.
- Venetian blind cords should be kept out of the reach of children.
- Be sure there are no small toys or objects in the bed/crib that could be swallowed.
- Be sure there are no large objects in the bed or crib that the child could stand on. The child might fall out of bed as a result.
- Keep all poisonous substances in a high place behind locked doors.

## Safety Precautions for the Aged

Abilities change as we age. Unfortunately, people often do not realize this fact. Therefore, they attempt tasks that they can no longer do safely. As a homemaker/home health aide, you should be aware of the capabilities of your particular client. In addition, there are general rules you should keep in mind.

- Be sure there is adequate lighting for every task.
- Be alert to sensory changes that may or may not have taken place.
- Protect your client from falling. Recovery from falls takes a long time.
- Protect your client from burns. Temperature sensation becomes less accurate as we age. Run cold water through a faucet after you run hot water. Then if your client touches the faucet, he will not burn himself. Test the bath water yourself (Fig. 9.26).
- If a confused client tells you he is going to do something that you know to be harmful, take him seriously and protect him.

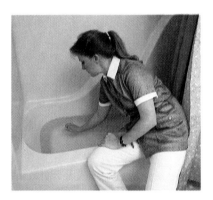

**FIGURE 9.26** Be sure water in the tub is well mixed to avoid hot or cold spots.

### Electricity

Electricity is a great help in our lives. If we misuse it, however, it can cause a great deal of damage (Fig. 9.27).

- Make sure all electrical equipment you use is in good condition.
- Be sure the cords are not frayed and that you are using the proper tool for the job.

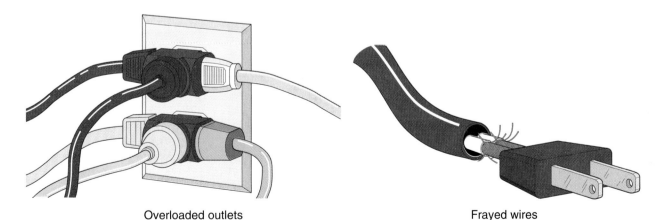

Overloaded outlets       Frayed wires

**FIGURE 9.27** Be familiar with misuses of electricity that exist in your client's home. Assist him with correcting them.

- Do not put electrical cords under rugs. They get frayed and can go unnoticed under a rug. This is a perfect place for a fire to start.
- Be sure your hands are dry before you use any electrical equipment.
- Do not change fuses or touch circuit breakers unless you are sure you know what you are doing.
- Do not run all household appliances at the same time in an effort to save time.

### Smoking

Many clients smoke. Many visitors smoke. If a client permits smoking in his home—unless it is not allowed due to a medical reason or the presence of oxygen—you will be asked to tolerate it. If you are uncomfortable in a house with cigarette smoke, discuss this with your supervisor. There are some rules you should keep in mind if people are smoking in the house (Fig. 9.28).

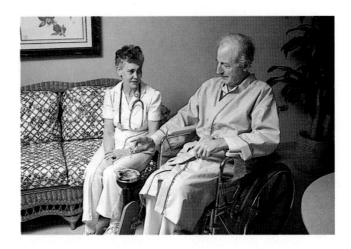

**FIGURE 9.28** During the stress of illness, many clients cannot stop smoking. Provide a safe environment for them and you.

- Be sure ashtrays are provided and that they are used.
- Never empty warm ashtrays into plastic bags, plastic wastebaskets, or containers. When you empty ashtrays, be sure the contents are cool. Wet the ashes if you are in doubt.
- A client who has been given a sedative should not smoke.
- A confused client should not smoke.
- A client in bed should not smoke unattended.
- Check chairs, upholstery, and blankets for ashes or cigarettes if your client is smoking.
- If a client has hand tremors, light his cigarette, and assist him as he smokes.

### Safety in the Kitchen

Some people cook in a hurry and think about many other things while they are cooking. This leads to various types of accidents common to the kitchen area. There are some basic safety rules you should keep in mind when you are in the kitchen.

- Keep a fire extinguisher in the kitchen.
- Do not leave grease on the stove. Clean it up.
- If you have a grease fire, do not put water on it. Use a chemical-type fire extinguisher or baking soda to smother it.

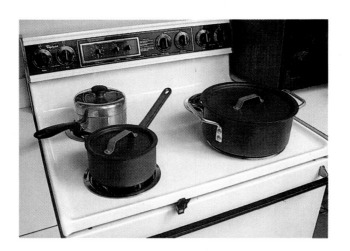

*FIGURE 9.29* Never leave pots of food cooking while you are unable to check on them frequently

- Do not leave cooking pots unattended (Fig. 9.29).
- Have good lighting in the kitchen.
- Be alert when carrying hot liquid.
- Keep paper towels, napkins, and pot holders away from the burner.
- Keep the kitchen floor clean and free of clutter and spills.
- Store knives so that blades are protected.
- Electric cooking does not produce a visible flame, so be sure to check that the dial is at the setting you want or at OFF.
- If you or the client has a pacemaker, stay out of the kitchen when a microwave oven is working.

### Safety in the Bathroom

Many accidents occur in the bathroom. Young and old alike have these accidents. You must be alert to potential hazards that exist due to conditions in the room and your clients' abilities.

- Is the toilet secure to the floor? Is the seat secure to the toilet?
- Can your client get up and down safely? Can he sit without additional support?
- Are the hot and cold water faucets correctly marked?
- Is the tub very deep, and can your client get in and out safely?
- Does your client get weak while bathing?
- Is there ventilation in the bathroom?
- Are the floor tiles slippery when wet? Is there a secure bathmat on the floor?
- If there are grab bars, are they secure in the wall? Towel bars were not designed to support weight. Special bars are necessary!
- If you must use electrical equipment, such as hair dryers or shavers, be sure your hands, body, and feet are dry.

### Proper Storage

Dispose of articles in well-ventilated containers. Do not keep used rags in closed containers. They can catch fire by a process called **spontaneous combustion**. This means they will burn as a result of their own heat. Get rid of the rags before this happens!

Do not store **flammable** liquids near any source of heat. Flammable liquids are those that can burn. Keep them in the garage but away from cars. Use flammable liquids in a well-ventilated area. This reduces the risk of fire and the risk of illness due to the fumes.

**spontaneous combustion** process of catching fire as a result of the heat of the chemicals that are burning

**flammable** substance that will burn quickly

Do not keep piles and piles of newspapers. Make arrangements for them to be given to a recycling plant.

## FIRE AND SAFETY PREVENTION

Fire safety means three things:

1. Preventing fires
2. Doing the right things if fire should occur
3. Protecting your client and yourself (Fig. 9.30)

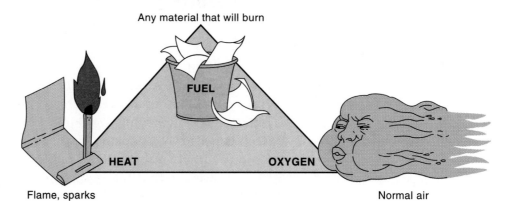

**FIGURE 9.30** By removing one of the needed elements, you can prevent a fire.

Fires start because of:

- Smoking and matches
- Misuse of electricity
- Defects in heating systems
- Spontaneous combustion
- Improper rubbish disposal
- Improper cooking techniques
- Improper ventilation

### Making a Fire Plan

As you meet your client and learn the layout of the home, ask yourself the following questions:

- Where are the exits from this house in case of fire?
- How would I remove the client from this house in case of fire?
- If the client is bedbound, how would I remove him from the fire scene?
- Are there fire extinguishers in this house—one for grease fires and one for other types of fires?
- Are there smoke detectors in this house? Do they work?

### What to Do in Case of Fire

Seal off the fire! If the fire is behind a closed door, do not open it! (Fig. 9.31a) Take another route out of the building to safety. If you must go through a smoke-filled room, put a cloth (a wet one if you can get it) over your mouth and nose and one over your client. Crawl along the floor to safety or keep your client as low to the ground as possible (Fig. 9.31b).

### Actions in Case of Fire

- Get your client out of the house.
- Call the fire department from a neighbor's house. Do not reenter the house for any reason.

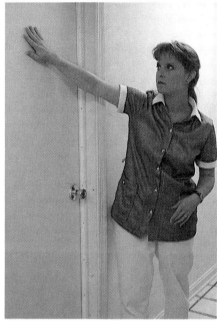
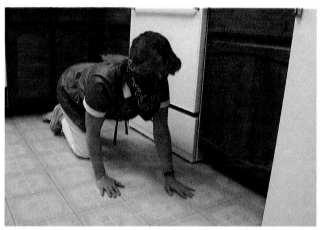

FIGURE 9.31 (a) Feel the door BEFORE you open it. If it is hot, the fire is close. Stay in the room. (b) Heat and smoke rise. Crawling increases your ability to reach safety.

- Keep your client warm and comfortable.
- Stay with your client.

## POISONS

Children frequently swallow things that are not meant to be swallowed. This is considered poisoning. Clients often forget that they took their medication and take additional doses of it. This, too, is considered poisoning. A confused client may take one medication when he really wanted another one. This, also, is considered poisoning.

Prevention is the best treatment for poisoning.

- Keep all poisons and medications locked away from children and confused clients.
- Never keep food products near poisons or cleaning products.
- Make it a habit to read labels each time you pick up any container.
- Call the poison control center for assistance if you have any suspicion a poisonous substance has been swallowed or an overdose of medication taken.
- There are instructions for antidotes on the bottles of many potentially dangerous substances; unfortunately, these antidotes are not always correct. Do not use them. Call the poison control center and follow their instructions.

## OXYGEN SAFETY

Clients may have oxygen prescribed to them for many different reasons. They may be instructed to use the oxygen in different ways, but the safety rules are always the same.

- There is never any smoking in the room where the oxygen tank is kept (Fig. 9.32). This is true if the tank is open or shut.

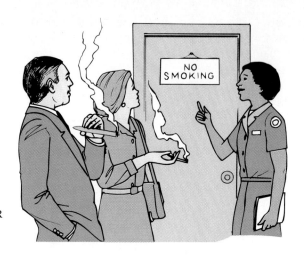

**FIGURE 9.32** There is NEVER any smoking or open flame in the area when oxygen is in use.

- Do not use electrical appliances such as heating pads, hair dryers, or electric shavers near oxygen. Keep the plugs out of the wall while the oxygen is running. If a plug is pulled from the outlet while the oxygen is running, a spark could cause an explosion.
- Remove cigarettes, matches, and ashtrays from the room.
- Do not use candles or open flames in the room.
- Oil, alcohol, and talcum powder should not be used to rub the client while the oxygen is running.
- Avoid combing a client's hair while he is receiving oxygen. A spark of electricity from his hair can set off an explosion.
- Wool blankets, nylon, and some synthetic fabrics can cause **static electricity,** an electric spark sent into the air. Remove these from the client's room. Use cotton items when possible.
- Check the equipment regularly for leaks and proper functioning.
- Ask for careful instructions as to which valves you may touch and which valves should not be moved.
- All oxygen tanks are painted green.

**static electricity** electrical discharges in the air

# Section 4  Making Your Own Equipment

**Objectives: What You Will Learn to Do**

- When it is necessary to improvise some basic pieces of equipment
- How to make a backrest
- How to make a bed table
- How to make a bed cradle
- How to make a foot support

 *Introduction: Making Your Own Equipment*

There are times when you will want to make your client more comfortable or to provide him with items that will help him become more independent. Many of these items cost money and may be an expense the client cannot afford or does not want. Many of these items will not be used for long and therefore the family does not wish to buy them. If the equipment will not be used frequently or for a long period, or the client does not wish to purchase the item, suggest to him that you **improvise** and make some of the needed items. The client may help in this task. The members of the family may help. Their assistance will be important because they will feel they are part of the client's care, and they will know how to construct the item when you are not in the house.

**improvise** to make do with the tools or equipment at hand; to use an item for a task for which it was not originally designed

### BACKREST

Backrests are used in client's beds to prop them up when they eat, take part in their care, visit with people, or read or watch TV. When a client is propped up, it is important to remember that:

- He should be able to support himself in that position and not fall or slip out of bed or into an uncomfortable position.
- He should be able to call for help to change position.
- He should be comfortable in that position, and the position should be permitted by his physician.
- You will be able to secure the backrest so that it does not slip in the bed.

## Procedure 9: Making a Backrest

*FIGURE 9.33*

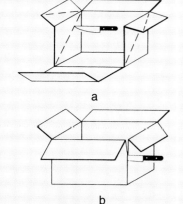
a

b

1. Gather the equipment you will need:
   A clean sturdy cardboard box about 24 inches by 24 inches by 18 inches
   A pair of scissors or sharp knife
   String, tape or cord to secure the ends
2. Position the box on a flat surface with the wide side toward you.
3. Cut the right and left seams from the top to the bottom. The box will now be open and the front will be lying flat (Fig. 9.33a).
4. Make a cut (score) through the inside layer of the cardboard on the side flaps as shown in the figure (Fig. 9.33b).
5. Fold the ends toward the middle of the box along the scoring lines (Fig. 9.33c).
6. Fold the front of the box (the part that has been laying flat) up to cover the triangles.
7. Fold the top down and tie or tape (Fig. 9.33d and e).

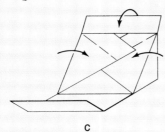
c

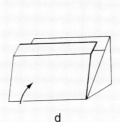
d

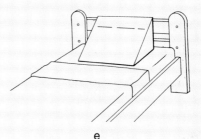
e

## BED TABLES

A bed table can be used by the client during meal time, during personal care, and for recreation activities such as cards or reading. Having a light, easy-to-use bed table available encourages the client to be more independent. A table at the side of the bed, much like the ones in the hospital, can be improvised by standing an adjustable ironing board near the bed, adjusting the height, and locking it in place.

## Procedure 10: Making a Bed Table

1. Gather the equipment you will need:
   A clean sturdy cardboard box about 10 inches by 12 inches by 24 inches
   A sharp knife or pair of scissors
   A pencil
2. Cut off the four top flaps of the box along the seams (Fig. 9.34a).
3. Draw a curved opening on both wide sides of the box. Be sure the opening is large enough to fit over the client's legs. Be sure there is enough cardboard left on the side, at least 2 inches, to support the weight of the items you will put on the tray.
4. Cut out the opening along the lines you have drawn (Fig. 9.34b).
5. Cut small openings in the side near the top for handholds.
6. Cover the table with adhesive-backed plastic or wallpaper to protect it and to make it more attractive (Fig. 9.34c).

FIGURE 9.34

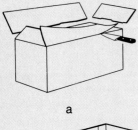

a

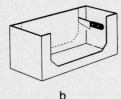

b

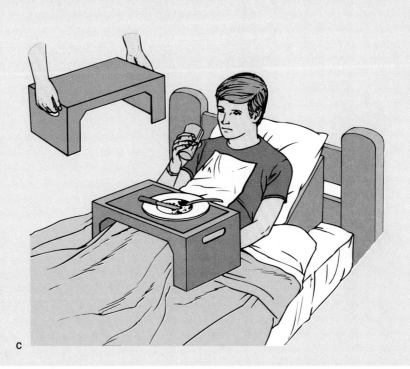

c

**bed cradle** frame placed over a body area to hold bedclothes away from the body part

**foot board** a flat piece of wood or cardboard placed at the end of the bed, under the covers so that the client can rest his feet flatly against it

**foot drop** a contraction of the foot due to a shortening of the muscles in the calf of the leg. The foot falls forward and cannot be held in proper position

## BED CRADLE

A **bed cradle** is used under the blankets and sheets and over the client's legs so that the covers do not touch the skin. This relieves the knees, the legs, and the feet of the pressure of the covers. Use the same procedure to make a bed cradle as you would to make a bed table. Be sure, however, that the box you choose is big enough to provide space for the client to move his legs.

## FOOT BOARD

A **foot board** is used to support the covers so that they do not touch the client's toes, and to provide a place where the client can rest his foot. If the possibility of **foot drop** exists, this is a necessary piece of equipment.

### *Procedure 11: Making a Foot Board*

1. Gather the equipment you will need:
   A piece of wood that is just about as long as the bed is wide and high enough to keep the covers at least 2 inches off the client's feet
   A piece of board that is about the same size, which will slip under the mattress
   Two blocks of wood for added support
   Sandpaper, nails or screws, hammer or screwdriver
2. Sand the edges of the boards so that they are smooth and will not cause splinters or tear the bed covers.
3. Secure the two pieces of wood at right angles to each other (Fig. 9.35a).
4. Position the support on the bed under the bed covers (Fig. 9.35b).
5. Instruct the client and family as to the function of the support.

*FIGURE 9.35*

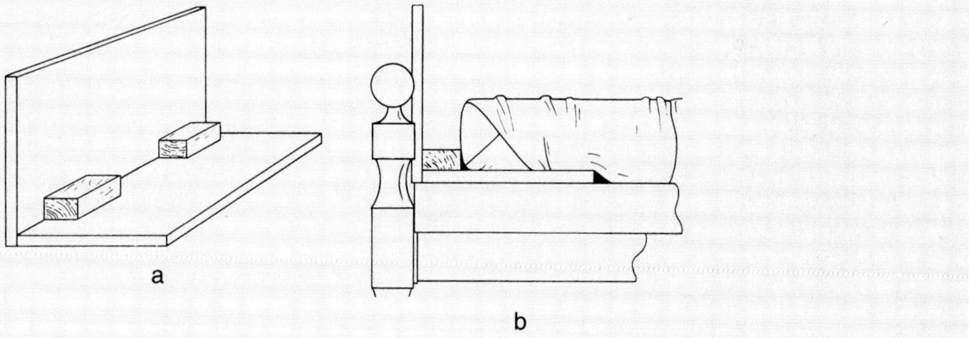


## *Topics for Discussion*

1. Discuss your feelings about doing the housekeeping tasks that may be part of your assignment.
2. What are some of the differences between making a hospital bed and making a regular bed?
3. List common safety hazards in your home. How would you change them? How would you point out safety hazards in your client's home as you notice them?

# Chapter 10

# Planning, Purchasing, and Serving Food

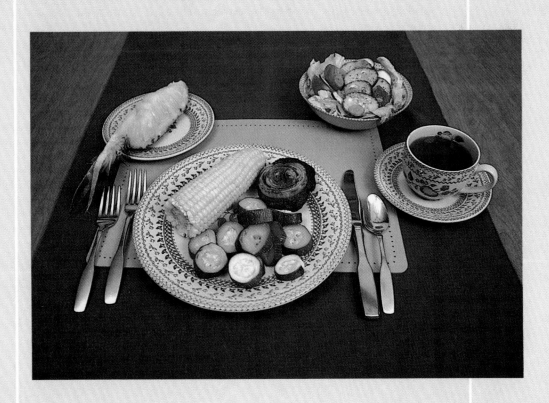

# Section 1  Basic Nutrition

## Objectives: What You Will Learn to Do

- Define a well-balanced diet.
- Discuss the food pyramid and what it means.
- List food sources of each nutrient.

### *Introduction: Basic Nutrition*

**nutrition** that which nourishes; food

Eating properly is important to all people. Good **nutrition** is especially important for a person whose body is in a weakened condition. Food gives us energy to carry out the day's activities and is necessary to rebuild body tissue. Eating is also a social activity. In some homes it is the only time when all family members come together.

**nutrients** food substances that are required by the body to repair, maintain, and grow new cells

**Nutrients** are substances that our bodies need to repair, maintain, and grow new cells. Each nutrient comes from many sources. It does not matter from which sources you get the nutrient as long as you get it in sufficient supply. When a person is unable to get the proper amount of a nutrient from his food, he will take supplements. It is necessary for proper bodily function that a balance be kept among all nutrients—not too much of one or the other.

*FIGURE 10.1*

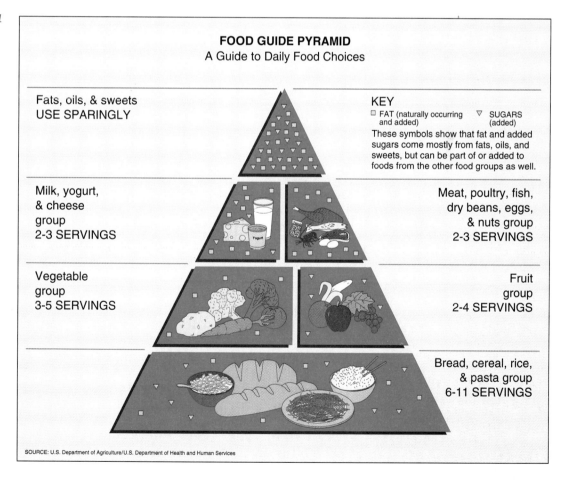

**FOOD GUIDE PYRAMID**
A Guide to Daily Food Choices

Fats, oils, & sweets
USE SPARINGLY

KEY
□ FAT (naturally occurring and added)     ▽ SUGARS (added)
These symbols show that fat and added sugars come mostly from fats, oils, and sweets, but can be part of or added to foods from the other food groups as well.

Milk, yogurt, & cheese group
2-3 SERVINGS

Meat, poultry, fish, dry beans, eggs, & nuts group
2-3 SERVINGS

Vegetable group
3-5 SERVINGS

Fruit group
2-4 SERVINGS

Bread, cereal, rice, & pasta group
6-11 SERVINGS

SOURCE: U.S. Department of Agriculture/U.S. Department of Health and Human Services

| NUTRIENT CLASS | BODILY FUNCTION | FOOD SOURCES |
|---|---|---|
| CARBOHYDRATES | Provides work energy for body activities, and heat energy for maintenance of body temperature. | Cereal grains and their products (bread, breakfast cereals, macaroni products), potatoes, sugar, syrups, fruits, milk, vegetables, nuts. |
| PROTEINS | Build and renew body tissues; regulate body functions and supply energy. Complete proteins: maintain life and provide growth. Incomplete proteins: maintain life but do not provide for growth. | Complete proteins: Derived from animal foods — meat, milk, eggs, fish, cheese, poultry. Incomplete proteins: Derived from vegetable foods — soybeans, dry beans, peas, some nuts and whole-grain products. |
| FATS | Give work energy for body activities and heat energy for maintenance of body temperature. Carrier of vitamins A and D, provide fatty acids necessary for growth and maintenance of body tissues. | Some foods are chiefly fat, such as lard, vegetable fats and oils, and butter. Many other foods contain smaller proportions of fats — nuts, meats, fish, poultry, cream, whole milk. |
| MINERALS Calcium | Builds and renews bones, teeth, and other tissues; regulates the activity of the muscles, heart. nerves; and controls the clotting of blood. | Milk and milk products except butter; most dark green vegetables; canned salmon. |
| PHOSPHORUS | Associated with calcium in some functions needed to build and renew bones and teeth. Influences the oxidation of foods in the body cells; important in nerve tissue. | Widely distributed in foods; especially cheese, oat cereals, whole-wheat products, dry beans and peas, meat, fish, poultry, nuts. |

*FIGURE 10.1 continued*

**protein** one of the nutrients necessary to all animal life

**calories** unit for measuring the energy produced when food is oxidized in the body

**food groups** the division of nutrients into four categories of dairy products, vegetables and fruits, meat and fish, and bread and cereal products

Dietary requirements are different at different stages of life. Children need more **protein** and **calories** than older persons need, but older persons need more of other nutrients.

All foods have been divided into basic **food groups:** milk, yogurt and cheese; vegetables; meat, poultry, fish, eggs, and nuts; breads, cereals, rice and pasta; fruit; oils and fats. The food groups are presented in a pyramid that indicates the recommended daily servings of each group (Fig. 10.1). If you eat the correct number of servings from each food group, you will get the correct amount of each nutrient. Although diet will often be as important to the

| NUTRIENT GLASS | BODILY FUNCTIONS | FOOD SOURCES |
|---|---|---|
| MINERALS (continued)<br>Iron | Builds and renews hemoglobin, the red pigment in blood which carries oxygen from the lungs to the cells. | Eggs, meat, especially liver and kidney; deep–yellow and dark green vegetables; potatoes, dried fruits, whole–grain products; enriched flour, bread, breakfast cereals. |
| Iodine | Enables the thyroid gland to perform its function of controlling the rate at which foods are oxidized in the cells. | Fish (obtained from the sea), some plant–foods grown in soils containing iodine; table salt fortified with iodine (iodized). |
| VITAMINS<br>A | Necessary for normal functioning of the eyes, prevents night blindness. Ensures a healthy condition of the skin, hair, and mucous membranes. Maintains a state of resistance to infections of the eyes, mouth, and respiratory tract. | One form of vitamin A is yellow and one from is colorless. Apricots, cantaloupe, milk, cheese, eggs, meat organs, (especially liver and kidney), fortified margarine, butter fish-liver oils, dark green and deep yellow vegetables. |
| B Complex<br>$B_1$ (Thiamine) | Maintains a healthy condition of the nerves. Fosters a good appetite. Helps the body cells use carbohydrates. | Whole–grain and enriched grain products; meats (especially pork, liver and kidney). Dry beans and peas. |
| $B_2$ (Riboflavin) | Keeps the skin, mouth, and eyes in a healthy condition. Acts with other nutrients to form enzymes and control oxidation in cells. | Milk, cheese, eggs, meat (especially liver and kidney), whole grain and enriched grain products, dark green vegetables. |

**FIGURE 10.1** continued

health of your client as his medication or exercise regime, the client and his family may not understand this. Discuss with your supervisor ways to teach the family the importance of food and the proper diet.

## PERSONAL PREFERENCE

Everybody has foods he likes and those he dislikes or will not eat. Sometimes a client will not eat a food for a cultural reason, a religious reason, or a reason that is unexplainable. You must respect these

| NUTRIENT CLASS | BODILY FUNCTIONS | FOOD SOURCES |
|---|---|---|
| VITAMINS (Continued) Niacin | Influences the oxidation of carbohydrates and proteins in the body cells. | Liver, meat, fish poultry, eggs, peanuts; dark green vegetables, whole–grain and enriched cereal products. |
| $B_{12}$ | Regulates specific processes in digestion. Helps maintain normal functions of muscles, nerves, heart, blood — general body metabolism. | Liver, other organ meats, cheese, eggs, milk, leafy green vegetables. |
| C (Ascorbic Acid) | Acts as a cement between body cells, and helps them work together to carry out their special functions. Maintains a sound condition of bones, teeth, and gums. Not stored in the body. | Fresh, raw citrus fruits and vegetables — oranges, grapefruit, cantaloupe, strawberries, tomatoes, raw onions, cabbage, green and sweet red peppers, dark green vegetables. |
| D | Enables the growing body to use calcium and phosphorus in a normal way to build bones and teeth. | Provided by vitamin D fortification of certain foods, such as milk and margarine. Also fish–liver oils and eggs. Sunshine is also a source of vitamin D. |
| WATER | Regulates body processes. Aids in regulating body temperature. Carries nutrients to body cells and carries waste products away from them. Helps to lubricate joints. Water has no food value, although most water contains mineral elements. More immediately necessary to life than food — second only to oxygen. | Drinking water, and other beverages; all foods except those made up of a single nutrient, as sugar and some fats. Milk, milk drinks, soups, vegetables, fruit juices. Ice cream, watermelon, strawberries, lettuce, tomatoes, cereals, other dry products. |

FIGURE 10.1 *continued*

preferences and plan meals and diets taking these personal wishes into consideration. Discuss these situations with your supervisor so that you will be able to include all the nutrients in the client's meals and still adhere to his wishes.

# Section 2 Planning, Shopping, and Serving a Meal

## Objectives: What You Will Learn to Do

- List the factors a homemaker/home health aide must take into consideration when purchasing food.
- Become aware of ways to conserve energy when cooking.
- List ways of making mealtime pleasant and therapeutic.

## Introduction: Planning

Mealtime is important. It should be a pleasant change in a client's day. The atmosphere and the way the food is served is important in stimulating an appetite. Try to serve a client in a room that is free from unpleasant odors. Keep the room at a comfortable temperature and with a minimum of noise. It is often helpful to let the client decide what foods he wishes to eat. Mealtime is more pleasant when the food served is food that is liked.

### PLANNING A MENU

As the homemaker/home health aide you may find it necessary to purchase food for the client. First, develop a menu of what foods will be prepared. Be sure the menu is planned from the client's diet. Take into consideration the recommended servings from the four food groups and vitamins and minerals. Check the ingredients the client has on hand. Then make a shopping list. A list will help avoid unnecessary trips to the store for forgotten ingredients. It will also prevent duplicate buying of foods already on hand, and if grouped by types of food, avoid extra steps in the market. When planning a meal, remember:

- *Variety.* A well-balanced diet consists of getting nutrients from many different kinds of food. No one food is perfect.
- *Texture.* Combining crispy foods with smooth soft foods makes each texture seem more interesting. Unless the client is on a special diet where the texture of the food is controlled, try to choose different types of texture within each meal served.
- *Flavors.* If all foods in the meal have a strong distinctive taste, they will compete with one another and overwhelm the client's taste buds. Keep the strong-flavored foods as the spotlight and milder-tasting foods as the background in a meal.
- *Temperature.* Cook the food at the correct temperature. Ask the client at what temperature he prefers his food. Not everyone enjoys food very hot or very cold.
- *Taste.* Cook the meal to the taste of the client. Discuss with the family the spices they like and how they usually season their food.
- *Shape.* Prepare the food with familiar shapes. Some families always slice their tomatoes, some cut them into chunks. Ask what is prepared in this house.

■ *Color.* Give each meal eye appeal by keeping the colors compatible. A sprig of parsley, radish roses, olives, or carrot curls may make an interesting dash of color to an otherwise drab-looking meal.

■ *Cost.* Most clients are not free to spend an unlimited amount of money on their food, so plan meals that are within their budgets.

All the food eaten during a day is included in the planning. The food may be eaten at three traditional meals or as snacks throughout the day. Plan meals as close to the client's usual eating habits as possible.

When a client's diet is changed, special care should be taken to try to keep this new diet as close to the diet of the other family members as possible. For example, food for a client on a salt-free diet should be separated from the other family members' food before salt is added, but the food may be the same.

Food habits can also be influenced by the religious beliefs or ethnic background of the client. In some Jewish households, a kosher kitchen may be kept. This means that utensils and equipment used for meat products are kept separately from those used for dairy products. Meat and dairy products may not be eaten at the same meal. The degree to which a client keeps a kosher home should be discussed with the family.

People who have strong bonds with their ethnic background may choose foods that are not familiar to the homemaker/home health aide. Frequently, clients will not keep to a prescribed diet but eat foods that are more familiar to them. Encourage the client to stay on his therapeutic diet, and notify the supervisor. Most of the time your client's therapeutic diet can be adapted to his ethnic preferences. If you are unfamiliar with the dietary habits of your client, discuss this with your supervisor. Then you will learn, and you will be able to help your client within his ethnic tradition.

## Purchasing Food Wisely

When purchasing packaged food, *read the labels.* The listing of ingredients on labels is critical to a person on a special diet. People on a salt-free diet should read the product label and see if salt was used in preparing the food item. Clients whose diet restricts the use of sugar can tell by reading the label if sugar has been used in the product. People who are sensitive to certain types of foods or chemicals will find the label's list of ingredients helpful in planning what to eat.

Labels also provide information on the amount in the container. On some labels the number of servings and the amount of the serving is listed. Often the labels contain the calories per serving of the products. This information might be important to a client whose caloric intake is being monitored. The label may also list the kind of nutrients in the food and the amount of the nutrient (Fig. 10.2).

Products that contain more than one ingredient, such as spaghetti in meat sauce, must list all the ingredients used in making the product. The ingredient that is found in the greatest amount is listed first. In comparing two different brands of spaghetti in meat sauce, it might be easy to see that the can that listed meat first and flour last would have more meat than the can that listed flour first and meat last.

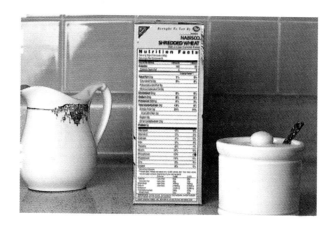

**FIGURE 10.2** Learning to read labels will help you plan meals and budget money.

## SHOPPING FOR YOUR CLIENT

Before you go shopping for your client, be sure your supervisor knows that you are leaving the home. Usually, clients and their families will be encouraged to assume the responsibility of shopping for themselves and of managing their own budget. Sometimes, however, you will be asked to help with shopping for a client within the family's budget.

Before you go shopping:

■ Prepare a list, and discuss it with the client.
■ Discuss the size of the purchase, money available, likes and dislikes, and favorite stores.
■ Be sure your client will be safe while you are out.

After you shop:

■ Save all receipts.
■ Carefully write down how much money you were given, how much you spent, and how much change you brought back.

## UNIT PRICING

Unit pricing is another tool sometimes available to help make wise purchases. **Unit pricing** tells the customer what the cost is by a particular quantity. This can be determined by weight (for example, a box of cereal might read 72 cents per pound) or by pieces (for example, a bag of soap bars might read 25 cents per bar). This information is given in addition to the amount you will be charged for the product at the checkout counter.

The unit price can be displayed in a variety of ways. One way can be a poster that tells all the prices for the food in this section of the store. Another way might be a label on the edge of the shelf where the food is displayed. A third way might be on the price sticker that is put on each item (Fig. 10.3).

Convenience foods (those foods with some of the preparation already done) generally cost more than those made from scratch. But if only one or two people are eating the food, the ingredients for the scratch process might spoil before they are completely used. The decision as to which is most practical must be made individually.

Purchasing larger quantities of an item is generally cheaper than buying small quantities. But if the item is rarely used or if storage is difficult, it may have to be discarded before it is finished. Discuss this with your client before you go to the store so you will not have to make this decision in the supermarket.

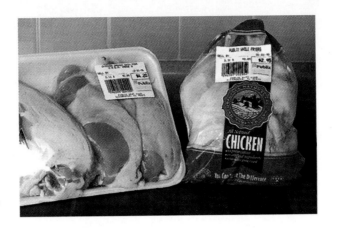

**FIGURE 10.3** Use the unit price to decide which item is the best buy.

### Good Buys

Foods in season are almost always a good buy. Menus should be planned with seasonal foods in mind. The cost will be less and the selection greater.

In selecting foods, the best quality is not always necessary. In choosing tomatoes for a salad, the most attractive and usually the most costly would be desirable. However, in selecting tomatoes for tomato sauce, a less expensive product with perhaps a blemish on the skin might be considered a better buy.

When buying foods high in protein, you can reduce the cost by:

- Using poultry when it is cheaper than meat
- Considering cuts of meat that may cost more per pound but give more servings per person
- Learning to prepare less tender cuts of meat in casseroles or pot roasts
- Serving egg or egg substitutes
- Substituting dried bean and pea dishes for higher-cost meats
- Using fillers such as bread crumbs or pasta to make a meat dish serve more

### STORING FOOD

After shopping for food economically, it is essential to store it properly. Proper storage prevents the loss of nutrients and possible food poisoning.

### General Storage Hints

- Do not buy more food than you can safely store.
- Keep refrigerators operating properly by defrosting when needed.
- Check the expiration date on food before purchasing it. Choose the food with the longest time before expiration.
- Rotate food at home using the most recently purchased food last.
- Dry ingredients such as flour, sugar, cereal, and pasta products should be stored in tightly covered containers.

### Tips for Specific Foods

- *Meats.* Refrigerate all meats. Ground meat and variety meats spoil more quickly than others, so use them soon after purchase.
- *Fruits and vegetables.* Keep most fresh fruits and vegetables in the refrigerator in plastic bags, tightly covered containers, or the crisper.

- *Bread.* If wrapped properly, bread can be frozen to keep it most efficiently for a long time.
- *Milk.* Instant nonfat dry milk can be used in many of the same ways as whole milk and can be stored for much longer periods without refrigeration.
- *Canned foods.* Store in a cool, dry place.
- *Frozen foods.* Keep in freezer at 0°F temperature.

## *Preparing a Meal*

When preparing foods, be aware of the amount of energy you are using. By doing this you will save time, money, and indicate your concern for the client's resources.

- Use the oven to prepare more than one food at a time.
- Do not preheat the oven longer than necessary.
- Put the pot on the correct-size burner. The burner should be as close to the size of the pan as possible. Too big a burner wastes fuel (Fig. 10-4).
- Cover pots when they are cooking.
- Make one-dish meals.
- Make enough food for more than one meal and reheat the remaining servings.
- If you are using an electric range, turn off the heat a few minutes before the food is ready.
- Use the correct appliance for the job. Use small toaster ovens for small jobs and the big oven for big jobs.

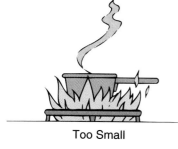

Too Small

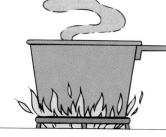

Too Big

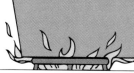

Correct

**FIGURE 10.4** Choosing the correct size pot is an important safety measure.

### Methods of Cooking

*Bake or roast:* to cook with dry heat in a confined space, such as an oven.

*Boil:* to cook in a liquid that is hot enough for bubbles to break on the surface.

*Braise:* a long, slow cooking method that makes use of moist heat in a tightly covered vessel at a temperature just below boiling. The cooking liquid should just barely cover the food to be braised. Braising is a good way to cook tough meats and vegetables as the long cooking breaks down their fibers.

*Broil:* to cook directly under or above a source of heat.

*Fry:* to cook food in fat or oil. When only a small amount of fat is used, the process is called pan frying or sautéing. When larger amounts of fat are used—enough to cover the food—the process is called deep frying or deep fat frying.

*Poach:* a method of cooking used to preserve the delicate texture and prevent the toughening of foods. The food is covered by water or some other liquid. Depending on the type of food being cooked, the liquid may be either at the boil or at the boiling point.

*Steam:* a method of cooking in which the food is exposed to the steam of boiling water. The food must be above the liquid, never in it. The container is kept closed during cooking to let the steam accumulate. Steaming keeps a high proportion of the original flavor and texture of the foods because the nutrients are not dissolved in the cooking liquid as is the case with boiling or poaching. Steaming is a more time-consuming way of cooking, however.

*Stew:* a process of long, slow cooking of food in liquid in a covered pot with seasoning. Good for tougher cuts of meat.

Serve the client in an orderly and friendly fashion. Prepare small portions, especially if the client has a poor appetite. A great deal of food will only cause him to be uncomfortable. Serve the meal as the client wants it. Some people want their soup first; some want their salad first. Accommodate the client unless there is a health reason why you may not. The place people eat is very important. If a client enjoys eating in the living room, serve him there. If he would rather eat in his bedroom and there is no reason not to, serve him there.

An important part of serving a client a meal are the observations made about the client at mealtime:

- How is the client's appetite?
- Does he eat foods on his diet?
- What foods does the client avoid?
- Is there any discomfort associated with eating?
- Does the client drink fluids?
- Does the client eat several big meals, or does he eat all day long?
- Who serves the client when you are not there?

## Serving a Meal

A poor appetite does not mean that the body's need for food is lowered. The sick person's body is in a weakened condition. The client needs as much food as ever—if not more—to return to health. The surroundings and the food served should be as cheerful, attractive, and appetizing as possible. The sight and aroma of food often make a person hungry. You can increase a client's appetite by showing him what he will be eating. Also, people have a better appetite for foods they especially like. Therefore, if a client asks for a particular food (and if he is permitted to have it), serve it to him.

Mealtime often is one of the highlights of the day for a convalescent client or a client who is not extremely sick. Mealtime is a break in the often boring routine. It gives the client something to look forward to.

- Tell the client you will be serving him a meal.
- Most people enjoy company during mealtime. Visitors and family members should be encouraged to remain with the client.
- Before or after the meal offer the client the bedpan or urinal.
- After the meal offer the client oral hygiene.

# Section 3    Therapeutic Diets

**Objectives: What You Will Learn to Do**

- Explain what is meant by *therapeutic diet*.
- Describe various kinds of therapeutic diets.
- Explain the purpose of each type of therapeutic diet.

**therapeutic** an act which helps in the treatment of disease or discomfort

The type of diet will be determined by the doctor. The supervisor or dietitian will help the client plan his diet. The **therapeutic** diet will be planned to incorporate the client's likes and dislikes, his ethnic background, and his budget.

It is your responsibility to follow the diet plan when preparing the client's meals. Assist the client and his family with incorporating the therapeutic diet into the family's usual eating habits. If there are any questions about the diet or its preparation, call your supervisor. If the client is not eating the food on the diet, the supervisor should also be notified.

## Introduction: Chemotherapy and Radiation

**chemotherapy** the regime of taking drugs to treat a malignancy

**radiation therapy** the use of X rays to treat a tumor or a condition

Many people who are receiving **chemotherapy** and **radiation therapy** change their eating habits due to periods of nausea, vomiting, appetite loss, and/or constipation. It is helpful to consult with your supervisor so that the best possible diet can be planned, taking nutrients from the four food groups and the minerals and vitamins.

Here are some helpful hints:

- Decrease intake of red meats; many people prefer fish, chicken, turkey, and other foods high in protein.
- Use plastic utensils, as some people complain of a bitter taste from metal utensils.
- Maintain adequate fluid intake of cool, clear liquids. Set a goal each day and drink before or after meals.
- Eat small, frequent meals; chew food well; eat warm, not hot food.
- Decrease intake of sweets and fried or fatty foods; this will decrease nausea and decrease intake of empty calories.
- Remain in a sitting position for two hours after meals.
- Eat nongas-producing foods.
- Discuss the fiber intake with your supervisor.
- Provide a pleasant, quiet atmosphere.
- Vary the diet.
- If the client has difficulty eating by himself or being neat as he eats, protect his clothes without making him feel like an infant.

**Types of Diets Given to Patients: What They Are and Why They Are Used**

| Type of Diet | Description | Common Purpose | Foods Often Recommended | Foods to Avoid |
|---|---|---|---|---|
| Normal regular | Provides all essentials of good nourishment in normal forms | For clients who do not need special diets | | |
| Soft (mechanical) | Same foods as on a normal diet, but chopped or strained | For clients who have difficulty in chewing or swallowing | | |
| Bland | Foods mild in flavor and easy to digest; omits spicy foods | Avoids irritation of the digestive tract, as with ulcer and colitis clients | Puddings, creamed dishes, milk, eggs, plain potatoes | Fried foods, raw vegetables or fruit, whole-grain products |

| Type of Diet | Description | Common Purpose | Foods Often Recommended | Foods to Avoid |
|---|---|---|---|---|
| Low residue | Foods low in bulk; omits foods difficult to digest | Spares the lower digestive tract, as with clients having rectal diseases | | Whole-grain products, uncooked fruits and vegetables |
| High calorie | Foods high in protein, minerals, and vitamins | For underweight or malnourished clients | Eggnog, ice cream, frequent snacks, peanut butter, milk | |
| Low calorie | Foods low in cream, butter, and fats; cereals; low-fat desserts | For clients who should lose weight | Skim milk, fresh fruit and vegetables, lean meat, fish | Fried foods, sauces, gravies, rich desserts |
| Low fat | Limited amounts of butter, cream, fats, and eggs | For clients who have difficulty digesting fats as in gall bladder, cardiovascular, and liver disturbances | Veal, poultry, fish, skim milk, fresh fruits, and vegetables | Bacon, butter, cheese, fried foods, liver, whole milk, ice cream, chocolate |
| Low cholesterol | Low in eggs, whole milk, cheese, and meats | Helps regulate the amount of cholesterol in the blood | Fruits, vegetables, cereals, grains, nuts, vegetable oil | Brains, organ meats |
| Diabetic | Balance of carbohydrates, protein, and fats, devised according to the needs of individual clients | For diabetic clients: matches food intake with the insulin and nutritional requirements | Fresh fruits and vegetables, low-sugar products | High-sugar foods, alcohol, carbonated beverages |
| High protein | Meals supplemented with high-protein foods, such as meat, fish, cheese, milk, and eggs | Assists in the growth and repair of tissues wasted by disease | Milk, meat, eggs, cheese, fish | |
| Low sodium (salt) | Limited amount of foods containing sodium; no salt allowed at the table | For clients whose circulation would be impaired by fluid retention; with certain heart or kidney conditions | Puffed wheat/rice or shredded wheat, fruits, fruit juices | Canned vegetables, ham, luncheon meats, frankfurters, most cheeses |
| Salt-free | Completely without salt | | Most fresh or frozen vegetables | |

# Section 4   Feeding a Client

## Objectives: What You Will Learn to Do

■ List safety factors important in feeding a client.
■ List emotional factors that are important in feeding a client.
■ Know the proper technique for feeding a client.

## Introduction: Why Clients Must Be Assisted with Eating

Some clients are not able to feed themselves and therefore will have to be fed. The reason might be:

- The client cannot use his hands.
- The doctor wants the client to save his strength and to be on complete bed rest.
- The client may be too weak to feed himself.

Usually, it is hard for an adult to accept the idea of not being able to feed himself. Because a client is unable to feed himself, he may feel resentful and depressed. Be friendly and natural. Talk pleasantly, but not too much. Encourage him to do as much as he can (Fig. 10.5).

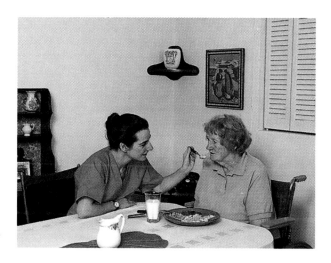

**FIGURE 10.5** Feed a client in a quiet atmosphere. Both you and the client should be comfortable.

### WHEN FEEDING A CLIENT

- Allow clients to feed themselves as much as possible; only give assistance as needed.
- Do not rush the feeding; sit if possible.
- Be gentle with forks and spoons; straws may help in feeding liquids.
- Keep the conversation pleasant and make the meal a highlight of the day.
- Feed the foods separately rather than mixed together.
- When offering a glass or cup, first touch it to the lips.
- Record the intake and output.
- Record your observations about the client when you were feeding him.

### SAFETY FACTORS

Be sure a client is able to swallow before you put food in his mouth. Some clients will be able to swallow one food and not another. Pay special attention to the temperature of food. If a food is hot, tell the client and then offer him a small amount. If the food is cold, do the same. Keep food on a table away from the client's bed so that the client can change position without spilling the food. If a client is blind, name each mouthful before you offer it to him.

## Topics for Discussion

1. What would you do if a client refused to eat the meal you had prepared?
2. Suppose your client is alone. How would you plan for his meals when you are not in the house?

# Chapter 11

# Basic Body Movement and Positions

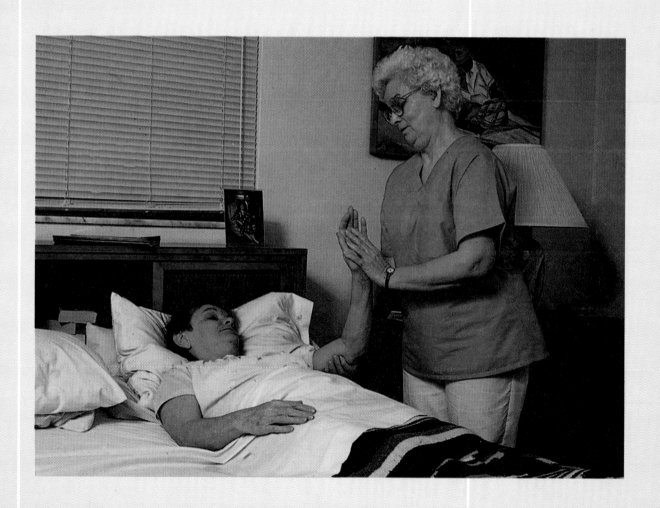

## Objectives: What You Will Learn to Do

- Discuss the basic ideas of good body mechanics.
- Apply good body mechanics during activities on and off the job.
- Explain to someone else (client or caregiver) how to use good body mechanics.

### Introduction: Body Mechanics

**body mechanics** proper use of the human body to do work, to avoid injury and strain

The term **body mechanics** refers to the way of standing and moving one's body so as to prevent injury, avoid fatigue, and make the best use of strength. You should understand the rules of good body mechanics and learn to apply them to your work and everyday life. You will find you will be less tired and will feel better at the end of the day. Once you understand how to control and balance your body, you will understand how to control and balance your client's body. This is a major safety factor for both of you.

Remember, low-back problems are one of the leading causes of employee sick time. It is most important that you learn good body mechanics to protect your back and your job.

### BASE OF SUPPORT

**base of support** part of the body that bears the most weight

The **base of support** determines how stable your balance will be. Try standing with both feet together. How far can you reach forward? Sideways? You probably lost your balance very quickly. Now stand with your feet separated about 6 to 8 inches with one foot a half step ahead of the other. Repeat reaching forward and sideways. You reach farther this time before losing your balance. That is because by separating your feet you made your base of support larger and your balance more stable (Fig. 11.1).

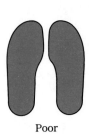
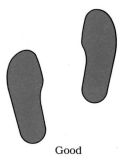

Poor                    Good

FIGURE 11.1 Providing the proper base of support for each activity will allow you to work in a safe manner and be less tired at the end of the day.

### CENTER OF GRAVITY

**center of gravity** point at which, when held, you will have the greatest control over an object

The **center of gravity** of any object is the point at which, when held, you will have the greatest control over the object with the least amount of effort. A person's center of gravity is located around the pelvic area (Fig. 11.2). When moving or assisting a client, support him through his center of gravity. By holding a client close to his cen-

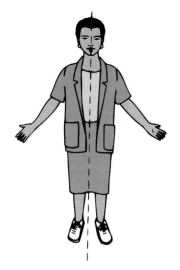

**FIGURE 11.2**  Be aware of your center of gravity and your base of support as you work.

ter of gravity and your center of gravity, you will have the greatest amount of control with the least amount of effort. The client will also feel that you have control and will be more likely to trust you and follow your directions.

### BALANCING

When you must lift heavy objects, spread your feet apart and bend your knees. This will lower your center of gravity, increase stability, and broaden your base of support. For people to balance themselves, their center of gravity must remain within their base of support. Getting up from a sitting position is one example. Some people have difficulty getting up from a sitting position because they are afraid to lean forward far enough, so their center of gravity is not balanced over their base of support. If you help them move their buttocks out over their feet (properly positioned), they will usually balance quite well and learn to lose their fear.

### STRONGEST MUSCLES

Generally, the muscles that flex (bend) the joints are the strongest. In your arms, the greatest power and control is when you are lifting with your palms facing up. In your leg, your hip flexors and your knee flexors are strongest. This is why you bend your hips and knees slightly when using good body mechanics. This puts the muscles in the best position to do heavy work. Your strongest muscles are not in your back, so do not expect your back to do heavy work.

## *Guidelines: Good Body Mechanics*

**align** to put the body into its proper anatomical position

- When an action requires physical effort, try to use as many groups of muscles as possible. For example, use both hands rather than one hand to pick up a heavy piece of equipment.
- Use good posture. Keep your body **aligned** properly. Keep your back straight. Have your knees bent. Keep your weight evenly balanced on both feet.
- Check your feet when you are going to lift something. They should be at least 12 inches apart. This will give you a broad base of support and good balance.
- If you think you may not be able to lift the load, if it seems too large or heavy, get help.
- Lift smoothly to avoid strain. Always count "one, two, three" with the person with whom you are working. Do this with both the client and with other helpers.
- If you have to move or lift a heavy object or person, use a lumbar support. A support can be obtained from your agency, or you may prefer to purchase one of your own so it is always available to you.
- When you want to change the direction of movement:
  a. Pivot (turn) with your feet.
  b. Turn with short steps.
  c. Turn your whole body without twisting your neck and back.
- Get close to the load that is being lifted.

- When you have to move a heavy object, it is better to push it, pull it, or roll it rather than lift and carry it.
- Use your arms to support the object. The muscles of your legs actually do the job of lifting, not the muscles of your back (Fig. 11.3).

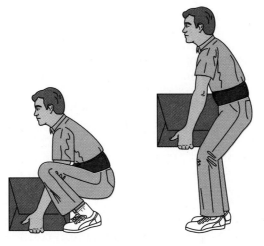

**FIGURE 11.3** Use your longest and strongest muscles, close to your center of gravity and base of support as you lift and move objects.

- The muscles that bend your elbow are stronger than the ones that straighten it out—your greatest lift power is in pulling.
- When you are doing work, such as giving a back rub, making a corner on a bed, or exercising a client, work with the direction of your efforts, not against them.
- When working with a client in a hospital bed (bathing, dressing, exercising, etc.) raise the bed to a comfortable position for you. Also, move the client close to the side of the bed where you are working.
- When working with a client in a bed that does not raise up, if you must stand, put one foot up on the lowered side rail or on a footstool to relieve the pressure on your lower back. Remember, the same rules of a broad base of support, using the strongest muscles for the work and keeping your center of gravity close to your work apply when you are working with a regular bed.
- Avoid twisting your body (or your client's body) as much as you can.

Remember:

- Knowing how your body balances means you will know how your client's body will balance.
- Use proper body mechanics—protect your back, it is the only one you have.
- Proper body mechanics need to be used *whenever* you stand or move. It cannot be *only* on-the-job behavior.
- An injured back is painful, inconvenient, and costly.

# Section 2 Client's Daily Level of Ability

## Objectives: What You Will Learn to Do

- State why you must check your client's level of ability.
- Demonstrate the proper technique to check daily level of ability.

---

**daily ability level** the capability of the client to perform an activity on a given day

**activity tolerance** the most activity the client will be able to do

### *Introduction: Daily Ability Level*

Each client is different. Depending on many factors, such as age, disability, weather, and family pressures, a client may be totally or partially dependent on you, or fully independent. Activities performed one day may not be possible the next. It is your responsibility to check the **daily ability level** of the client before you ask him to perform an activity. Observe the client's **activity tolerance** each day. Note if it decreases or increases.

### CHECKLIST

- Can the client hear and understand you?
- Can the client follow directions?
- How much can the client do alone?
- How does the client look?
- What are his vital signs?
- Will pain be a factor in this activity?
- Are joint motions limited?
- Does the client tire easily?

Your role is to help the client complete the activity, not do it for him. Because you are not in the house all the time, the client and his family must know how to give care when you are not there. They will learn from your supervisor and your example. By setting a good example, you will teach and will assist the client and his family in accepting whatever limitations remain.

### *Guidelines: Assisting Clients*

- Expect the client to do as much as possible.
- Help only when needed.
- Work at the client's level and speed.
- Direct activity instead of asking for it. For example, "It is time to stand, Mrs. N." instead of "Do you want to stand up, Mrs. N?" If Mrs. N says "No!", what do you do then?
- Plan ahead. Gather all equipment, and put it in place before you begin the activity.
- Know your own capabilities.

- Give the client short, simple directions.
- Praise the client for following directions. If he does not do something correctly, stop the activity and redirect him until the correct activity is done. That way the client will get used to doing the activity the correct way only.
- Your body language (your tone of voice, facial expression, the way you touch, etc.) will be received more strongly than the meaning of the words you use. Make sure your nonverbal messages fit the words you use.
- Touch is the most important of the senses. You will be giving contact care to your client. If you are comfortable with this, they will be too.
- Always use smooth, steady motions with clients. Avoid sudden jerking movements.

# Section 3  Positioning a Client in Bed

## Objectives: What You Will Learn to Do

- Be familiar with the words physical therapists use in their work.
- Be familiar with the principles taken into consideration when positioning a client in bed.
- Demonstrate the proper techniques for moving and positioning clients in bed.

### *Introduction: Body Support and Alignment*

Many of your tasks require lifting and moving clients. Some clients will be able to help you. Some will not. A bedridden client must have his position changed at least once every two hours. Proper support and alignment of the client's body are important.

**body alignment** arrangement of the body in a straight line, placing of body parts in correct anatomical position

The client's body should be straight and properly supported; otherwise, his safety and comfort might be affected. The correct positioning of the client's body is referred to as **body alignment** or bed positioning. Arrangement or adjustment of the client's body is made so that all parts of the body are in their proper positions in relation to each other. Proper body alignment can be seen as proper standing posture. When people lie in bed, it is often necessary to use pillows and rolled-up towels to keep this alignment. Some conditions and injuries, as well as special client care treatments, make it difficult or even dangerous for a client to be in a certain position. You will be told as to any special positions that your client requires.

A client who is unable to move needs to have his position changed every two hours to:

- Minimize the possibility of muscle tightness
- Reduce the chance of skin breakdown
- Maintain proper body alignment
- Make the client comfortable
- Avoid delaying rehabilitation

If a client is not properly positioned during the first part of his illness, it can create problems that must be taken care of before rehabilitation can begin. This often prevents or delays exercises and activities that would allow a client to function more fully. For example, if a client who is not properly positioned in bed develops a decubitus, or bedsore, it will have to heal before he can start exercises.

## USING THE CORRECT TERMS

**involved** body part undergoing therapy or part of a disease process

**uninvolved** body part which is not affected by the disease process

Clients who need physical therapy, or any other types of assistance, usually have some type of disability. They may have a weakness on one side or an injury. This side is not the bad side. There is nothing bad about it. Refer to it as the **involved** side. This means it is involved in the treatment. Refer to the other side as the **uninvolved** side. To point out continually to your client the fact that you, too, call his weak side the bad side will only discourage him from using it. If your client understands the concept of right and left, refer to his limbs in those terms. At times you will have to touch the arm or leg you want him to move. You may also have to demonstrate the activity first.

**functional** able to be used

You will hear the words *functional* and *nonfunctional*. **Functional** describes the usefulness of something. It may be an activity or a body part. An activity such as folding clothes, making salad, or combing one's hair is a functional activity, because it produces a desired result. **Nonfunctional** body parts will not perform a useful activity. You can see that words are important and describe the way you feel and the way you see the client and his disability.

**nonfunctional** having no use; not able to be used

## MOVING CLIENTS IN BED

For good positioning, the client must be up at the head of the bed. If your client can stand, even briefly, have him sit over the edge of the bed. Help him to stand and move his buttocks up toward the head of the bed. Repeat the process until he is in a good position to lie back down with his head at the top of the bed. In this way you not only have your client back where you want him, but he will have exercised his muscles, heart, balance system, and coordination system all at the same time. You also have taught him a valuable activity that he can use in the future when he is stronger.

**pull sheet** a sheet or piece of cloth placed under the client and used by the caretaker to facilitate moving the client in the bed

For those clients who cannot move themselves, a **pull sheet** can help you move the client in bed more easily. A regular extra sheet folded over many times and placed under the client can be used as a pull sheet. The cotton draw sheet can also be used as a pull sheet. When moving the client, roll up the pull sheet tightly on each side next to the client's body. Grip the rolled portion underhand to slide the client into the desired position. By using the pull sheet, you avoid friction and irritation to the client's skin that touches the bedding.

## COMMONLY USED POSITIONS

A client can be positioned on the back, stomach, either side, or a position halfway between side lying and stomach lying. It will depend on the client's diagnosis, condition, and comfort which one you choose to use. Also, remember that just because a client cannot move without help when asked does not mean that he will stay for two hours in the correct position. Keep checking your client for proper position.

# GENERAL POSITIONING RULES

▨ A rolled-up washcloth makes an excellent support for the hand.

▨ If an arm or leg is swollen, try to keep the part higher than the heart. Gravity will help the extra fluid drain from the limb.

▨ Any open skin will heal more quickly if pressure is reduced and air is allowed to circulate around it.

▨ Position and support only nonfunctional parts of the body. The rest should be left free to move. This will help the blood to circulate.

▨ Proper positioning can help a client maintain or recover his best possible state of health.

## POSITIONING A CLIENT ON HIS BACK

▨ Place:
a small comfortable pillow under the client's head
a small hand towel folded under the shoulder blade of the weak side
a bath towel folded under the hip on the weak side
a washcloth rolled up in the hand on the weak side
a weak arm and elbow on a pillow higher than the heart
a small pillow under the calf of the weak leg with the heel hanging off the mattress edge (Fig. 11.4).

▨ Loosen the top sheet so pressure is removed from the toes.

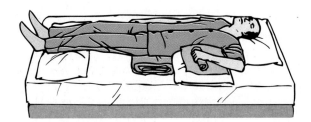

*FIGURE 11.4* Be sure the client is both safe and comfortable as you place the towels and pillows.

## POSITIONING A CLIENT ON HIS UNINVOLVED SIDE

A ▨ Place a small pillow under the head. Keep the head in alignment with the spine.

▨ Roll a large pillow lengthwise, and tuck it in at the client's back to prevent him from rolling and to give him support.

▨ Place:
a pillow in front to keep the arm the same height as the shoulder joint
a medium pillow between the client's knees (the top knee may be slightly bent or both may be bent)
a small pillow between the ankle and feet (Fig. 11.5)

B ▨ Place:
a small pillow under the head
a large pillow under the involved arm to keep it level with the shoulder joint
a large pillow at the stomach area (if the client wishes) for the client to roll onto

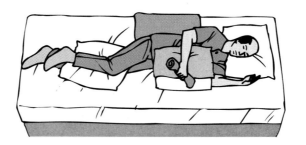

FIGURE 11.5 Remember, the client also has a center of gravity and must be in proper alignment when he is in bed.

## POSITIONING A CLIENT ON HIS INVOLVED SIDE

The same principles of positioning are used as listed, plus:

- The client's comfort will be the key to how and where support should be used.
- Change the client's position more frequently than when he is positioned on the uninvolved side.
- With disability can come a lessened sense of pain and pressure. Check the involved side for signs of pressure and skin irritation.

## Procedure 12: Moving a Client Up in Bed with His Help

1. Wash your hands.
2. Tell the client you are going to help him move up in the bed.
3. Lock the wheels on the bed.
4. Raise the whole bed to a height best for you.
5. Remove the pillow. Put the pillow on a chair or at the foot of the bed.
6. Put the side rail in the up position on the far side of the bed.
7. Put one hand under the client's shoulder. Put your other hand under the client's buttocks.
8. Tell the client to bend his knees and brace his feet firmly on the mattress.
9. Tell the client to put his hands on the mattress to help push.
10. Have your feet 12 inches apart. The foot closest to the head of the bed should be pointed in that direction.
11. Bend your knees. Keep your back straight.
12. Facing the client and turned slightly toward the head of the bed, bend your body from your hips (Fig. 11.6).
13. At the signal "one, two, three," have the client pull with his hands toward the head of the bed and push with his feet against the mattress.
14. At the same time, help him to move toward the head of the bed by sliding him with your hands and arms.
15. Put the pillow back in place. Reposition the client correctly.
16. Make the client comfortable. Lower the bed to his lowest horizontal position.

FIGURE 11.6

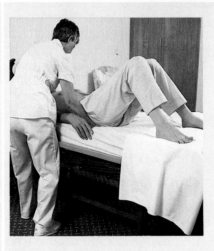

17. Wash your hands.
18. Chart your observations of the client during this procedure.

## Procedure 13: Moving a Client Up in Bed, Two People

1. Ask another person to work with you.
2. Wash your hands.
3. Tell the client you and your partner are going to move him up in bed. Say this even if he appears to be unconscious.
4. Remove the pillow from the bed. Place it on a chair.
5. Lock the wheels on the bed.
6. Raise the whole bed, if possible, to a height good for you.
7. Stand on one side of the bed. The person assisting will stand on the opposite side.
8. Both of you should stand slightly turned toward the head of the bed. Your feet should be about 12 to 14 inches apart. The foot closest to the head of the bed should be pointed in that direction. Bend your knees. Keep your back straight.
9. Use of a draw, pull, or turning sheet is always preferred for moving a client up in bed. This avoids friction between the client's skin and bedding. It will prevent irritation of the skin.
10. You will be sliding the client's body when you move him up in bed. Roll the draw sheet up to the client's body and grab underhand. Shift the weight of your body from your back leg to your front leg up near the head of the bed. By keeping your back and arms "locked" in position when you shift your weight, your legs will help you use your body weight to your advantage and pull the client up.
11. Explain step 10 to both your assistant and the client. Count to three as prearranged. You and your partner will move together to slide the client gently toward the head of the bed (Fig. 11.7).

**FIGURE 11.7** When a family member helps you, review the process with him BEFORE you move the client.

12. Replace the pillow. Position the client correctly. Raise the side rails (if necessary). Replace the bed to the original horizontal position.
13. Wash your hands.
14. Chart any observations you may have made while doing this procedure.

## Procedure 14: Moving a Client Up in Bed, One Person

1. Wash your hands.
2. Tell the client you are going to move him up in bed. Say this even if he appears unconscious.
3. Ask the visitors to leave, if appropriate.
4. Remove the pillow from the bed. Place it on a chair.
5. Lock the wheels on the bed.
6. Raise the whole bed, if possible, to a height that is comfortable for you.
7. Stand at the head of the bed. One foot should be in close to the bed, the other slightly behind.
8. Reach over the top of the draw sheet. Roll the edge and grab it.
9. On a count of three, "lock" your arms and back into one unbendable unit and shift your weight to your back leg. The client will slide easily to the top of the bed with the sheet. Make sure you do this slowly and use good body mechanics (Fig. 11.8).
10. Replace the pillow. Position the client correctly. Raise the side rails. Replace the bed to its original horizontal position.
11. Wash your hands.
12. Chart your observation of the client during the procedure.

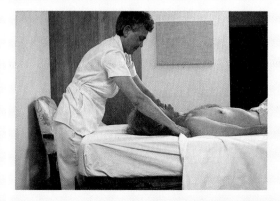

FIGURE 11.8 Use the sheet and good body mechanics to move the client.

## Procedure 15: Moving a Client to One Side of the Bed on His Back

1. Wash your hands.
2. Tell the client you are going to move him to one side of the bed on his back without turning him.
3. Lock the wheels on the bed.
4. Raise the whole bed to the highest position best for you.
5. Lower the backrest and footrest, if this is allowed.
6. Put the side rail in the up position on the far side of the bed.
7. Loosen the top sheets, but do not expose the client.
8. Place your feet in good position—one in close to the bed and one back. Slide both your arms under the client's back to his far shoulder, then slide the client's shoulders toward you by rocking your weight to your back foot (Fig. 11.9).

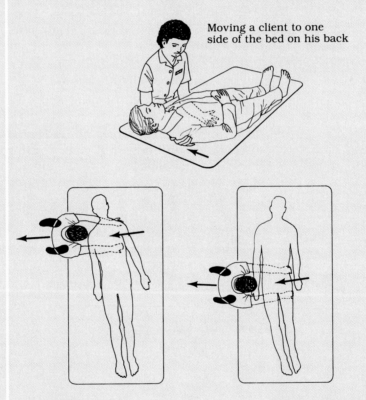

Moving a client to one side of the bed on his back

**FIGURE 11.9** As a safety measure, do this before turning the client so that when he is turned to his side, he'll be in the center of the bed.

9. Keep your knees bent and your back straight as you slide the client.
10. Slide both your arms as far as you can under the client's buttocks, and slide his buttocks toward you the same way. Use a pull (turning) sheet whenever possible for helpless clients.
11. Place both your arms under the client's feet and slide them toward you.
12. Replace and adjust the pillow, if necessary.
13. Remake the top of the bed.

14. Make the client comfortable. Lower the bed to its lowest horizontal position.
15. Wash your hands.
16. Chart your observations of the client during this procedure.

## Procedure 16: Rolling the Client (Log Rolling)

1. Wash your hands.
2. Tell the client you are going to roll him to his side as if he were a log.
3. Lock the wheels on the bed.
4. Raise the whole bed to the best height for you.
5. Raise the side rail on the far side of the bed.
6. Remove the pillow from under the client's head, if allowed.
7. Move the client to your side of the bed as in the previous procedure. While moving a client to one side of the bed on his back:
8. Raise the side rail closest to the client, and go to the other side of the bed and lower that rail.
9. By holding the client at his hip and shoulder, roll the client toward you onto his side. Turn him gently (Fig. 11.10).
10. Place the client in a good bed position, and remake the top covers of the bed.
11. Wash your hands.
12. Chart your observations of the client during this procedure.

FIGURE 11.10

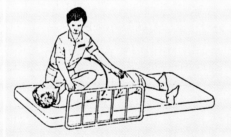

Toward you—better control; client will know if he rolls too far. Your body will stop him from rolling off the bed.

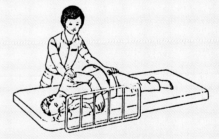

Away from you—be careful the client does not roll into the side rail.

## Procedure 17: Raising the Client's Head and Shoulders

1. Never pull on a client's arm to lift him up. If assistance is required, slide your arm under the shoulder blade to lift. Or raise the head of the bed, if possible.

2. If a client has some strength in one or both arms, "plant" your feet in the proper position, hold your arm out steady, and let the client pull up on you. That way you remain stationary while the client does the work. You then have one hand free to adjust the pillow, and so on (Fig. 11.11).

3. Remember, good body mechanics are important to your success.

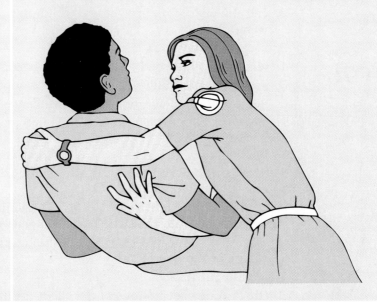

**FIGURE 11.11** Client's hand should be under your armpit and placed on your shoulder or across his waist.

### ▬ Topics for Discussion

1. What would you do if you were unable to move a client by yourself and there was nobody available to help you?

2. Describe the steps you would take before moving a client to prevent injury to you and to the client.

3. Discuss how you think a client feels when he is being moved. Does he feel helpless? Does he feel embarrassed? Does he feel that he deserves being cared for?

# Chapter 12

# Skin Care

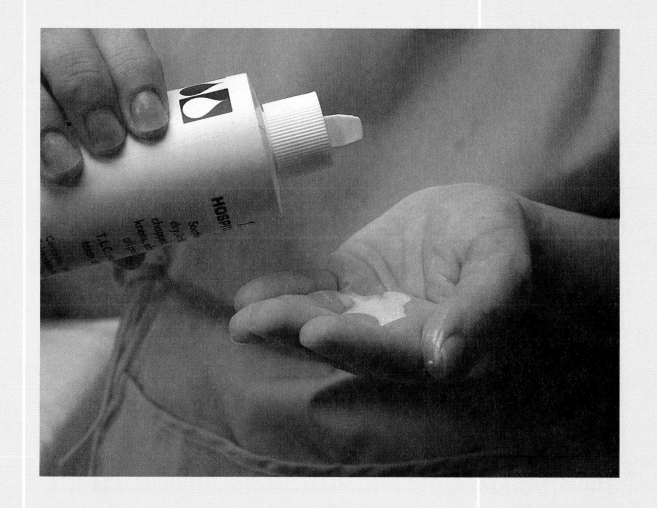

# Section 1  Basic Skin Care

## Objectives: What You Will Learn to Do

- List the basics of good skin care.
- List the conditions that increase the risk of skin breakdown.
- Discuss the effects of aging on the skin.
- Demonstrate special considerations when caring for an elderly client.
- Demonstrate ways of decreasing pressure to body areas.
- Discuss the effects of medication and chemotherapy on the skin.

## Introduction: Providing an Environment for Good Skin Care

Good skin care is one of the prime responsibilities of the homemaker/home health aide. It is much easier to prevent skin deterioration than to heal a decubitus ulcer. The skin must be inspected daily for changes, reddened areas, tender places, sore areas, or areas of breakdown. It is important to recognize the client who is at risk of skin breakdown and protect him from the danger of the formation of decubiti. Besides being very observant of your client's skin condition, you must be able to provide a safe environment for your client. By protecting him, you prevent injury to his skin. Be alert to your activities.

### GENERAL FACTORS AFFECTING SKIN

Many conditions working together affect the health of your client and the condition of his skin. Your client's:

- Disease process
- Exercise and mobility
- Medication
- Health habits
- Nutrition
- Financial resources
- Assistance in his home when you are not with him

When you accept your assignment, discuss with your supervisor how these factors will affect your client's skin and how your care will be affected by them.

### HIGH-RISK FACTORS

**bony prominences** areas of the body where the bones are close to the skin surface and subject to decubiti

**decubitus ulcer** bedsore; open wound which occurs from lack of blood supply to an area usually located on a bony prominence

The primary cause of skin breakdown is pressure on body parts, especially the **bony prominences**. These are places where the bones are close to the skin. Pressure on these areas decreases the circulation leading to **decubitus ulcer** formation. These areas are the shoulder blades, elbows, knees, heels, ankles, and backbone. Because these are the areas covered by thin layers of skin that receive a smaller blood supply than other areas, they are at high risk of bedsores (Fig. 12.1).

Obese clients tend to develop decubiti where body parts rub together, causing friction. Places to check on such clients are the folds of the body where skin touches skin, such as under the breasts, between the folds of the buttocks, and between the thighs.

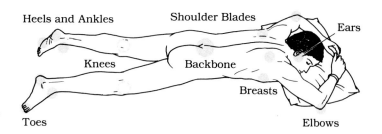

*FIGURE 12.1* Check each day for any irritation.

**shearing** the action of skin being moved in one direction while underlying tissue and/or bone is moved in another direction

**Shearing** is another force that can cause skin breakdown. Shearing occurs when the skin moves one way and the bone and tissue under the skin moves another (Fig. 12.2). When this happens, the skin is pinched, the tiny blood vessels are pinched, and the blood supply to the skin is decreased. This leads to skin damage.

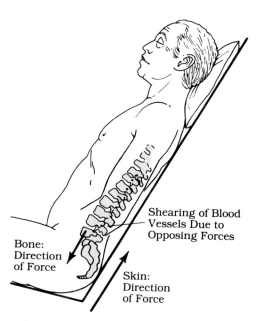

*FIGURE 12.2* Moving and positioning clients correctly eliminates shearing.

## SKIN CARE OF THE ELDERLY

Skin care of the elderly client is an important aspect of your daily care. The elderly are especially susceptible to skin problems. With aging there is a gradual loss of skin tone. This includes loss of the natural oils, leading to dry, itchy, scaly, or rough skin. As the skin loses its underlayer of fat, the skin becomes thin, fragile, and unable to sense temperature accurately. With aging there is also a decrease in circulation to the skin. This condition often slows the healing process.

## WAYS OF DECREASING PRESSURE TO BODY AREAS

You may be instructed to reduce the pressure to the back under the base of the spine or leg using an air cushion (Fig. 12.3). If you use an air cushion, do not fill it more than half full.

You may also use sheepskin. These special pads should be placed against the skin and should be washed and dried frequently. An egg-crate mattress placed on the mattress and under the sheet will also

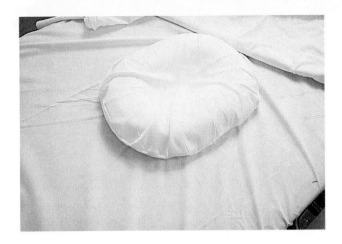

**FIGURE 12.3** Use an air cushion to reduce pressure to the back.

decrease the pressure on the back and permit air to circulate. An air mattress or a water-filled mattress redistributes the weight of a patient and is placed over the regular mattress and under a loosely fitting sheet (Fig. 12.4). Do not use safety pins to anchor the mattress. If your client has a special mattress, be sure to ask how you should care for the equipment.

To reduce the pressure on the heel and elbows, sheepskin booties and elbow pads can be used.

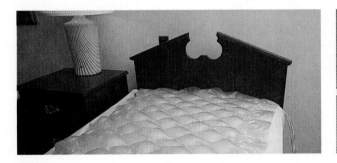

a

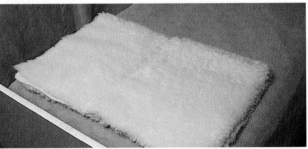

b

**FIGURE 12.4** Special mattresses : (a) water-filled mattress; (b) sheep skin pad; (c) elbow protector; (d) wheelchair cushion; (e) heel protector.

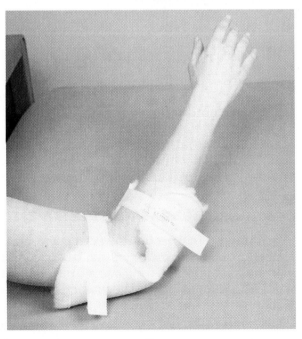

c

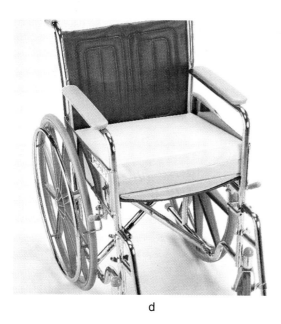

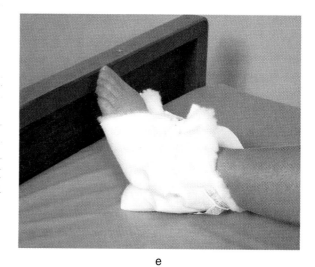

d

e

Bed cradles are used under blankets and sheets and over the client's legs so that the covers do not touch the client's skin (Fig. 12.5).

Another trick is to put cornstarch directly on the sheets. Then the patient will slide in the bed without as much friction.

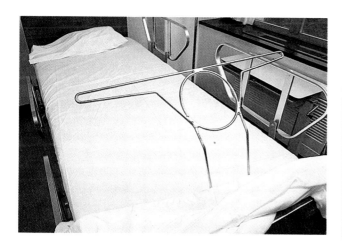

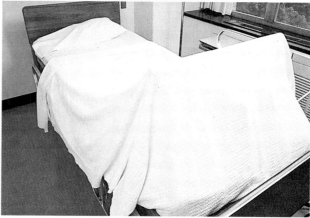

**FIGURE 12.5** Secure the cradle to the bed so that neither the covers nor the cradle touch the client's toes and feet.

## Guidelines: Basic Skin Care

▓ Care for the skin gently. A simple act, such as accidentally scratching the skin, can introduce bacteria and lead to infection. Accidentally stubbing a toe can cause many weeks of discomfort. Protect your client and his skin from all injuries.

▓ Protect your client from exposure to the sun and the elements, such as wind, cold, or rain. If your client insists on sitting in the sun, encourage him to use a protective lotion with a sunscreen in it.

▓ Keep the client's body as clean and dry as possible. Clients need not bathe daily unless they exercise heavily or perspire heavily. It is important to keep their perineum clean and dry, but a complete bath is often unnecessary on a daily basis. Use a mild soap to wash clients, and be sure to dry each body area thoroughly. Do not use perfumes, bubble-bath crystals, or bath salts. They tend to dry the skin and cause the tub to become very slippery. If itchy skin is a problem, discuss with your supervisor what can be added to the bath water or put on the client's skin.

**incontinence** the inability to control one's bowel movements or urination

■ If the client is **incontinent**, keep him clean and dry no matter how often you must wash him and change the bed. If you do not have enough linen in the house, report this to your supervisor. Do not put the client in rubber pants, as they are very irritating to the skin. To protect the bed and to make cleaning the client easier, use a disposable bed protector. This allows the area that is soiled to be cleaned easily and often. These pads protect the linen on which the client lies. Change the bed immediately when it becomes wet, and be sure that the plastic side of the protector never touches the client's skin.

■ There are many new types of disposable products. Some are better than others; some are useful for specific types of clients and some are not. Before you request that your client purchase any product, discuss with your supervisor which product would be most appropriate and fit within the family budget.

■ Use lotion on the skin to prevent contact with any bodily discharges or drainage from a wound. Use powder and cornstarch sparingly, and be sure to wash it all off when you bathe the client.

■ Turn the client often. You should change the client's position at least every two hours. The family should follow this schedule when you are not there. Move the client slowly so as not to cause sheet burns or shearing.

■ Be careful when using bedpans. Pressure from sitting on the rim causes friction when getting on and off the pan, and this can worsen the skin condition. Never leave your client on the bedpan longer than necessary. Use care when removing the bedpan. Avoid spilling urine on the skin, as urine can irritate and cause skin damage. Padding the rim of the bedpan can reduce some pressure. Powdering the rim will also minimize friction.

■ Keep linen wrinkle free and dry at all times.

■ Remove crumbs, hairpins, and any other hard objects from the bed promptly.

■ Do not let clients lie on catheters.

■ If your client's skin is dry and flaky, discuss with your supervisor the best lotion or cream to replace the lost natural oils.

■ Be alert to the effects that medications have on the skin.

■ Do not rub the skin hard. Always rub the skin with lotion and in a circular motion. Rubbing stimulates the circulation of blood to the skin. But hard rubbing can damage skin that is fragile.

■ Keep walkways clear of furniture so the client will not bump his toes or legs.

■ Avoid pressure on any part of the body.

■ Encourage good eating habits and the adequate intake of fluids.

■ Rinse all soap off clients after bathing. Soap has a drying effect on the skin.

# Section 2   Decubitus Ulcers (Bedsores)

## Objectives: What You Will Learn to Do

- Recognize signs of decubiti.
- Demonstrate ways to prevent further skin breakdown after decubiti formation.
- Discuss your role as a homemaker/home health aide once decubiti have formed.

## Introduction: Decubitus Ulcers

**bedsores** decubiti

**pressure sore** decubitus

Decubitus ulcers, **bedsores,** or **pressure sores** are areas where the skin has broken because of pressure. Both external and internal factors affect the skin's breakdown. External factors may be abrasions, scratches, burns, or chemicals. Internal factors may be swelling, abscesses, or allergic reactions. Disease may also cause skin breakdown. An elderly or very ill client may have poor circulation as part of his disease process, which leads easily to decubitus formation. The pressure can also come from the weight of the body lying in one position too long or from splints, casts, or bandages. Even wrinkles in the bed linen can cause a decubitus ulcer. Bedsores are often made worse by continued pressure, heat, moisture, and lack of cleanliness. Irritating substances on the skin, such as perspiration, urine, feces, wound drainage, or even soap, tend to make decubiti worse. If a decubitus ulcer is not treated, it will quickly become larger, very painful, and even infected.

Once a decubitus ulcer has formed, it is the responsibility of the entire health team. Therefore, as the homemaker/home health aide, you have to know how to recognize them when they occur. Report the first sign of decubiti to your supervisor so that steps can be taken to prevent further damage.

### SIGNS OF DECUBITI

The signs of a decubitus are warm areas of skin, redness, tenderness, discomfort, and a feeling of burning. After this, the skin often gets gray in color. This means that the blood supply to the area is greatly decreased. If the condition is allowed to continue, a blister will form, and finally the skin will actually break and a wound will appear (Fig. 12.6). If you notice any one of these signs, alert your supervisor and remove the pressure to the area. By doing this you may well prevent further skin breakdown. When the skin is broken, a decubitus ulcer has formed.

### CARE OF A DECUBITUS ULCER

Specific treatment for a decubitus is prescribed by a doctor. The wound, however, must be kept clean, and the rules of asepsis must be followed. The client must be positioned so that pressure is removed from the decubitus.

If the care of the decubitus is simple nonsterile dressing, you may be assigned to clean the area and cover it. Be sure you understand the

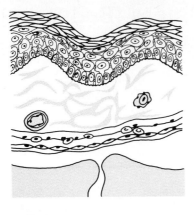

Inflammation or redness of the skin which does not return to normal after 15 minutes of removal of pressure. Edema is present. It involves the epidermis. Skin may or may not be broken.

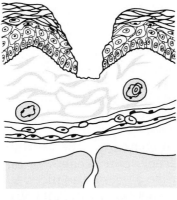

Skin blister or shallow skin ulcer. Involves the epidermis and dermis. Looks like a shallow crater. Area is red, warm and may or may not have drainage.

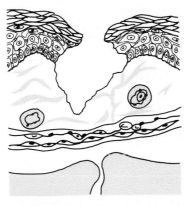

Full thickness skin loss exposing subcutaneous tissue, may extend into next layer. Edema, inflammation and necrosis present. Drainage present which may or may not have an odor.

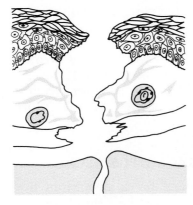

Full thickness ulcer. Muscle and/or bone can be seen. Infection and necrosis is present. Drainage present, which may or may not have an odor.

*FIGURE 12.6*

procedure. Ask your supervisor to advise you of the best place to fasten the tape. Alternate the site so that the tape does not cause skin irritation.

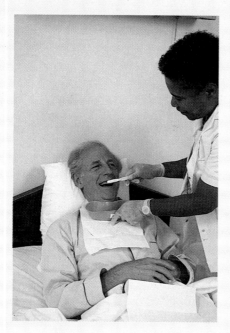

FIGURE 13.1

8. Hold the emesis basin under the client's chin so he can spit out the water (Fig. 13.1).

9. Put toothpaste on the wet toothbrush.

10. Offer the toothbrush to the client if he is able to brush his own teeth. If he is unable, you must do it. Use a gentle motion, starting above the gum line and going down the teeth. Repeat this until you have brushed all the teeth.

11. Offer the client water to rinse his mouth.

12. Offer the client mouthwash if he likes it.

13. Make the client comfortable.

14. Clean and put away the equipment.

15. Wash your hands.

16. Make a notation on the client's chart that you have completed this procedure. Also note anything you observed about the client during this procedure.

## ORAL HYGIENE FOR CLIENTS WHO WEAR DENTURES

**dentures** false teeth

Clients who wear **dentures** (false teeth) also require oral hygiene. Pieces of food must be removed from gums and the tongue. The gums must also be stimulated to ensure good circulation. Gums should be stimulated with a *soft* toothbrush whenever dentures are removed. Dentures need not be cleaned each time they are removed if the client removes them several times a day. They can, however, be soaked in a cleansing solution each time. They should be brushed thoroughly at least once every twelve hours.

Be careful while you are handling dentures. They are expensive and difficult to replace. Always put them in a carefully marked denture cup. Do *not* wrap them up in tissue, put them under a pillow, or leave them on a night table. They could be thrown out by accident.

## Procedure 19: Oral Hygiene for Clients Who Wear Dentures

1. Assemble your equipment:
   Tissues
   Denture cup
   Small basin or emesis basin
   Toothbrush or denture brush
   Denture-soaking solution
   Towel
   Denture toothpaste
   Mouthwash (optional)

2. Wash your hands.

3. Ask visitors to step out of the room if appropriate.

4. Tell the client you wish to clean his dentures.

5. Spread the towel across the client's chest to protect his bedclothes.

6. Ask the client to remove his dentures. Have tissue in the emesis basin ready to receive the dentures. Help the client if he cannot remove them himself.

7. Take the dentures to the sink in the basin. Hold them securely.

8. Line the sink with a paper towel or washcloth so that if the dentures slip out of your hand, they will be cushioned as they fall. Fill the sink with water.

9. Apply toothpaste or denture cleanser to the dentures. With the dentures in the palm of your hand, brush them until they are clean. *Do not use kitchen cleanser or abrasive cleansers* (Fig. 13.2).

FIGURE 13.2

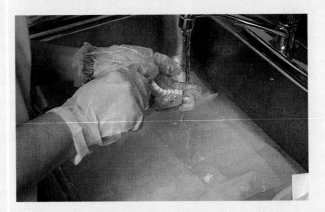

10. Rinse the dentures thoroughly under cool water.

11. Fill the denture cup with denture soaking solution, cool water, or some mouthwash and water. Place the dentures in the cup, and cover it.

12. Help the client rinse his mouth with water and/or mouthwash.

13. Have the client replace the dentures in his mouth if that is what he wants. Be sure the dentures are moist before replacing them. Ask the client if he uses denture adhesive.

14. Leave the labeled denture cup with the clean solution where the client can easily place the dentures if he takes them out between cleanings.

15. Clean your equipment and replace it in the proper place.

16. Wash your hands.

17. Make a notation on the client's chart that you have completed this procedure. Also note anything you have observed about the client during this procedure.
*Note:* It is a safety precaution to label a denture cup so that no one throws the dentures out accidentally.

 ## *Oral Hygiene for the Unconscious Client*

Be very careful not to overlook mouth care of your client if he is unconscious. A responsible homemaker/home health aide always remembers to give frequent and thorough oral hygiene to unconscious clients. By doing this, you will prevent the oral tissues from cracking and bleeding. If you share the care of a client with family members, be sure they observe you giving oral hygiene. This way they will learn, by your example, the necessity of this procedure.

## *Procedure 20: Oral Hygiene for the Unconscious Client*

*Do not put water into the client's mouth.*

1. Assemble your equipment:
   Towel
   Small basin or emesis basin
   Special disposable mouth care kit—if such a kit is not available, you will need a:
   Tongue depressor, padded with several gauze squares. (Be sure they are securely fastened to the tongue depressor.)
   Lubricant, such as glycerine or a solution of glycerine and lemon juice

2. Wash your hands.

3. Ask visitors to step out of the room if appropriate.

4. Tell the client what you are going to do. Even though the client seems to be unconscious, he may still be able to hear you.

5. Stand at the side of the bed, and turn the client's face toward you.

6. Support the client's face on a pillow covered by a towel.

7. Put a small basin on the towel under the client's chin.

8. Place the mouth care equipment near you so you do not have to move.

9. Wipe the client's entire mouth (roof, tongue, and inside the lips and cheeks) with the swab or the tongue depressor dipped in solution. *Do not put your fingers in the client's mouth. He may close his mouth and injure you* (Fig. 13.3).

FIGURE 13.3

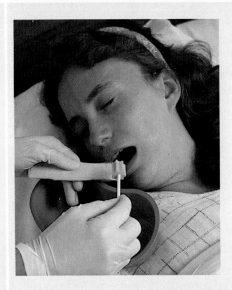

10. Put the used swabs in the basin. The swabs will leave a coating of glycerine solution on the entire mouth and tongue. This will protect and lubricate the oral tissues.
11. Dry the client's face with a towel.
12. Using a clean applicator, put a small amount of lubricant on the client's lips.
13. Make the client safe and comfortable.
14. Clean your equipment, and put it in the proper place.
15. Wash your hands.
16. Make a notation on the client's chart that you have completed this procedure. Note your observations of the client during the procedure.

# Section 2   Assisting a Client to Dress

**Objectives: What You Will Learn to Do**

■ Demonstrate the proper way to assist a client with dressing and undressing.

### Introduction: Assisting a Client to Dress and Undress

Allow a client to choose his own clothes if he wishes to do so. If a client is in his bed most of the day, bedclothes are preferred (be sure they are not wrinkled). If a client spends most of the day out of bed, encourage him to dress in street clothes.

If a client has a method of dressing himself that suits him and is safe, allow him to continue using his personal method. For example, some clients may not zip up their dresses all the way or always leave the top button on a shirt unbuttoned. The following procedure is to be used as a guide. Individualization is always necessary.

Remember not to expose the client unnecessarily as you assist him. In this way you will avoid chilling the client and embarrassing him.

inflexible unbending, rigid

*Remember:* An injured or **inflexible** (rigid) arm or leg is first into the garment and last out.

## Procedure 21: Assisting a Client to Dress and Undress

1. Assemble your equipment:
   Clean clothes
2. Wash your hands.
3. Ask visitors to leave the room if appropriate.
4. If the client is able to sit on the edge of the bed, assist him into this position. Avoid exposing him. If the client must remain in bed, assist him into a flat position on his back.
5. Put on underwear and trousers or pajamas. If a leg is injured, place it into underwear or pajamas first, followed by the other leg.
6. Ask the client to stand up, if possible, and pull the pants to his waist. If the client is in bed, have him lift his buttocks and you pull up his pants.
7. To put on an over-the-head type of shirt (or other garment), place an injured arm into the shirt first. Then put the neck of the shirt over the client's head. Finally, guide the other arm into the shirt.
8. To put on a button-type shirt, place the sleeve over an injured arm first. Bring the shirt to the back of the client and guide the other arm into the sleeve (Fig. 13.4).
9. Assist the client with socks or stockings. Do not use round garters, as they decrease circulation.

*FIGURE 13.4*

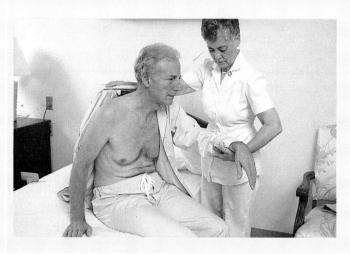

10. Assist the client with shoes. Be sure they fit well and give support. Look for any blisters or red areas on the feet.
11. Make the client comfortable.
12. Wash your hands.
13. Make a notation on the client's chart that you have completed this procedure. Also note anything you have observed about the client during this procedure.

# Section 3  Bathing a Client

**Objectives: What You Will Learn to Do**

- Discuss the reasons for bathing a client.
- Demonstrate a complete bed bath.
- Demonstrate a partial bath.
- Demonstrate the proper technique for assisting a client with a shower or tub bath.

## Introduction: Helping a Client to Bathe

There are several important reasons for bathing a client:

- Bathing takes waste products off the skin.
- Bathing cools and refreshes the client.
- Bathing stimulates the skin and improves circulation.
- Bathing requires movement of the muscles.
- Bathing provides a good opportunity for the homemaker/home health aide to observe the client.
- Bathing provides an opportunity to talk with the client.

Clients at home may not need to have a complete bath each day. They may prefer to have a partial bath at times. Most people are used to bathing themselves privately. Some clients are embarrassed by having another person do this for them. Demonstrate your understanding of the client's feelings by keeping him covered and not exposing him, and by bathing him in a professional and reassuring manner. Clients who tire easily may prefer to have a different part of the body bathed each day. The frequency of your client's bath will depend on climate, need, skin condition, and the client's diagnosis. Discuss your client's preference with your supervisor, and try to meet the client's preference.

There are four types of baths. When you are given your client assignment, your supervisor will indicate which type of bath to give. Do not change the type of bath unless you check with your supervisor and discuss the change.

1. *The complete bath.* This is usually given in bed. If the client is weak or unable to bathe himself, it is your responsibility to bathe him. When you are giving the bath, the client will usually give you little or no assistance.

2. *The partial bath.* A client may be able to take care of some of his own bathing requirements. When this is the case, you will be responsible for bathing only the areas that are hard for him to reach (back, feet, or genitalia).

3. *The tub bath.* This is given in a tub and requires a special order from the doctor. Do not give a client a tub bath until you have checked with your supervisor. Sometimes you will be asked to help the client with a bath into which he puts medication. Be sure that the client or his family can assume the responsibility for the medication.

4. *The shower.* The client is bathed under running water. This, too, requires a special order from the doctor.

## Guidelines: Bathing a Client

- Usually the complete bath is given as part of morning care. However, if your client enjoys his bath at another time of day, try to follow his request.
- Take everything to the bedside *before* you start the bath.
- Always cover the client with a bath blanket before giving the complete bath. If you do not have a bath blanket, a thin blanket, big towel, or terrycloth bathrobe can be used.
- Use good body mechanics. Keep your feet separated, stand firmly, bend your knees, and keep your back straight.
- When you are using soap, keep it in the soap dish, not the basin of water.
- Observe safety rules.
- Use lotions and creams the client usually uses. Do not ask him to buy the one you prefer. Deodorant is used only if the client requests it and then after the entire bath is completed.
- Check the client's bedclothes for personal items before putting them in the laundry.
- Talk to the client as you bathe him.
- Keep the client's body in proper alignment.
- Change the water as often as you need to so that you have warm clean water at all times.
- Continually observe the client for distress. If he appears to be tired or uncomfortable, stop the bath.

## Procedure 22: The Complete Bed Bath

1. Assemble your equipment:
   Soap in a soap dish
   Washcloth
   Several bath towels
   Wash basin
   Powder, deodorant
   Clean gown or pajamas
   Bath blanket

Orange stick for nail care if used by your agency
Lotion for back rub
Comb and hairbrush

2. Wash your hands.
3. Ask visitors to step out of the room if appropriate.
4. Tell the client you are going to give him a complete bed bath.
5. Offer the bedpan or urinal.
6. Assist the client with oral hygiene.
7. Take the bedspread and regular blanket off the bed. Fold them loosely over the back of a chair, leaving the client covered with the top sheet.
8. Place the bath blanket over the top sheet. Ask the client to hold the blanket in place.
9. Remove the top sheet from underneath without uncovering (exposing) the client (Fig 13.5). Fold the sheet loosely over the back of the chair if it is to be used again; if not, put it in the laundry bag.

FIGURE 13.5

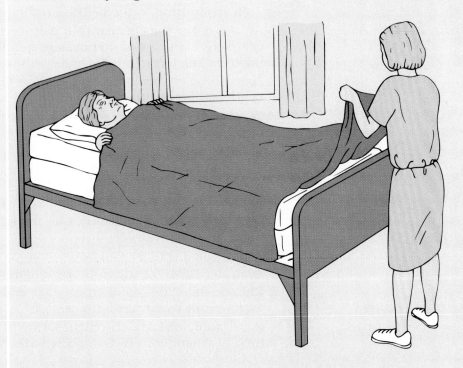

10. Lower the headrest and knee rest of the bed, if permitted. The client should be in a flat position, as flat as is comfortable for him and as is permitted.
11. Raise the bed to its highest horizontal position.
12. Remove the client's nightclothes and jewelry. Keep the client covered with the bath blanket. Place the gown in the laundry bag, and put the jewelry in a safe place.
13. Fill the wash basin two-thirds full of water. Ask your client how he likes the water—hot, warm, cool. Test it with your whole hand. Then let him test it with the inside of his hand.
14. Help the client to move to the side of the bed closest to you. Use good body mechanics.

FIGURE 13.6

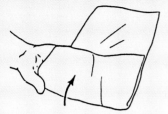

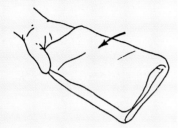

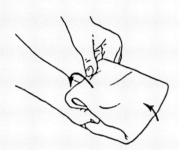

15. Put a towel across the client's chest and make a mitten with the washcloth (Fig. 13.6). Wash the client's eyes from the nose to the outside of the face. Be careful not to get soap in his eyes. Rinse and dry by patting gently with the bath towel.

16. Put a towel lengthwise under the client's arm farthest from you. This will keep the bed from getting wet. Support the arm with the palm of your hand under his elbow. Then wash his shoulder, armpit (axilla), and arm. Use long firm strokes. Rinse and dry the area well.

17. Place the basin of water on the towel. Put the client's hand into the water and let it soak. Be sure and support the arm and the basin. Wash, rinse, and dry the hand well. Place it under the bath blanket.

18. Wash, rinse, and dry the arm, hand, axilla, and shoulder closest to you in the same way.

19. Clean the client's fingernails with an orange stick if used by your agency.

20. Place a towel across the client's chest. Fold the bath blanket down to the client's abdomen. Wash and rinse the client's ears, neck, and chest. Take note of the condition of the skin under the female client's breasts. Dry the area thoroughly.

21. Cover the client's entire chest with the towel. Fold the bath blanket down to the pubic area. Wash the client's abdomen. Be sure to wash the umbilicus (navel) and in any creases of the skin (Fig. 13.7). Dry the client's abdomen. Then pull the bath blanket up over the abdomen and chest and remove the towels.

FIGURE 13.7

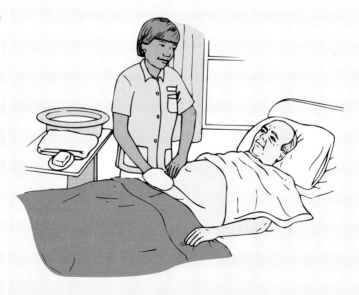

22. Empty the dirty water. Rinse the basin and refill it.

23. Fold the bath blanket back from the client's leg farthest from you.

24. Put a towel lengthwise under that leg and foot.

FIGURE 13.8

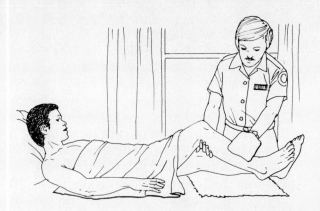

25. Bend the knee and wash, rinse, and dry the leg and foot. Support the leg if the client is unable to do so. Take hold of the heel for more support when flexing the knee (Fig. 13.8).

26. If the client can easily bend his knee, put the wash basin on the towel. Then put the client's foot directly into the basin to wash it. Support his leg and the basin. Protect the ankle area from too much pressure on the basin.

27. Observe the toenails and the skin between the toes for general appearance and condition. Look especially for redness and cracking of the skin. Take away the basin. Dry the client's leg and foot and between the toes. Cover the leg and foot with the bath blanket and remove the towel.

28. Repeat the entire procedure for the leg and foot closest to you. Empty the basin, rinse and refill it with clean water.

29. Ask the client to turn on his side with his back toward you. If he needs help in turning, assist him.

30. Put the towel lengthwise on the bottom sheet near the client's back. Wash, rinse and dry the back of the neck behind the ears, his back, buttocks with long, firm, circular strokes. Give the client a back rub with warm lotion. The client's back should be rubbed for at least a minute and a half. Give special attention to bony areas (for example, shoulder blades, hips, and elbows). Look for red areas. Dry the client's back, remove the towel, and turn him on his back.

31. Offer the client a soapy washcloth to wash his genital area. Give him a clean, wet washcloth to rinse himself well. Give him a dry towel for drying himself. If he is unable to do this for himself, it is your responsibility to wash the client's genital area. Provide for privacy at all times.

32. Put a clean gown or pajamas on the client. *Note:* Usually, the client's hair is combed and the bed is changed; however, this depends on the needs of *your* client.

33. Arrange the bed so that your client is comfortable and safe.

34. Clean your equipment, and put it in its proper place.

35. Wash your hands.

36. Make a notation on the client's chart that you have completed this procedure. Note your observations of the client during this procedure.

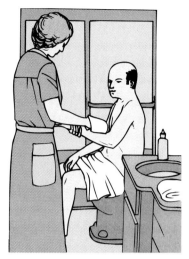

FIGURE 13.9  Assisting a client with a partial bath.

## The Partial Bath

Your clients should be encouraged to take as active a part in their care as their medical condition allows. It may be easier, faster, and more efficient for *you* to bathe your client, but do not let the client know how you feel. Remember, as a homemaker/home health aide, you will have to leave the client after a period of service. It is your responsibility to help him gain his independence so he can function when you are gone. He will gain this independence and self-confidence only if you encourage him to take an active part in his care. A partial bath routine must be individualized to suit the needs of your client. However, there are certain rules to always keep in mind—safety and client ability.

- Assist the client with establishing a bathing routine to save his energy.
- Allow the client to bathe as much of his body as he can safely reach.
- Bring a basin to his bed, or assist the client to the bathroom.
- Take a chair into the bathroom, or have the client sit on the toilet covered by a towel (Fig. 13.9).
- Be very observant of safety while the client is bathing.
- Give the client privacy as he bathes.

## The Tub Bath and Shower

Several of your clients will want a tub bath. Some houses do not have showers. Some clients are used to taking baths rather than showers. Some baths are prescribed for therapeutic reasons. Remember, you must have specific instructions from your supervisor to give a client a tub bath, and you, as the homemaker/home health aide, must be sure that you can carry out this procedure.

## Procedure 23: The Tub Bath

1. Assemble your equipment:
   Bath towels
   Nonskid bathmat on the bathroom floor
   Washcloths
   Soap
   Nonskid bathmat to be used in the tub
   Chair for client to sit on, or use the commode
   Clean gown or pajamas
   Equipment to wash the tub before and after your client's bath
2. Check the tub. Wash it if necessary.
3. Wash your hands.
4. Ask visitors to leave the room if appropriate.
5. Tell the client that you would like to assist him with his tub bath.
6. Assist the client to the bathroom.

7. For safety, remove all electric appliances from the bathroom. Check grab bars. Check to see that there is proper ventilation.

8. Fill the bathtub half full with water. Ask your client how he likes the bath water—warm, hot, or cool. Run cold water through the faucet last so it will be cool if the client should touch it. Test the water for temperature. Have the client test the water.

9. Assist the client in getting undressed and into the bathtub (Fig. 13.10).

FIGURE 13.10

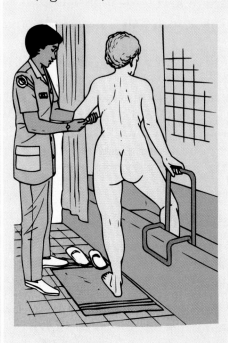

10. Let the client stay in the bathtub as long as permitted, according to your instructions. Give him privacy as is safely permitted.

11. Help the client wash himself as needed.

12. Empty the tub. It is easier to get out of an empty tub than a full one.

13. Put one towel across the chair or the commode. Have the client sit on this.

14. Allow the client to dry as much of his body as he can. Assist him with putting on clean bedclothes or street clothes.

15. Assist the client out of the bathroom to his bed or chair. Make him comfortable.

16. Return to the bathroom. Clean the tub and bathroom as necessary.

17. Remove all used linen, and put it in the proper place.

18. Wash your hands.

19. Make a notation on the client's chart that you have completed this procedure. Also note anything you have observed about the client during this procedure.

## Procedure 24: Assisting a Client with a Shower

1. Assemble your equipment:
   Bath towels
   Nonskid bathmat on the bathroom floor
   Soap
   Shower cap (optional)
   Washcloth
   Nonskid bathmat in the shower
   Clean pajamas or street clothes
   Equipment to clean the shower before and after your client's shower
2. Check the shower. Wash it if necessary.
3. Wash your hands.
4. Ask visitors to leave the room if appropriate.
5. Tell the client that you would like to assist him with his shower.
6. Assist the client to the bathroom.
7. For safety, remove all electrical appliances from the bathroom. Check grab bars. Check ventilation.
8. Turn on the shower and adjust the water temperature. Ask your client how he likes the water—hot, warm, or cool.
9. Assist the client into the shower.
10. Give the client as much privacy as is safely permitted.
11. When the client is finished washing, turn off the water and assist the client out of the shower. Assist the client with washing and drying those body areas he finds difficult to reach.
12. Help the client to dress as needed. Assist the client out of the bathroom to his bed or a chair. Make him comfortable.
13. Return to the bathroom. Clean the shower and bathroom as necessary.
14. Remove all used linen, and put it in the proper place.
15. Wash your hands.
16. Make a notation on the client's chart that you have completed this procedure. Also note anything you have observed about the client during this procedure.

## Section 4 Giving a Back Rub

### Objectives: What You Will Learn to Do

- List the reasons for giving a back rub.
- Demonstrate the correct technique for giving a back rub.

## Introduction: The Back Rub

Rubbing a client's back refreshes him, relaxes his muscles, and stimulates circulation. Because of pressure caused by the bedclothes and lack of movement to stimulate circulation, the skin of a client who spends a great deal of time in bed needs special attention.

Back rubs are usually given as part of morning care after the client's bath. They are also given in the evening before a client goes to sleep and during the day whenever a client changes position or requires this procedure.

Some clients do not enjoy having their back rubbed. Respect their wishes unless this procedure is ordered to increase circulation. Then discuss this problem with your supervisor. Do not take it personally if a client refuses a back rub. He just may not enjoy this.

## Procedure 25: Giving a Client a Back Rub

1. Assemble your equipment:
   Towels
   Lotion of the client's choice
   Basin of warm water (optional)
2. Wash your hands.
3. Ask visitors to leave the room if appropriate.
4. Tell the client you are going to give him a back rub.
5. Raise the bed to its highest horizontal position. Ask the client to turn on his side or abdomen so that you can easily reach his back. Have him positioned as close to the side of the bed where you are working as possible.
6. Keep the side rail up on the far side of the bed, but remove them on the side of the bed where you are working.
7. Warm the lotion by placing it in a basin of warm water. Also warm your hands by running warm water over them.
8. Expose the client's back and buttocks. Do not overexpose him.
9. Pour a small amount of lotion into the palm of your hand.
10. Rub your hands together, using friction to warm the lotion.
11. Apply lotion to the entire back with the palms of your hands. Use firm long strokes from the buttocks to the shoulders and the back of the neck and shoulders.
12. Use proper body mechanics. Keep your knees slightly bent and your back straight.
13. Exert firm pressure as you stroke upward from the buttocks toward the shoulders. Use gentle pressure as you move your hands down the back. Do not lift up your hands as you massage.
14. Use a circular motion on each bony area. This rhythmic rubbing motion should be continued for one to three minutes (Fig. 13.11).
15. Dry the client's back by patting it with a towel.
16. Assist the client in putting on a gown or pajamas.
17. Reposition the client. Make him comfortable.

FIGURE 13.11

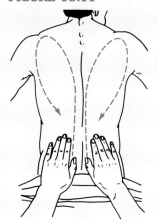 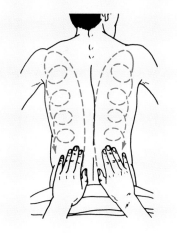 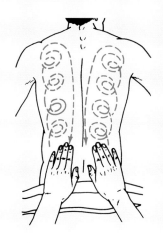

18. Arrange the top sheet of the bed neatly.
19. Arrange the bed so that your client is safe and comfortable.
20. Put your equipment back in its proper place.
21. Wash your hands.
22. Make a notation on the client's chart that you have completed this procedure. Also note anything you have observed about the client during this procedure.

## Section 5 Hair Care

**Objectives: What You Will Learn to Do**

■ Demonstrate the proper technique for a bed shampoo.
■ Demonstrate the proper technique for a sink shampoo.
■ Demonstrate the proper technique for combing a client's hair.

### Introduction: Shampooing a Client's Hair

It is important to keep your client's hair neat and clean. This prevents scalp and hair breakdown, improves the client's appearance, improves circulation to the scalp, and improves the client's general feeling about himself.

There are various methods of washing a client's hair:

■ Bed shampoo
■ Shampoo at the sink
■ Shampoo in the shower (usually done by the client)
■ Dry shampoo

Before you wash a client's hair, there are several things to consider:

■ Has your supervisor given you specific instructions to wash the client's hair?
■ Can the client safely remain in the required position during the procedure?

■ Keep the client free of drafts.

■ Never cut a client's hair.

■ Never color a client's hair.

■ Never give a client a permanent.

■ Never use a hot comb or curling iron on a client's hair.

■ Style the client's hair as *he* or *she* is accustomed to have it.

## Procedure 26: Giving a Shampoo in Bed

1. Assemble your equipment:
   Client's comb and brush
   Client's shampoo
   Conditioner (optional)
   Several containers of warm to hot water, as client prefers
   Chair
   Pitcher
   Large basin or pail to collect dirty water
   Bed protectors
   Several large bath towels
   Wash cloth
   Water trough or 1 1/2 yards of 60-inch-wide plastic to make one
   Cotton balls (optional)
   Bath blanket
   Waterproof pillow (optional)
   Electric blow dryer (optional)
   Curlers (optional)

2. Wash your hands.

3. Ask visitors to leave the room if appropriate.

4. Tell the client that you are going to shampoo his hair in bed.

5. Raise the bed to the highest horizontal position. Lower the headrest and the side rail on the side you are working. Ask the client what water temperature he prefers.

6. Place a chair at the side of the bed near the client's head. The chair should be lower than the mattress.

7. Inspect the client's hair for knots and lice. If the client has knots, carefully comb them out. If the client has lice, stop the procedure and report this to your supervisor. Lice are tiny black insects that live on hair and scalp.

8. Place a towel on the chair. Place the large basin or pail on the towel.

9. (Optional) Remove the pillow from under the client's head. Cover the pillow with a waterproof case. Have the pillow under the small of the client's back so when he lies on it his head is tilted backward.

10. Put the bath blanket on the client. Fanfold the top sheets to the foot of the bed without exposing the client.

11. Ask the client to move across the bed so that his head is close to where you are standing.

12. Place the bed protectors on the mattress under the client's head.

13. Put small amounts of cotton in the client's ears for protection.

14. Place the shampoo trough under the client's head. A trough can be made by rolling up the sides of the plastic sheet. This makes a channel for the water to run into the pail. Three sides must be rolled to make the channel. The top edge should bc rolled around a rolled bath towel. Place the edge with the rolled towel in it under the client's neck and head. Have the open edge hanging into the pail on the chair.

15. Loosen the pajamas so the client is comfortable and no clothing is in the trough.

16. Ask the client to hold the washcloth over his eyes (Fig 13.12).

*FIGURE 13.12*

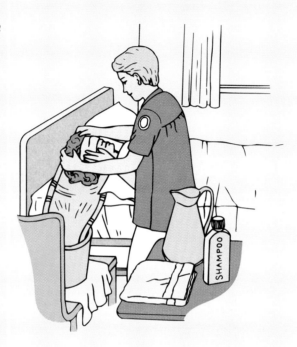

17. Pour some water over the client's hair. Use a pitcher or a cup. Repeat until the hair is completely wet.

18. Apply shampoo and, using both hands, wash the hair and massage the scalp with your fingertips. Avoid using your fingernails, as they could scratch the client's scalp.

19. Rinse the shampoo off by pouring water over the hair. Have the client turn from side to side. Repeat this until the hair is free of soap.

20. If the client uses a conditioner, apply it after reading the directions.

21. Dry the client's forehead and ears.

22. Remove the cotton from the client's ears.

23. Raise the client's head, and wrap it in a bath towel.

24. Rub the client's hair with a towel to dry it as much as possible.

25. Remove the equipment from the bedside. Be sure the client is in a safe, comfortable position before you leave.

26. Comb the client's hair as he is accustomed to having it done. You may leave a towel spread over the pillow under the client's head as his hair dries or you may set the client's hair. If an electric blow dryer is available, use it on cool.

27. Remove the bath blanket, and at the same time, bring up the top sheets to cover the client.

28. Lower the bed to its lowest horizontal position, and raise the siderails.

29. Make the client comfortable.

30. Clean your equipment, and put it in its proper place.

31. Wash your hands.

32. Make a notation on the client's chart that you have completed this procedure. Also note anything that you have observed about the client during this procedure.

## SHAMPOOING A CLIENT'S HAIR AT THE SINK

If a client is able to sit with his head over the sink, this procedure is preferable to a bed shampoo. It is faster and easier.

## Procedure 27: Shampooing a Client's Hair at the Sink

1. Assemble your equipment:
   Client's comb and brush
   Client's shampoo
   Pitcher for water (optional)
   Chair that allows the client to sit comfortably facing the sink
   Several towels
   Washcloth
   Cotton balls (optional)
   Electric blow dryer (optional)
   Curlers (optional)

2. Wash your hands.

3. Ask visitors to leave the room if appropriate.

4. Assist the client to the sink. Be sure a chair is available for him to sit on if he gets tired.

5. Place a towel around the client's shoulders.

6. Inspect a client's hair for knots and lice. If the client has knots, carefully comb them out. If the client has lice, stop the procedure and report this to your supervisor.

7. Put a small amount of cotton in the client's ears for protection.

8. Give the client a washcloth to cover his eyes.

9. Ask the client what temperature he prefers the water. Adjust it.

10. Ask the client to lean forward so that his head is over the sink.

11. Wet his head thoroughly.

12. Apply shampoo, and using both hands, wash the hair and massage the scalp with your fingertips. Avoid using your fingernails as they may scratch the client's scalp.

13. Rinse the shampoo off by pouring water over the hair.

14. Dry the client's forehead and ears. Have him assume a comfortable position. Raise the client's head, and wrap it in a towel.

15. Remove the cotton from the client's ears.

16. Rub the client's hair with a towel to dry it as much as possible.

17. Comb the client's hair as he is accustomed to having it done. You may leave a towel around the client's shoulders while his hair is drying. Leave a towel under the client's head if he prefers to lie down as his hair dries. You may also set the hair and use the electric blow dryer set on cool.

18. Make sure that the client is comfortable and safe following this procedure.

19. Clean your equipment and the area you used.

20. Wash your hands.

21. Make a notation on the client's chart that you have completed this procedure. Also note anything you have observed about the client during this procedure.

### COMBING A CLIENT'S HAIR

As with other types of personal care, a client may be unable to take care of his own hair. When this is the case, it is your responsibility to comb and brush his hair. This almost always makes him look better and feel better.

*Procedure 28: Combing a Client's Hair*

1. Assemble your equipment on the bedside table:
   Towel
   Paper bag
   Comb or brush
   Any hair preparation the client usually uses
   Hand mirror, if available

2. Wash your hands.

3. Ask visitors to leave the room if appropriate.

4. Tell the client you are going to brush or comb his hair.

5. If possible, comb the client's hair after the bath and before you make the bed. Some clients prefer to have their hair combed while sitting in a chair (Fig 13.13).

FIGURE 13.13

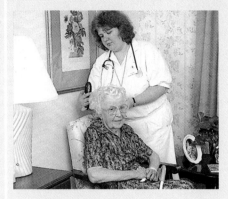

6. Lay a towel across the pillow, under the client's head. If the client can sit up in bed, drape the towel around his shoulders.

7. If the client wears glasses, ask him to take them off before you begin, unless this makes the client uncomfortable. Be sure to put the glasses in a safe place.

8. Part the hair down the middle to make it easier to comb.

9. Brush or comb the client's hair carefully, gently, and thoroughly in his usual style.

10. For the client who cannot sit up, separate the hair into small sections. Then comb each section separately, using a downward motion, starting at the loose end and working up toward the head. Ask the client to turn his head from side to side. Or turn it for him so that you can reach the entire head.

11. Arrange the client's hair the way he wants it.

12. If the client has long hair, suggest braiding it to keep it from getting tangled.

13. Be sure you brush the back of the head.

14. Remove the towel when you are finished.

15. Let the client use the mirror.

16. Make the client comfortable.

17. Wash your hands.

18. Make a notation on the client's chart that you have completed this procedure. Also note anything you have observed about the client during this procedure.

# Section 6  Shaving a Client

## Objectives: What You Will Learn to Do

■ Demonstrate the proper technique for shaving a client's beard.

## Introduction: Shaving a Client's Beard

A regular morning activity for most men is shaving the beard. A client is often well enough to shave himself. In this case, you will give him the help that is necessary, such as being sure he has the equipment he needs. Sometimes, however, clients are unable to shave themselves. In such cases, you will do it. Before shaving any client's face, be sure you have been instructed to do so by your supervisor. Certain clients may not be permitted to shave or be shaved.

**safety razor** razor provided with a guard to prevent cutting the skin

Shaving can be done only with an electric razor or a **safety razor.** Electric razors should never be used if the client is receiving oxygen.

## Procedure 29: Shaving a Client's Beard

1. Assemble your equipment at the bedside:
   Basin of water, very warm to hot
   Shaving cream
   Safety razor
   Face towel
   Mirror
   Tissues
   Aftershave lotion (optional)
   Face powder (optional)
   Washcloth
2. Wash your hands.
3. Ask visitors to leave the room if appropriate.
4. Tell the client that you are going to shave his beard.
5. Adjust a light so that it shines on the client's face but not in his eyes.
6. Raise the head of the bed if allowed.
7. Spread the face towel under the client's chin. If the client has dentures, be sure they are in his mouth.
8. Put some warm water on the client's face, or use a damp warm washcloth to soften his beard.
9. Apply shaving cream generously to the face.
10. With the fingers of one hand, hold the skin taut (tight) as you shave in the direction that the hair grows. Start under the sideburns and work downward over the cheeks. Continue carefully over the chin. Work upward on the neck under the chin. Use short firm strokes.
11. Rinse the razor often in the basin of water.
12. Areas under the nose and around the lips are sensitive. Take special care in these areas.
13. If you nick the client's skin, report this to your supervisor.
14. Wash off the remaining shaving cream when you have finished.
15. Apply aftershave lotion or powder as the client prefers.
16. Make the client comfortable.

17. Clean your equipment, and put it in its proper place.
18. Wash your hands.
19. Make a notation on the client's chart that you have completed this procedure. Also note anything you have observed about the client during this procedure.

# Section 7  Assisting a Client with Toileting

## Objectives: What You Will Learn to Do

■ Demonstrate the proper technique for assisting a client with a bedpan.
■ Demonstrate the proper technique for assisting a client with a urinal.
■ Demonstrate the proper technique for assisting a client with a bedside commode.

 *Introduction: Assisting a Client with Toileting*

Toileting is usually an activity that is private, and one that is not openly discussed. The clients you care for will now have to perform this activity with varying amounts of assistance. They may be embarrassed. You may be embarrassed. Your role is to assist the client with this important and normal bodily function in a way that is both acceptable to him and safe to you both. There are often special words associated with elimination. Knowing these words may make the communication between you and your client easier. Try to keep to the schedule and way the client usually toilets, as this will help when you are not there.

Elimination of body waste is important if the body is to maintain its health and function. You will be asked to report on the elimination of your client. Often this information will provide an indication of your client's health status. Report the following:

■ Frequency of elimination
■ Color
■ Odor
■ Any pain with elimination
■ Ability to control elimination
■ Any foreign material, such as blood or mucus

**urinal** container into which male clients can urinate; women use female urinals

**bedpan** container into which a person defecates or urinates while in bed

**defecate** to have a bowel movement

Some clients are unable to get out of bed to use the bathroom. For these clients a urinal and a bedpan are required (Fig. 13.14). The **urinal** is a container into which the male client urinates. The **bedpan** is a pan into which he **defecates** (moves his bowels). The female client uses the bedpan for urination and defecation. There are times, however, when a female urinal must be used. You should always cover the bedpan and remove it from the client's bedside to the bathroom as quickly as possible after use. At this time you would collect a specimen if required. You would also measure the urine if necessary.

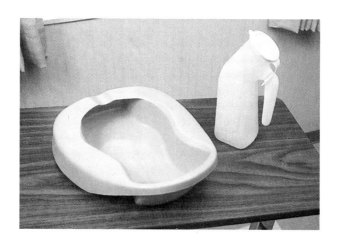

**FIGURE 13.14** A bedpan and male urinal.

**commode** a portable frame, with pan or pail, into which client's urinate or defecate

Some clients are able to get out of bed but unable to walk to the bathroom. For these clients, your supervisor will arrange to have a portable **commode** brought to the house. Whenever the client uses it you will be responsible for cleaning it just as if he had used the bedpan or urinal.

When a client is told he may go to the bathroom, you will be responsible for assisting him to the bathroom, observing all the rules of safety that you have been taught. Do not take a client to the bathroom unless your supervisor says that you may do so.

# Procedure 30: Offering the Bedpan

1. Assemble your equipment:
   Bedpan and cover, or fracture bedpan and cover
   Toilet tissue
   Wash basin with water or wet washcloth
   Soap
   Talcum powder or cornstarch
   Hand towel
2. Wash your hands.
3. Ask visitors to leave the room if appropriate. You may, however, wish to demonstrate this procedure to the family members.
4. Ask the client if he would like to use the bedpan.
5. Warm the bedpan by running warm water inside it and along the rim. Dry the outside of the bedpan with paper towels and put talcum powder or cornstarch on the part that will touch the client. If the client is going to move his bowels and a specimen is not needed, place several sheets of toilet tissue or a slight bit of water in the bedpan. This will make cleaning it easier.
6. Raise the bed to the highest horizontal position.
7. Lower the side rail on the side where you are standing.
8. Fold back the top sheets so that they are out of the way.
9. Raise the client's gown, but keep the lower part of his body covered with the top sheets.

FIGURE 13.15

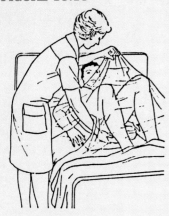

10. Ask the client to bend his knees and put his feet flat on the mattress. Then ask the client to raise his hips. If necessary, help the client to raise his buttocks by slipping your hand under the lower part of his back. Place the bedpan in position with the seat of the bedpan under the buttocks (Fig. 13.15).
11. Sometimes the client is unable to lift his buttocks to get on or off the bedpan. In this case, turn the client on his side with his back to you. Put the bedpan against the buttocks. Then turn the client back onto the bedpan (Fig. 13.16).

FIGURE 13.16

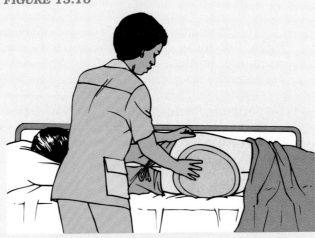

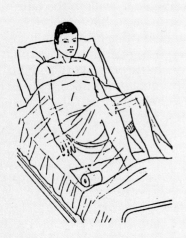

12. Replace the covers over the client.
13. Raise the backrest and knee rest, if allowed, so the client is in a sitting position.
14. Put toilet tissue where the client can reach it easily.
15. Ask the client to signal when he is finished.
16. Raise the side rails to the up position.
17. Leave the room to give the client privacy. Wash your hands if you are going to do another task.
18. When the client signals, return to the room.
19. Wash your hands.
20. Help the client to raise his hips so you can remove the bedpan.
21. Help the client if he is unable to clean himself. Turn the client on his side. Clean the anal area with toilet tissue.
22. Raise the side rails. Cover the bedpan immediately. You can use a disposable pad or a paper towel if no cover is available (Fig. 13.17).
23. Take the bedpan to the client's bathroom.
24. Return to the client. Offer the client the opportunity to wash his hands in the basin of water.
25. Make the client comfortable.
26. Note the excreta (feces or urine) for amount, odor, color.

FIGURE 13.17

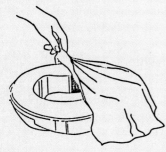

27. If a specimen or sample is required, collect it at this time. Measure the urine if necessary.

28. Empty the bedpan into the client's toilet.

29. Clean the bedpan, and put it in the proper place. Cold water is always used to clean the bedpan. You may also use a toilet brush, if available.

30. Wash your hands.

31. Make a notation on the client's chart that the client has used the bedpan. Also note anything you have observed about the client during this procedure.

## Procedure 31: Offering the Urinal

FIGURE 13.18

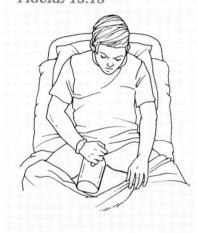

1. Assemble your equipment:
   Urinal and cover
   Basin of water or wet wash cloth
   Soap
   Towels
   Disposable gloves (optional)

2. Wash your hands.

3. Ask visitors to leave the room if appropriate. You may, however, wish to demonstrate this procedure to family members.

4. Ask the client if he wishes to use the urinal.

5. Give the client the urinal. If the client is unable to put the urinal in place, put his penis into the opening as far as it goes. If the client is unable to hold it in place, you will have to do so. Raise the head of the bed if the client prefers (Fig. 13.18).

6. Ask the client to signal when he is finished.

7. Leave the room to give the client privacy. Wash your hands.

8. When the client signals return to the room.

9. Take the urinal. Be careful not to spill it. Cover it, and take it to the client's bathroom.

10. Return to the client. Help him wash his hands in the basin of water or wet wash cloth.

11. Make the client comfortable.

12. Check the urine for color, odor, and amount.

13. Measure the urine if that is necessary. Collect a specimen or sample at this time if necessary.

14. Empty the urinal into the toilet. Rinse the urinal with cold water.

15. Clean it as is your agency policy, and return it to the proper place.

16. Wash your hands.

17. Make a notation on the client's chart that he has used the urinal. Also note anything you have observed about the client during this procedure.

## Procedure 32: Assisting the Client with a Portable Commode

FIGURE 13.19

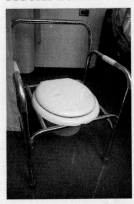

1. Assemble your equipment:
   Portable bedside commode
   Toilet tissue
   Basin of water or wet washcloth
   Soap
   Towel

2. Wash your hands.

3. Ask visitors to leave the room if appropriate. However, you may want to demonstrate the procedure to family members.

4. Tell the client you are going to assist him onto the commode.

5. Put the commode next to the client's bed in a safe position for him to transfer to (Fig 13.19).

6. Using proper body mechanics and transfer techniques, assist the client onto the commode.

7. If you do not have to collect a specimen, leave a small amount of water in the bottom of the pail. This will make cleaning it easier.

8. If the client is safe, leave the room to give him privacy.

9. Wash your hands if you are going to do another task.

10. When the client signals you that he is finished, wash your hands and return.

11. Offer the client toilet tissue to clean himself. If he is unable to do so, it is your responsibility to clean him.

12. Assist the client back to his bed.

13. Offer the client a basin of water or the wet washcloth to wash his hands.

14. Make the client comfortable.

15. Remove the pail from the commode. Cover it and carry it to the bathroom.

16. Check the excreta (feces or urine) for color, amount, and odor.

17. Measure output if that is ordered. If a specimen or sample is required, collect it at this time.

18. Empty the pail into the toilet, and clean it according to your agency policy.

19. Put the pail back into the commode.

20. Wash your hands.

21. Make a notation on the client's chart that he has used the commode. Also note anything that you observed about the client during this procedure

# Section 8  Perineal Care

## Objectives: What You Will Learn to Do

- List the reasons you will be asked to give peri-care to a client.
- Demonstrate the correct procedure for giving peri-care.

### Introduction: Care of the Perineal Area

**Perineal care** cleansing of the perineal area

**Perineum** area between the anus and the external genital organs

**Perineal care** or peri-care is the gentle cleansing of the perineal area or **perineum**. This may be necessary following the birth of a child, following surgery, or when a female client does not take a full bath but wishes to clean the genital area. This procedure is done to promote healing, prevent infection, and refresh the client. The use of a squeeze bottle—or peribottle—is encouraged rather than cleansing the area with a washcloth. The bottle directs a stream of water so that it removes waste or drainage without damaging the skin. The use of the bottle also enables clients to clean themselves even if they cannot reach the area with their hands.

## Procedure 33: Care of the Perineal Area

1. Assemble your equipment:
   2 peribottles or squeeze bottles
   Mild soap
   Clean dressings or peripads and undergarments
   Towels
   Garbage bag for soiled dressings
   Warm water
2. Wash your hands.
3. Ask visitors to leave the room if appropriate.
4. Tell the client what you are going to do and what you expect.
5. Remove old peripads or dressings, and discard in a paper or plastic bag. Note the drainage, color, amount, and odor.
6. Assist client onto commode, toilet, or bedpan.
7. Fill one bottle with warm soapy water and the other with warm clean water.
8. Place the bottle filled with soapy water parallel to the perineum. Let the water drain over the perineum. Move the bottle so that the whole perineal area is cleansed. Do this for at least two minutes. You may have to refill the bottle.
9. Rinse the perineum with plain warm water.
10. Assist the client to stand up or to get off the bedpan.

11. Pat the area dry.
12. Assist the client with clean dressings and undergarments. Make the client comfortable.
13. Clean the equipment and commode.
14. Wash your hands.
15. Make a notation on the client's chart that you have completed this procedure. Also note anything you observed about the client during this procedure.

# Section 9  Postpartum Care

## Objectives: What You Will Learn to Do

- Recognize the first physical changes that occur after childbirth.
- Discuss some of the emotional changes experienced by women after childbirth.
- List the changes that would require medical attention.
- Discuss some of the changes families experience after the birth of a child.

### Introduction: The Postpartum Period

The first several weeks after childbirth are considered the postpartum period. This is the time when a woman is getting used to being a mother for the first time or getting used to this baby. She is bonding with the child and getting acquainted with it. Her body is changing rapidly. Women also experience emotional changes as their role changes, as their hormones change, and as their bodies return to their prepregnancy state.

Families react to the addition of a new child in many ways. Families have cultural practices that dictate how they react to the new mother. Some families react differently when the child is a girl or when the child is a boy. Some families lavish gifts and attention on the child. Some lavish gifts and attention on the mother. Some do neither.

### Changes for Family Members

There are changes for all members of the family. Husbands or significant others either become fathers for the first time or learn to balance emotions for one more child. Sometimes the new responsibility is assumed with ease. Sometimes the man becomes frightened and does not know how to respond. It takes time to learn the role of father. Be patient. Refer to role models the man may have seen as he grew up. He will be able to identify those behaviors he liked as a child and those he did not. By thinking about those things, he will better be able to pattern his behavior to support his child.

Learning to relate to a woman who has become a mother also takes time. Encourage the new mother and father to talk about their needs and feelings with each other. If they need professional assistance, contact your superior for a referral.

Children learn to adjust to a new sibling. The presence of a new brother or sister can affect each child differently. Respect each child's way of adjusting to the new family member. If you have any questions about the meaning of behaviors, discuss it with your supervisor. Remember, children are all individuals. Do not compare one child with another.

- Some children assume extra responsibility.
- Some children return to very childish behaviors, such as talking baby talk, sucking their thumbs, or even wetting their beds.
- Some children may refuse to go to school, leave their house, or leave their parents.
- Some children ignore the new baby.
- Some children are anxious to take part in the care of the new baby.

## Emotional Changes for the New Mother

It is difficult to predict how a woman will react to a new baby. Each woman is different, and each birth experience is different. Usually however, there are several shared experiences. When emotional concerns prevent the woman from taking part in the care of the new baby or from having any interest in her family, this should be reported to your supervisor so that a complete assessment can be made and a plan of care formulated that will help the woman through this difficult period of time.

- Women usually experience some mood swings. This occurs as a result of the hormonal changes and the fact that the woman is assessing her new role and planning how to adjust. Some women are weepy. Some are euphoric and have a great deal of energy.
- Women may want friends around or they may want to be alone. Be sensitive to the wish of your client. If she wants to be alone, gently tell friends and family that perhaps they should call before coming to visit or they should come and stay for short periods of time. Designating a time to visit is helpful so that the client and the visitor know the time frame that has been set for the visit.
- Getting used to a body that is changing continuously is difficult for some women. It takes about six weeks until the internal organs return to prenatal status. It may take six months for the woman to lose weight and regain her prenatal appearance. Support her as she tries to exercise, change diet, and become familiar with her changing needs. Encourage her to discuss exercise regimes with her physician before any new activity is started.

## Physical Changes

The first six weeks after birth, a woman's body is continuously changing. During the first two to three days, a reddish, bloody discharge from the vagina is to be expected. This is called lochia. About the fourth day this discharge changes to yellowish and continues for another week. Usually, all discharge stops about the twenty-first day. The discharge is normal, and the woman should wear whatever peripads she wishes. It is usually recommended that they be deodorant free. Tampons are not worn. Dispose of the used pads as you would any dressing in a paper or plastic bag. The perineum should be cleaned and washed with warm soapy water after each bowel movement and voiding. The peripads should be changed at that time too.

Usually the woman looses the fluid she accumulates during pregnancy between the second and fifth day postpartum. Encourage her to continue to drink fluids throughout this period as water and fruit juices will help with the process and prevent dehydration.

It is important that bowel function be regular during this time. Because the perineal area may be sore, bowel movements may be uncomfortable. If this is the case, encourage your client to discuss this with her physician so that stool softeners can be prescribed. A diet that has sufficient fiber and fluid usually prevents most discomfort. If you have concerns that regular bowel function is not occurring, discuss this with your supervisor.

## Diet

During this period a balanced diet is important. It helps with maintaining a feeling of well-being, regulating bowel and bladder function, and helping the body return to prenatal status. If the woman is nursing, additional calories and fluids will be required. During the postpartum period a woman should be encouraged to eat regularly and enjoy her food. This is not the time to start crash diets or decrease fluids in an attempt to lose weight.

## Contraception

Sexual relations following the birth of a child are a very personal activity. Sometimes there is a change in the pattern of sexual activity. This change will be discussed between the client and her partner. Often, if questions or concerns remain, she should be encouraged to discuss this with her physician.

Remind your client that pregnancy can occur shortly after the birth of a child. Pregnancy can occur while a women is nursing a child. Pregnancy can also occur before normal menstrual periods have resumed. Contraception or abstinence is recommended if another pregancy is to be avoided.

## Breast Care

The decision to breast feed a baby is a personal one. If your client has made a decision that is different from the one you would have made, respect her decision and support her. Sometimes, even when a woman decides not to breast feed, her breasts fill with milk. Encourage her to call her physician if this happens. Breasts should always be supported with a good bra until they return to prenatal size. They should be kept clean at all times.

## Guidelines: Postpartum Care

Document the normal activities of the household including:

- activity level
- sleep patterns of the client

- emotional status
- diet and fluid intake
- lochia: amount, color, odor
- bowel and bladder function
- family dynamics

Call your supervisor if:

- The client experiences temperature and/or chills.
- There is any discomfort, pain, or discoloration of limbs or abdomen.
- There is any difficulty breathing or speaking, or general anxiety.
- The lochia is excessive and/or foul smelling.
- The client has difficulty urinating or voiding is painful.
- There is a sudden change in the client.

## Your Role as a Homemaker/Home Health Aide

You will be asked to support the client during this time of change. The way in which you respond to her emotional needs and her physical changes will signal to the client and her family whether her actions are normal and acceptable. Every family reacts to childbirth differently. You will be asked to reinforce the family's culture and their customs in dealing with the new baby and the new mother. If you do not understand some of the actions, ask your supervisor to explain them. If you feel that some actions are not safe or are contrary to your assignment, discuss this with your supervisor immediately. You may suggest changes in a routine or action that in your experience has worked. Do not be offended if the family chooses not to adopt your suggestion. There are often many ways to accomplish the same goal, and each family must set up a system that is comfortable for them when you leave.

## Topics for Discussion

1. Discuss the proper order for offering complete care to a client who is bedbound.
2. What would you do if your client refused personal care?
3. Invite an experienced homemaker/home health aide to present some real cases to you. Then try and make a plan as to which procedure you would do first, second, and so forth. Give your reasons for each decision.
4. Discuss how you would feel and what you would do if a family treated a new baby and a new mother in a way that you had not seen before.
5. What would you do if you did not have the proper equipment to give personal care:
   - a basin
   - a bath blanket
   - hot water
   - clean sheets
   - soap

# Chapter 14

# Rehabilitation of the Client

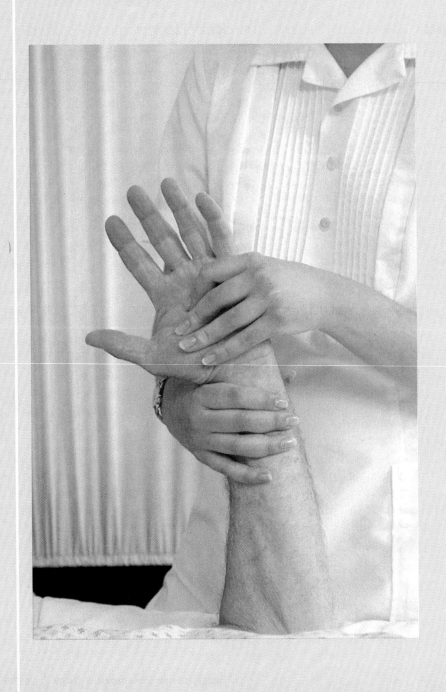

# Section 1 Introduction to Rehabilitation

## Objectives: What You Will Learn to Do

▓ Define *rehabilitation.*

▓ Discuss the many things that therapists take into consideration when they establish a program for your client.

## *Introduction: What Is Rehabilitation?*

**rehabilitation** process by which people who have been disabled by injury or sickness are helped to recover as many as possible of their original abilities and live with the remaining disabilities

**Rehabilitation** is the process of relearning how to function, in the best possible way, as an independent person despite a disability. Rehabilitation is not easy and not always pleasant, but with proper direction and encouragement, the client can accomplish his goals. Sometimes a client will use a brace or support for an injured body part. Be sure you completely understand the care and use of this piece of equipment. The way in which you assist the client will communicate to him if you really believe he will succeed or if you feel his attempts are useless. Be alert to your verbal and nonverbal communications.

### ESTABLISHING A REHABILITATION ROUTINE

Before a therapist establishes a routine for the client, she reviews the whole client profile, including his environment. Your objective reporting during this assessment will help establish a useful individualized program for your client. Some of the factors taken into consideration during this assessment are:

▓ How much active motion does the client have?

▓ How much passive motion does the client have?

▓ Symptoms of all medical diagnoses that may affect function.

▓ Sensory deficits in vision, hearing, speech, touch, balance, or proprioception (knowledge of limb position in space with eyes covered).

▓ How does the client see his situation? his disability?

▓ *Attitude:* Is he depressed, euphoric, angry, cooperative, resentful, frustrated? Is he motivated: Does he want to try to do things for himself?

▓ *Ability:* What can he do for himself? What does he attempt to do?

**dominant** stronger half of a pair

▓ *Previous level of function:* Which limb is **dominant** (used for most activities)? What did he do before he became disabled? If a person did not have the desire to do something before an illness, he may not be motivated to do it afterward.

**priority** giving something more importance than another

▓ *Priorities:* A **priority** is something the client wants to do. Often the priority is something that we might not feel is important, but achieving it makes the client feel less handicapped. It could be a little thing like putting on makeup, setting hair, shaving, tying shoes, using the telephone, or signing checks.

▓ *Equipment:* What is the client using now, and what does he need to help him function: hospital bed, commode, crutches, catheter, walker, cane, brace, splints, or adaptive equipment, such as built-up spoons or dressing sticks?

■ *Environmental barrier:* Those things in the client's home that make it difficult for him to care for himself: a second-floor bathroom when a client cannot climb stairs, throw rugs that can trip him, narrow doorways that prevent him from moving from room to room in a wheelchair, heavy furniture that he cannot pass in a walker or with crutches or a cane, a bed without side rails to help him sit up.

■ *Support system:* The people involved in the care of a client. Besides the homemaker/home health aide, are there family members or friends who will assist him to regain functional independence?

# Section 2   Working with a Physical Therapist

**Objectives: What You Will Learn to Do**

■ Explain the principles of range-of-motion exercise.
■ Demonstrate the proper techniques for complete or partial range of motion with a client.
■ Lift, hold, or transfer a client using good body mechanics.
■ Demonstrate several types of client transfers.
■ Discuss the proper type of chair for client use.
■ Demonstrate various ways of assisting your client with ambulation.

 ## *Introduction: Muscles, Joints, Movement*

Joints are where two or more bones meet to form a movable area of the skeletal frame. Muscles move the bones. If muscles are not used, they can shorten and tighten. This makes the joint motion painful and limited. Muscle shortening can happen in a short time. Therefore, it is important that clients are helped to use their muscles. This is done by encouraging them to do normal daily activities and their prescribed exercises (Fig. 14.1).

### RANGE-OF-MOTION EXERCISES

**range of motion** (ROM) exercises that take a body part through the entire ability of its motion

There are four types of **range-of-motion** (ROM) exercises. Each is ordered for a specific purpose.

| | Client | Helper |
|---|---|---|
| Passive | | Takes client through ROM<br>Client does not help |
| Active/assist | Active motion | Helps to make motion easier; moves part farther than client can |
| Active | Done totally by client | |
| Resistive | Active motion | Makes exercise harder by providing resistance to motion but allows completion of motion |

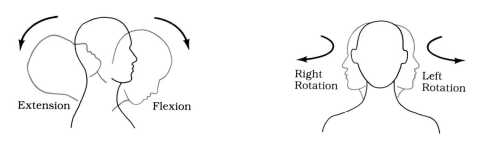

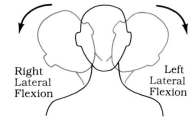

**FIGURE 14.1** Assist clients with proper exercises to keep muscles flexible.

## Guidelines: Assisting with ROM

▨ Do not start ROM exercises until you have received specific instructions for your particular client.

▨ Never take a client beyond the point of pain. Pain is a warning sign and should be heeded. Report client pain to your supervisor.

▨ Report to the supervisor if the client does not do the exercises when you are not in the house.

▨ Report to the supervisor if the client is finding the exercises harder to do rather than easier.

▨ Use the flat part of your hand and fingers to hold the client's body parts. Do not grip with your fingertips. Some people are sensitive to pressure. Some people are ticklish.

▨ If you forget what to do, think of your own body and how it works.

▨ Talk to the client. Explain what is being done and why. Even if the person does not appear to understand, the tone of your voice and touch of your hands can help you communicate.

▨ Better communication greatly improves your chances for client cooperation.

▨ Do each exercise three to five times or as you have been instructed.

▨ Follow a logical sequence during the exercises so that each joint and muscle is exercised. For example, start at the head and work down to the feet.

▨ Be gentle—never bend or straighten a body part farther than it will go.

▨ Slow, steady movement of a tight muscle will help the muscle relax and so increase the joint range.

▨ Include the family or caregivers in the activity so they can learn and continue the exercises when you are not there.

# Procedure 34: Range of Motion

1. Wash your hands.
2. Explain to the client that you are going to help him exercise his muscles and joints.
3. Ask visitors to leave if appropriate.
4. Offer the client the bedpan or urinal.
5. Drape the client for modesty.
6. Raise the bed to the highest horizontal position.
7. Lower the side rail on the side you are working. Move the client close to you.
8. Proceed with the exercises as you have been instructed (Fig. 14.2).
9. Make the client comfortable.
10. Wash your hands.
11. Chart that you have completed the exercises. Also note anything you observed about the client during the procedure.

**FIGURE 14.2** Range of motion exercises.

**(a) Shoulder flexion**
With elbow straight, raise arm over head, then lower, keeping arm in front of you the whole time.

**(b) Shoulder abduction & adduction**
With elbow straight, raise arm over head, then lower, keeping arm out to the side the whole time.

**(c) Shoulder internal & external rotation**
Bring arm out to the side. Do NOT bring elbow out to shoulder level. Turn arm back and forth so forearm points down toward feet, then up toward head. With arm alongside body and elbow bent at 90°, turn arm so forearm points across stomach, then out to the side.

**(d1, d2) Shoulder horizontal abduction & adduction**
Keeping arm at shoulder level, reach across chest past opposite shoulder, then reach out to the side.

**(e) Elbow flexion & extension**
With arm alongside body, bend elbow to touch shoulder, then straighten elbow out again.

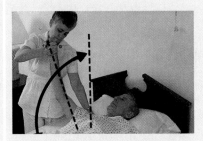

a

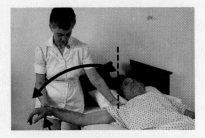

b

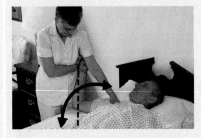

c

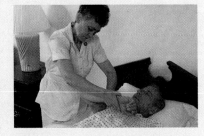

d1

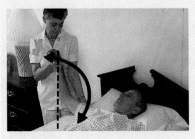

d2

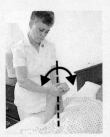

e

## Procedure 37: Helping a Client to Stand

1. "Move to the front of your chair or bed. Put your hands on the arms of the chair." This client is sitting over the edge of the chair or bed. Place one of your knees between his knees. Your feet should be in good position and you should be close to the bed. If the client has a weak knee, brace it with your knee.

2. "Put one foot in under you." This should be the strongest leg. Bend your knees and lean onto your forward foot to place the same side arm around the client's waist and place your other hand at the other side of the client's waist. You have now encircled the client and are holding him at his center of gravity (Fig.14.6a).

3. "On the count of three, push down with your arms, lean forward, stand up." Remember to count to three. It allows you both to know when to start the motion and work as a team. Hold the client closely. The more assistance needed, the closer you hold the client. On the count of three, rock your weight to your back foot (Fig. 14.6b).

*FIGURE 14.6*

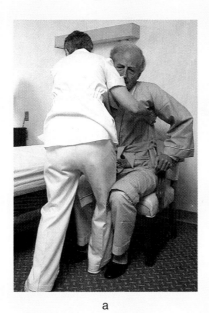 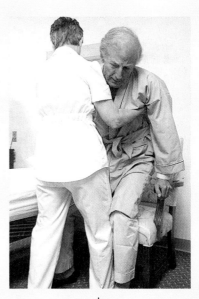

a                    b

## Procedure 38: Helping a Client to Sit

Your body mechanics and positioning are the same as in helping the client to stand. Just reverse the directions.

1. Be sure that the wheels on the bed or chair are locked.

2. Remind the client to feel the bed or chair with the back of his legs.

3. Direct the client to reach back for the arms of the chair or the bed.

4. You support and direct the activity as he sits down.

## Procedure 39: Pivot Transfer from Bed to Chair

1. Prepare the equipment. Place the wheelchair at a 45° angle to the bed. Place the chair so that the client will move toward his stronger side.

2. If you are transferring the client to a wheelchair, lock the wheels of the chair. If the bed has wheels, lock these wheels, too.

3. Wash your hands.

4. Tell the client what you are going to do.

5. Bring the client to a sitting position with his legs over the edge of the bed (Fig. 14.7a).

6. Place slippers or shoes on his feet.

7. Explain the procedure to the client:

   a. He will come to a standing position.

   b. He will then reach for the arm of the chair, pivot, and sit (Fig. 14.7b).

   c. You will remain in good support position and guide him.

   d. You will keep your foot near the client's foot for extra support (Fig. 14.7c).

   e. You will use good body mechanics to support him and prevent injury to yourself.

8. When you are sure that the client understands the procedure, perform the transfer.

9. Secure the client in the chair. Make him comfortable. Leave him in a safe place.

10. Wash your hands.

11. Chart any observations you may have made during this procedure.

FIGURE 14.7

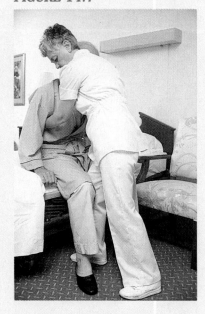
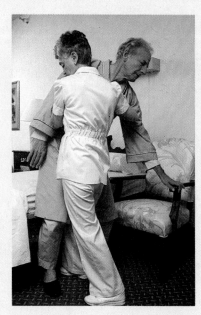
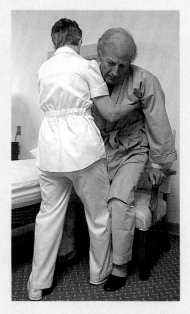

a          b          c

## Procedure 40: Transfer from Chair to Bed

1. Your body mechanics and positioning are the same as in helping the client into the chair. Just reverse the directions.
2. Wash your hands.
3. Prepare the bed.
4. Place the chair at a 45° angle to the bed so the client moves toward his stronger side.
5. If you are transferring the client from a wheelchair, lock the wheels of the chair. If the bed has wheels, lock these, too.
6. Get into a good position using a firm base of support and proper body mechanics.
7. Direct the client to come to a standing position.
8. Direct the client to reach for the bed and pivot. Help and guide him.
9. Make the client comfortable. Reposition the side rails.
10. Wash your hands.
11. Chart any observations you may have made during this procedure.

### MINIMAL ASSISTANCE

As the client gains strength and confidence, he will require less assistance. You will use the same basic body positioning but will not hold him. You may remain with him for directions and in case you are needed. When minimal assistance is needed, it is best to stand on the weaker side of the client and support him with a guarding belt. This way, as the client is changing position, you will be available if he falls or loses balance.

## Ambulation Activities

ambulate to walk

**Ambulation** refers to the action of walking. If the client requires a special gait or must learn a new way to walk, the physical therapist will set up a plan for the client and you to follow. However, the same basic assisting positions can be used for clients with all types of gaits.

- Use the proper procedure for the client to come to a standing position.
- Use a guarding belt for extra support.
- Stand on the client's weaker side and a little behind him.
- One hand should be on the guarding belt, the other hand in front of the collarbone on the weaker side.

## Assistive Walking Devices

Canes, crutches, and walkers are all used by people to help support them while walking (Fig. 14.8). Use of this equipment may be permanent or temporary. A client may use different pieces of equipment at different times. The decision as to which piece of equipment to use will take into consideration the needs and abilities of the client. Do not change the equipment or the way in which the client has been instructed to use it. If you have a suggestion or a concern as to safety, discuss it with your supervisor.

Each piece of equipment is prescribed by a physician and fit by a professional nurse or physical therapist to the client's unique needs. This individualized fit decreases the possibility of accidents. If a piece of equipment is borrowed, check it for fit and make sure that it is safe before it is used.

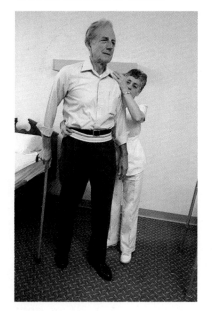 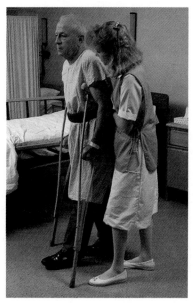 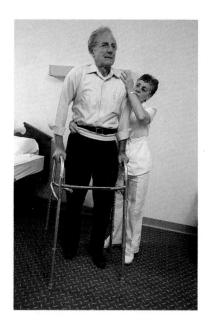

*FIGURE 14.8* Clients using assistive devices for walking: (a) cane; (b) crutches; (c) walker.

a                b                c

## Guidelines: Using Assistive Walking Devices

- Canes, crutches, and walkers must always be used with rubber tips on the ends.
- Tips should not be worn, wet, or torn.
- Screws and bolts should be securely in place. If one is lost, replace it. Do not use the device without the proper screws in place.
- Wooden canes and crutches should be smooth without cracks.
- Metal canes, crutches, and walkers should not have any sharp edges and should be straight.
- To go up stairs: Advance the strongest leg to the next step. Bring the cane or crutch and then the weaker leg to the step.
- To go down stairs: Advance the cane or crutches to the lower step, followed by the weaker leg and then the stronger one.
- The hand piece of each device should be level with the hip so that there is a slight bend at the elbow when the client is standing.
- All equipment is used after the client has come to a standing position.
- Do not come to a standing position pulling up walkers or canes.

### Canes

A client may use either a single-tipped cane, a tripod cane, or a quad-cane (Fig. 14.9). A cane is usually used on the stronger side. That way, the client's weight will be balanced between the cane and the involved side. The base of support will change from that of a normal walking gait.

The client walking with the cane will:

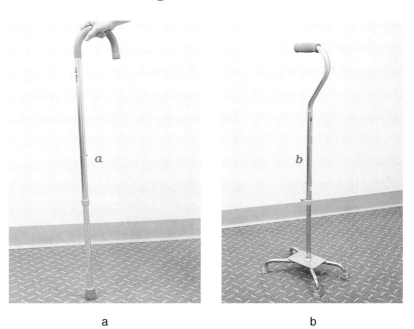

a                                        b

FIGURE 14.9  Two types of canes: (a) single-tipped cane; (b) quad-cane.

1. Place the cane about 12 inches in front on his stronger side (Fig. 14.10).
2. Bring the weaker leg forward so that it is even with the cane (Fig. 14.11).
3. Bring the stronger leg forward, just ahead of the cane (Fig. 14.12).

FIGURE 14.10            FIGURE 14.11            FIGURE 14.12

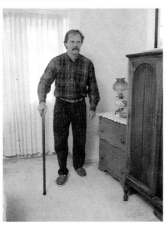
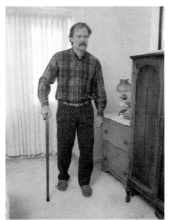
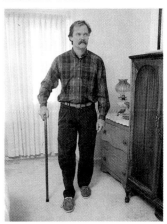

### Crutches

Crutches are used when the client is unable to put complete weight on one or both legs. Crutches are prescribed by a physician and fit by a professional nurse or physical therapist to the client's unique needs. This individualized fit decreases the possibility of accidents. If the client has a pair of crutches in the house or borrows them, be sure that they are checked for fit and that they are safe before they are used. Crutches may be made of wood or aluminum.

While using crutches, the body's weight is on the client's hands and arms, not on the top of the crutch under his arms. Sometimes clients will have to exercise their upper arms before they begin using crutches.

The physical therapist, nurse, or physician will teach the client how to use the crutches and which gait to use.

## Crutch Walking

| Gait | Features | Steps |
|---|---|---|
| Three-point gait One leg nonweight-bearing | | |
| Swing through (Fig. 14.13) | Strong upper arms Some weight bearing | 1. Place crutches 8 to 12 inches in front of body. 2. Swing body past crutches. |
| Swing to crutch | Strong upper arms Some weight bearing | 1. Place crutches 8 to 12 inches in front of body while bearing weight on strong leg. 2. Swing body to crutches. |
| Standard Three-point gait (Fig. 14.14) | One leg nonweightbearing Strong upper arms Client can balance well | 1. Place crutches 8 to 12 inches in front of body with weaker leg. 2. Bring strong leg forward in front of crutches. |
| Two-point gait (Fig. 14.15) | Weight bearing on both feet Client can balance well | 1. Bring right foot and left crutch 8 to 12 inches forward. 2. Bring left foot and right crutch 8 to 12 inches forward. |
| Four-point gait (Fig. 14.16) | Weight bearing on both feet Stable gait, slow | 1. Bring right crutch 8 to 12 inches forward. 2. Bring left foot in front of crutch. 3. Bring left crutch in front of left foot. 4. Bring right foot in front of left foot. |

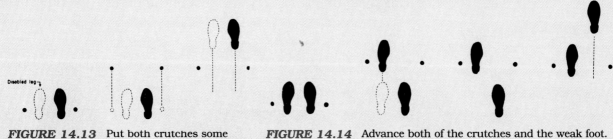

**FIGURE 14.13** Put both crutches some distance in advance with weight on stronger leg.

**FIGURE 14.14** Advance both of the crutches and the weak foot. Balance weight on both crutches then advance the stronger foot.

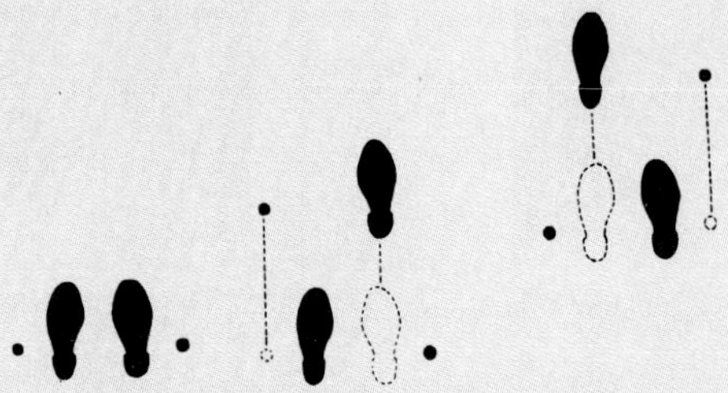

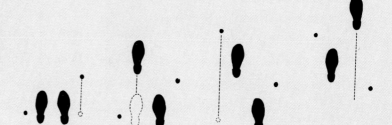

**FIGURE 14.15** Advance right foot and left crutch. Then advance left foot and right crutch simultaneously.

**FIGURE 14.16** Put right crutch forward and advance left foot. Then put left crutch forward and advance right foot.

### Walker

A walker is used when a person requires support because of greater imbalance or weakness (Fig. 14.17). The walker is safe to push down on only when all four legs are on the ground in a level position. If the walker is being moved, the client's feet should be stationary. If the walker is stationary, the client can move his feet. The walker should be picked up and moved, not slid along the ground.

*FIGURE 14.17*

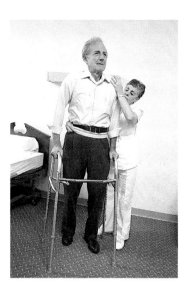

## Procedure 41: Going from a Standing Position to a Sitting Position Using Assistive Devices

1. Check to see that the chair is secure and safe. Brace it against a wall if possible.
2. The client will walk toward the chair and get close to it.
3. Direct the client to turn his back to the chair and feel it with the back of his legs.
4. Direct the client to let go of the assistive device and to reach for the arms of the chair and slowly lower himself into the chair. (*Note:* The client may need reassurance.)
5. Guide and support him as needed. Remain in front of the client and in good position to assist him.
6. Always use good body mechanics.

### Guidelines: As You Help Clients with Rehabilitation Therapy

- Always apply basic body mechanics.
- Be sure of your client's abilities before you attempt a procedure. Check each time.
- Use common sense.
- TCOB.
- Know your own abilities. Do not be ashamed to ask for help or additional instruction with a procedure.

- Communicate through words, gestures, and tone of voice.
- Set an example to the client and the family.
- Use the same procedure each time you assist the client. This will set up a routine with which you will both be familiar.
- Apply what you know from one procedure to help you with another one.
- Clothing should fit well and not block the client's view of the floor. Shoes should be flat with nonskid soles.

# Section 3 Speech and Language Therapy

## Objectives: What You Will Learn to Do

- Understand the different ways we can communicate.
- Understand the meaning of receptive and expressive aphasia.
- Understand the role of the homemaker/home health aide in working with the speech-language pathologist.
- Understand what the homemaker/home health aide may do to help the communication impaired client.

### Introduction: Working with a Speech-Language Pathologist

Speech and language therapy is one of the services provided by the home health team. The speech-language pathologist is the professional who evaluates the need for therapy and who plans the therapy program.

Speech and language therapy is given when the client has difficulty communicating. It is important to remember that there is more to communication than just speaking. Communication also means the ability to understand speech, to read, to write, and to gesture (Fig. 14.18).

*FIGURE 14.18*

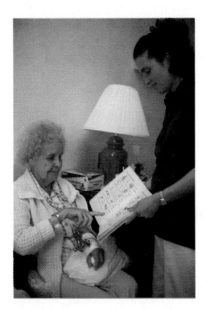

A client may need speech and language therapy if he has a disorder that affects parts of the brain, face, lips, tongue, or throat that are used to form words. Some examples of this kind of disorder are Parkinson's disease, cerebral palsy, and cleft palate. A person who has had cancer of the tongue or larynx (voice box) may need therapy after the surgeon has removed the cancer.

## APHASIA

Injury to the brain may cause a loss of speech or language abilities, which is called aphasia. Usually the injury is from a cerebrovascular accident (CVA), often called a stroke. **Cerebrovascular accident** means that a blood clot, hemorrhage, or vascular spasm in the brain has stopped oxygen from reaching some parts of the brain tissue. When those parts of the brain do not receive oxygen, they stop working. Damage to the brain may also be caused by a blow on the head or by a tumor.

**cerebrovascular accident** blockage of blood vessel within the brain leading to death of brain tissue

An aphasic person may have difficulty in all areas of communication. It may be hard for him to speak, understand speech, read, or write. Aphasia may be mild, moderate, or severe. The kind of aphasia is determined by where the brain injury occurs and how much damage is done to the parts of the brain. Aphasia does not mean that the person is unable to make judgments or think. Aphasia only means a person cannot communicate with words.

There are two types of aphasia, expressive and receptive. A client with **expressive aphasia** has difficulty expressing his thoughts and sometimes communicating in writing. Such a client may say things involuntarily. He may have difficulty:

**expressive aphasia** difficulty communicating in writing and orally

- Naming people and things
- Saying "yes" and "no" at the right time
- Spelling words
- Counting
- Telling time

Everyone has had the experience of having the name of a person or a thing "right on the tip of the tongue." The feeling of knowing what you want to say but not being able to think of the right word is what happens to an expressively aphasic person all day long.

A person with **receptive aphasia** has trouble receiving, or understanding, what he is hearing, seeing, or touching. For example, he can hear words clearly, but they do not have any meaning for him. It is as if he were listening to a foreign language. He might have the same problem whcn he looks at words. Some aphasic people even have trouble understanding the use of common objects. They might pick up a comb and not know what to do with it.

**receptive aphasia** inability to understand stimuli due to a deficiency within the brain

A person with receptive aphasia may have:

- No interest in watching television or listening to the radio
- No interest in reading the newspaper
- No ability to follow directions
- No ability to answer questions appropriately

The behavior of the aphasic person may seem rude or confusing at times. But think about how *you* might act if you could not say what you wanted to say or if you could not understand what people were saying to you. Always remember that the aphasic person is an intelligent adult. He is just as smart as he was before the injury to his brain. He simply cannot communicate easily. He will be most cooperative and least frustrated when you treat him like the adult that he is.

A client with aphasia:

- Tires very easily
- Laughs or cries frequently
- Uses profanity without meaning to
- Repeats the same word over and over

## Your Role as a Homemaker/Home Health Aide

Your role in working with the aphasic client is important. You will probably spend more time with the client than any other person on the home health team. So you will have a better chance to get to know the client and to help him adjust to his new schedule of exercises and activities.

There are two specific tasks the speech-language pathologist will ask you to do. The first will be to help the client practice speech or language activities. These activities are always taught first by the speech-language pathologist. Remember that the aphasic person may have trouble communicating in many different ways and with different degrees of severity. For this reason, it is always the job of the speech-language pathologist to determine which activities best fit the needs of a particular client. The speech or language activities you practice with one client must never be used with another.

If the client has difficulty understanding or using words, you may be taught how to use pictures and printed words to help improve communication. You may be shown how to help your client practice printing or writing. Sometimes the client may have weakened muscles of the face, lips, or tongue. The speech-language pathologist may teach specific exercises to help improve the strength and coordination of those muscles.

The second task will be to observe and report. It is important to observe how the client makes his needs known and how well he is able to perform the assigned practice tasks. You will want to note how the client makes his feelings known to you. Does he point? Shake his head? Use words? You will also want to keep a record of how often the assigned speech or language tasks are performed.

You will be with the client many more hours during the week than will the speech-language pathologist. So what you report will be very useful in planning the therapy program.

Here are some dos and don'ts to keep in mind when you are caring for an aphasic person.

### Do

- Get the attention of the client before starting to speak.
- Keep instructions and explanations simple. Speak slowly but naturally. Try to keep your conversation about the client's immediate needs or surroundings.
- Encourage the client to use common expressions, such as "hello," "goodbye," and "I want."
- Encourage the client to be as independent as possible. He is an adult; treat him like one.

- Ask direct questions requiring a simple "yes" or "no" answer. For example, "Did you eat lunch?" rather than "What's new?"
- Give the client time to reply.
- Give the client opportunities to hear speech, such as the radio and television.
- Meals and dressing times are good opportunities to encourage the client's attempts to speak. Let him ask for what he needs. He may say the word correctly sometimes and forget it at another time. This is usual for the aphasic person.
- Encourage the client to use whatever speech ability he has. Counting and singing are good activities. Words such as *up-down* or *push-pull* can be used during physical therapy exercises.
- Show the client understanding, but not pity. Help him verbalize his feeling of frustration ("I know it must be difficult for you.").
- By your body language, patience, and attitude of acceptance, create an air of relaxation for the client. Avoid directions, such as "Relax."
- Sometimes it will be impossible to understand what the client is saying. At such times tactfully try to change the subject or say, "Let's forget it now and come back to it later. The words will probably come when you're not trying so hard."

You also may encourage the client to learn the words that go with his personal care. When you are helping the client bathe, dress, or eat, say the name of each utensil or body part. For example, "Fork, you eat with a fork," or "Arm, I'm washing your arm." Your client may find that he is able to say some of the words with you. If he does, smile and let him know that he has succeeded. If he does not repeat the words, you must not force him. Remember, he wants to talk, and if he could, he would. Talking to him about these activities in the same way each day will help him to relearn what words mean, even if he cannot say them.

### Don't

- Answer for the client if he is capable of speaking for himself. Include the client in social conversations.
- Confuse the client with too much idle chatter or too many people speaking at once.
- Discuss the client's emotional reactions and problems in his presence.
- Interrupt the client or finish sentences for him. He may require extra time to think of the correct word.
- Show your concern about the client's speech either through word or facial expression. Do not under any circumstances put the client on display or force him to speak. Such remarks as "Say it for them" upset and embarrass the client.
- Ridicule or insist that the client give accurate responses, pronounce correctly, or "talk right." (There is nothing the client wants more than to do just that.)
- Speak to the client as if he were a child, deaf, or retarded. He is not deaf unless a definite hearing loss has been detected. His problem is generally one of understanding the meaning of your words, as though you were speaking a foreign language. Simplify or rephrase your wording without shouting. Treat him like the adult he is.

If you can show the client through your attitude and your work that you understand his problem and that you want to help him, you will often be rewarded by the gratitude of a more relaxed and comfortable client.

## Section 4 Dealing with a Hearing Loss

**Objectives: What You Will Learn to Do**

- Identify some common causes of hearing loss.
- Clean a hearing aid earmold.
- Identify common problems that may prevent a hearing aid from working properly.
- Identify the best ways to talk to a hearing-impaired person.

### Introduction: Hearing and Its Loss

Some of the people that you will work with may have some degree of hearing loss. Some are born with a hearing loss. Other people lose their hearing when they are exposed to loud noise over a long period of time. Head injuries or ear infections can also cause loss of hearing. Many people lose some of their ability to hear sounds clearly as they get older.

**hearing aid** mechanical device used to help a person perceive sounds

Whatever the cause of the hearing loss, it can be a frustrating problem. The person who is hard of hearing may feel that the speech of others is mumbled and unclear. He may have to work harder to understand what is being said. If it becomes too frustrating to try to follow a conversation, the hard-of-hearing person may begin to avoid social activities. A **hearing aid** can often be of great help to the hard-of-hearing person.

#### HEARING AID CARE

**earmold** an impression of the ear used with a hearing aide

The hearing aid **earmold** is custom-made to fit the ear. If the earmold does not fit snugly into the ear, there will be a high-pitched whistling noise when the aid is turned on (Fig. 14.19).

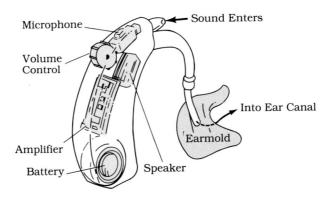

*FIGURE 14.19* Parts of a hearing aid earmold.

The earmold must be kept clean. If earwax or dirt is clogging the earmold, sound will not be able to pass through. The earmold and aid should be wiped with a dry tissue after each wearing. When not in use, the hearing aid should be kept in a safe place away from extreme heat or cold.

## Procedure 42: How to Clean the Hearing Aid Earmold

1. Assemble your equipment:
   Pan of warm water and mild liquid detergent
   Pipe cleaner or toothpick
2. Remove the earmold from the body of the hearing aid.
3. Wash the earmold gently with mild soap and water.
4. Carefully remove any earwax with the pipe cleaner or toothpick.
5. Dry thoroughly. Let it dry overnight, or blow air through the opening to be sure all water has come out of the tubing and earmold.

*Remember:* Wash only the earmold. Never put the body of the hearing aid in water. Never use alcohol or cleaning fluid on the earmold or the aid. Encourage your client to take the hearing aid off or protect it during rain and snow to prevent it from getting wet.

### Batteries Make the Hearing Aid Work

If the hearing aid does not work, the battery may be dead. To insert a new one, match the + on the battery to the + on the hearing aid case. One battery will last about 125 hours, or 10 days. The battery should be removed from the hearing aid whenever it is not being worn. This saves the batteries. Extra batteries should be stored in a cool, dry place, such as a dresser drawer.

### Precautions

- Keep the hearing aid away from heat, such as radiators or hair dryers.
- Do not get the hearing aid wet.
- Do not drop the hearing aid.
- Do not spray hairspray, perfume, or after shave lotion on the aid.
- Do not twist the tubing or wires.

If the hearing aid does not work, check to see if:

- The battery is put in correctly and that the case is closed tightly.
- The aid is turned on and the volume is loud enough.
- There is wax in the earmold.
- The tubing or wires are twisted.
- The battery is working.

If all of these things have been checked and the hearing aid still does not work, it should be taken to the hearing aid dispenser for repair.

### HOW TO TALK TO THE HEARING-IMPAIRED PERSON

- Get his attention before you start speaking.
- Talk face to face whenever possible. Your client will understand

more of what you say when he can see your face and expression.

- ■ Keep your hands away from your face so they do not block his view of what you are saying.
- ■ Do not chew food when you are speaking; it will make your words sound unclear.
- ■ Do not exaggerate your words. Speak at a normal rate of speed. You may be asked to speak louder. But do not shout.

The speech-language pathologist may teach you the following exercises to practice with the client. They are often used when the muscles used for speech are weaker. *Never* practice any exercise with a client that was not taught to him by the speech pathologist.

Name _____ Date _____

Do Each Exercise _____

### Lips:

1. Open mouth as wide as possible, stretch, close tightly and pucker, hold.
2. Pucker lips, hold, move lips to the left, hold, move lips to the right, hold.
3. Reach out with lower lip, hold. Reach out with the upper lip, hold.
4. Smile with lips closed, frown, repeat.
5. Press lips tightly as if you are saying *mm.*
6. Say *ma-me-mi-mo-mu* (as clearly and distinctly as you can).

### Tongue:

1. Put the tongue in the outer left corner of the mouth, move to the right and back. Work for speed and rhythm of movement.
2. Extend the tongue straight forward, then pull back vigorously with the whole tongue.
3. Open mouth wide, lift tongue tip up to the roof of the mouth, down. Do not move your jaw; lift your tongue.
4. Say *ta-te-ti-to-tu.* Do not move your jaw; lift your tongue.
5. Say *da-de-di-do-du.* Do not move your jaw; lift your tongue.
6. Say *la-le-li-lo-lu.* Do not move your jaw; lift your tongue.

### Throat:

1. Puff up cheeks. Hold air for five seconds—then release air as you blow out.
2. Suck in cheeks—then relax.
3. Puff up cheeks with air—move air from one cheek to the other without letting air escape lips. Alternate from one side to the other.
4. Drink liquids whenever possible through a straw.

# Section 5 · Working with an Occupational Therapist

## Objectives: What You Will Learn to Do

- Discuss your role while working with an occupational therapist.
- Discuss your role in assisting clients who are relearning daily living skills.
- Learn techniques to add to your basic knowledge of personal care.
- Know when and what to report to the OTR.

## Introduction: What Is Occupational Therapy?

For most of us, the skills/tasks we perform each day do not require conscious effort or awareness of how we do them. We get out of bed, go to the toilet, bathe, dress, prepare our meals, and feed ourselves. We do not think of the complex movements made by various parts of the body to push, pull, lift, close, zip, hook, and button clothing or to open or use various objects.

Many clients are unable to perform useful actions with a specific body part. This is called a **functional limitation**. A client with a functional limitation may have to concentrate to hold and lift a spoon to feed himself. Perhaps his grasp is weak. Perhaps he has lost sensation and cannot feel the spoon in his hand. Anyone who needs help with any or all such basic needs as toileting, bathing, dressing, feeding, grooming, or other day-to-day tasks is a candidate for occupational therapy. This training will help him improve his ability to function.

### Function of the OTR

The occupational therapy program focuses on increasing the functional ability of the client within his familiar environment. The trained person who administers this therapy is a registered **occupational therapist** (OTR). The client knows what household equipment he has to work with and will learn to adopt new skills in his own home. Being able to learn these skills at home shows the client that he is expected to take an active part in his care. Home is a nonthreatening place for relearning basic skills. An OTR can guide and instruct both the client and the homemaker/home health aide in ways to make the transition toward functional independence (Fig. 14.20).

General areas in which the OTR works with a homebound client include:

- *Mobilization:* teaching the client techniques that he can use to change position or to reach, grasp, turn while sitting, or maintain balance during an activity.
- *Daily living skills (DLS):* tasks we perform each day—toileting, bathing, dressing, feeding, grooming, homemaking, leisure activities.
- *Strength, coordination, and activity tolerance:* the ability to do something without tiring quickly. The client must learn techniques to conserve his energy, perform the skill task to his own satisfaction, and use his physical resources to the fullest.

**functional limitations** the inability to perform a task due to the deficit of a body part

**occupational therapist** trained person who assists people with performing their daily living tasks

**daily living skills** those tasks done each day to meet a person's basic needs

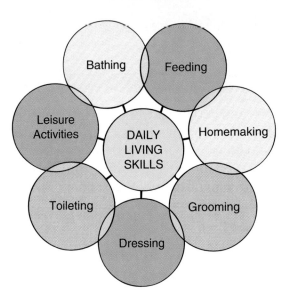

*FIGURE 14.20* Helping a client relearn daily living skills will aid him in his recovery and prepare him for independence.

## *Your Role as a Homemaker/Home Health Aide*

As you begin to assist clients in regaining their independence, your role as teacher, helper, and friend becomes very important. Remember:

- Your role in each task will be clearly defined by the OTR.
- If you do not understand what the client is supposed to do and what you are supposed to do, ask the OTR to explain more fully. If it is not clear to you, it will not be clear to the client. It is important for both of you to know what you are expected to do and why you are doing it.
- After each training session with the OTR, you and the client will have an opportunity to practice what has been demonstrated.
- If the client finds it difficult and says, "I can't," assist him with part of the routine to help him get started. Example: "You dress your involved arm, and I will help you put on the rest of the shirt."
- If the client shows sign of pain, being tired, or discomfort during the activity, stop the routine and report your observations to the OTR or the nurse supervisor.
- Observe which parts of each task the client is able and unable to do. Report your observations to the OTR on her next visit.
- Remember, the goal of the client, OTR, and homemaker/home health aide is to help the client become functionally independent, to take care of himself. As he achieves success with each task, your role will change.
- Do not attempt any technique that has not been taught to you and the client by the OTR. A method that was appropriate for a previous client may be wrong for your present client.
- Make the environment a safe and helpful one for your client (Fig. 14.21).
- As the client begins to regain skills, he also may become fearful that he will not be able to manage on his own as well as when you are there. Point out positive changes you have observed.

■ Discuss the outside world, the change of seasons, what is happening in the community, the specials at the grocery store, who won the ballgame. Bring the world into his home so he can begin to relate to it. Help him to realize that his disability does not have to be his whole world, that it no longer requires his total involvement.

■ On a day-by-day basis, try to determine the client's daily needs, such as his glasses, tissues, a glass of water, the newspaper, the TV. As early in his rehabilitation as possible, make these things accessible to him. Let him begin to assume responsibility for using them without your help.

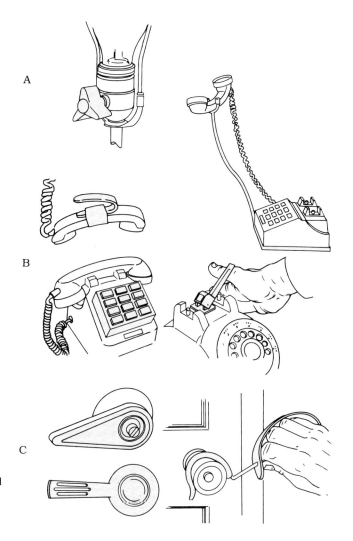

*FIGURE 14.21* Using adapted equipment on some everyday devices can help the client return to normalcy.

## Toileting

Taking care of one's own toileting needs is a basic and personal activity. When a person must rely on another person to help him with this, he often suffers a loss of self-esteem or dignity. If he is able to assume responsibility for this part of his personal care, he has taken the first step toward functional independence. This is usually the first skill a client wishes to learn. Follow the procedure established by the OTR.

Remember, you may assist the client with toileting, but do not attempt to change the place of toileting until you have been instructed to do so.

## Guidelines: Toileting in Bed

**pulling braid** a device used to assist a person in moving and/or sitting up in bed

▇ Tell the client what part of the procedure he will be doing and what you will do.

▇ Provide a **pulling braid.** A pulling braid is made from three 4-inch-wide strips of sheeting torn lengthwise and braided together. This braid is tied to the bed frame at one end. The other end is knotted and held by the client to assist him in sitting or turning in bed (Fig. 14.22).

▇ Place the bedpan where the client can reach it. Powder it to prevent the client's skin from sticking to it.

▇ Let the client do as much as he can himself. Assist only if he runs into difficulty.

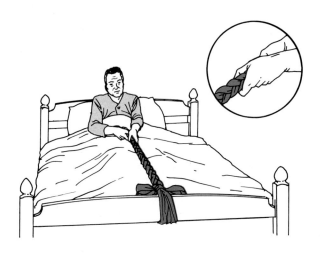

**FIGURE 14.22** A client using a pulling braid to sit up in bed.

## Guidelines: Toileting on a Commode

▇ Before he begins, explain to the client what he will be doing.

▇ Be sure the commode is standing securely.

▇ Place the commode in the position in which the client was instructed to use it.

▇ Assist the client out of bed as you have been instructed.

▇ Fasten the toilet paper to the commode. Tie the roll with a string or make a holder by stretching out a wire coat hanger and threading the roll onto it and hooking it to the frame. If you use a wire hanger, bend the ends and hook them over the front and back of the commode frame. Tape the ends so they do not scratch the client (Fig. 14.23).

▇ Place the roll on the client's uninvolved side. If he has general weakness, place it on his dominant (most used) side.

▇ Provide privacy.

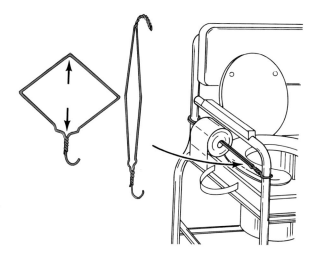

FIGURE 14.23 You can adapt a simple wire coat hanger to make the commode easier for the client to use.

![header icon] **Guidelines: Toileting in the Bathroom**

▓ Place the commode frame over the toilet as instructed or set the elevated toilet seat in place if the client uses such a device (Fig. 14.24). If using the commode frame, an 8-by-10-inch sheet of plastic, such as a piece from a garbage or trash bag, can be anchored between the commode seat and frame so it hangs down into the toilet bowl. This will serve as a baffle to prevent urine from splashing out of the toilet bowl. Rinse it off and replace it each time the client uses the toilet.

▓ Tell the client what he will do.

▓ Allow the client to do as much as he is safely able to do.

▓ Assist him with getting onto the toilet seat as you have been instructed.

▓ Provide privacy.

FIGURE 14.24

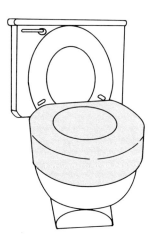
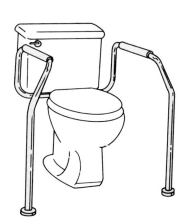

![header icon] **Bathing**

Bathing stimulates the body. The person who is bathing himself stimulates his involved extremities as he touches and rubs them. He becomes aware that the extremity "is there," even if he cannot really "feel" it. He may become aware that the involved extremity moves when

**hemiplegic** one who is paralyzed on one side of his body

he is using other parts of his body. As he bathes, he is moving many parts of his body together. He bends, stretches, reaches, grasps, balances, lifts his arms and legs, turns his head, and shifts his eyes.

For the **hemiplegic** (a person who is paralyzed on one side of his body), it is particularly important that he gives this stimulation to his involved extremities. As he rubs the affected part with the washcloth or towel, sensory nerves lying close to the skin may be aroused. The brain, receiving these sensations, may send a message down the motor pathways that could trigger an automatic response in the involved arm.

When you bathe the client, he does not use his own energy output. His body is not being involved with the automatic activity. Therefore, these responses may not be triggered.

The OTR may instruct the client to bathe in bed, seated on the commode, on a chair in front of a basin in his room, or seated on a chair or the toilet seat in the bathroom at the sink. As the client regains strength and mobility, the OTR may instruct him in tub bathing or showering using a bench or chair placed in the tub or shower stall. Some states permit the homemaker/home health aide to supervise and assist clients in showers and tubs. Some do not. You will be instructed according to the guidelines in your area.

## Guidelines: Bathing

- Do not attempt any technique that has not been taught to you and the client by the OTR. A method that was appropriate for a previous client may be inappropriate for your present client.
- Provide a safe environment.
- Assemble everything the client will need for bathing and dressing. Place them where he can reach them (Fig. 14.25).

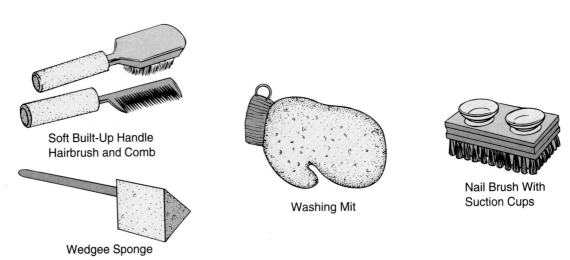

Soft Built-Up Handle
Hairbrush and Comb

Wedgee Sponge

Washing Mit

Nail Brush With
Suction Cups

**FIGURE 14.25** There is adapted equipment available to assist the client in bathing himself.

- Thin washcloths and small face towels may be easier for a weak or arthritic client to handle than thick cloths or large, heavy towels.
- Stabilize the wet soap by placing it on a dampened sponge, face cloth, paper towel, or rubber suction disk where it is less likely to slide.

- The client should remove his clothing as he was taught by the OTR.
- The hemiplegic should wash his involved arm first. He can drape a well-soaped washcloth over the palm of his involved hand, which should be resting palm up on his lap. Then he can lean forward and cradle his uninvolved arm in the hand and slide it back and forth to wash it.
- Remind your client to rinse off soap and dry each part of his body as he finishes washing it.
- Place nailbrush, bristles up, in the palm of his involved hand resting on his lap, palm up. Your client can rub his uninvolved fingers across the brush, pushing gently into the palm of the other hand to steady it.
- The client can also use the nailbrush on the fingers of the involved hand. He may lift the hand into the basin to rinse it, using the other hand for assistance if necessary.
- If the client is in bed, crank up the bed so that he is able to see his abdomen and legs. In a regular bed, prop him up with pillows.
- Place the washcloth and towel over the bed rail where the client can reach them. If he is in a regular bed, use a chair back or the head of the bed.
- Assist the client with transfers as necessary for safety.
- When the client is learning to turn on faucets and run water for himself, make sure he turns on the cold first and then the hot. Run cold water through the faucet last so it will be cool if the client touches it. With some diseases, a client's sense of heat and cold is affected and he cannot judge temperature. Check the water temperature with your hand before the client bathes.
- If your client cannot reach his back, he may use the foam rubber mop or back brush to extend his reach. If not, you should complete this task.

### TUB BATHING AND SHOWERING

By the time the client is able to bathe in a tub, he should have mastered such skills as balance, hip flexion, and transfers from sitting to standing with minimal assistance. Your role will be to provide a safe environment and provide assistance as the client requires it. Remind the client to transfer to the tub as he has been taught. Be alert for signs of fatigue or weakness.

By the time the client is able to shower, he will have mastered most skills necessary for this independent activity, but your role is to continue to remain close to provide assistance as needed. Be alert for signs of sudden weakness.

## Dressing and Grooming

The person who has been hospitalized or in bed for a long time often starts to feel better about himself when he is dressed in street clothes. He should be encouraged to get dressed for at least part of every day. Even the wheelchair-bound or partially bedbound person should be assisted to put on clothing other than sleepwear for some part of each day. When the dependent person is up and dressed, it affects not only his feelings of self-esteem, it also affects his family's and friends' perceptions about his health. Let him select what he would like to wear and do as much of the actual dressing as possible.

Dressing uses many muscle groups. By dressing himself, the client is helping to improve his coordination, balance, and mobility. Every piece of clothing presents some problem in dressing for the person with functional limitations. However, with careful attention to the types of clothing available and the skills needed to put them on, many problems may be lessened or eliminated.

## Guidelines: Assisting a Client to Dress

- Always dress the weak or most involved extremity first.
- Undress the weak or involved extremity last.
- Help the client select clothing that is roomy and will stretch or give when he is putting it on or taking it off. It is easier to put on a garment that opens all the way down the front than one which must be pulled over an involved arm and then pulled over the head.

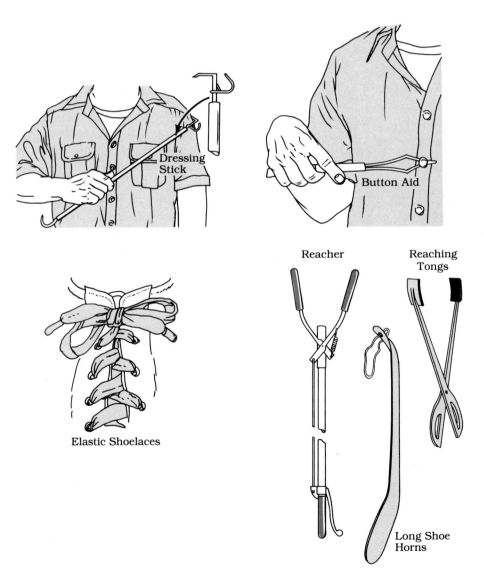

FIGURE 14.26 The client will become more self-sufficient when he learns to dress himself. Adaptive tools may be necessary.

- Position the client in front of a mirror. The client will become aware through his own eyes that he has missed a button, his collar is turned in, or his pants are pulled to the side.
- Lay out the clothing where the client can reach it in the order he will put it on.
- If the OTR has suggested the use of any special tools or adapted equipment for dressing, have them near the client's clothing (Fig. 14.26). Always use a shoehorn when putting on the client's shoes. He may use a dressing stick, a buttonhook, or a reacher when he begins to dress himself again.
- Follow the same procedure each time the client dresses and undresses.
- Follow the procedure that the OTR has established for your client.

## Laundry and Meal Preparation

For clients who live alone or are responsible for a family, it is important that they be able to care for their own basic needs. They should be able to prepare meals, or at least assist in their preparation, and to care for some aspects of housekeeping.

### LAUNDRY

Taking care of one's own laundry is a functional activity. Many clients need some encouragement to resume this function because they will not be able to do things as neatly and as easily as they once did. Assist the client with handwashing clothes, but let the client do as much as possible. Folding, sorting, and stacking clean clothes can be done slowly and should be adapted to the client's individual abilities. Folding socks and shirts obviously is easier than folding sheets. But stacking sheets is easier than stacking socks. These tasks should be shared as the family sees fit.

### MEAL PREPARATION

If the client must eventually take part in meal preparation, assist him to assume this responsibility slowly. Make use of the devices the OTR provides. Be sure the client is instructed by the OTR as to their proper use before he uses them. Supervise the client the first few times he attempts tasks in the kitchen. Praise him and offer support where needed. Point out the success he has. This increases his muscular control.

Include the client in all phases of meal planning and preparation. Use a cutting board with two stainless steel nails projecting from it to hold vegetables, fruits, or meats when paring, scraping, and cutting. Supervise as the client begins to place the food onto the nails, and help if he has difficulty turning it or removing it from the spikes.

Use small containers that are easy to handle. Do not fill containers all the way to the top. Use plastic containers instead of glass ones, if available. Let the client assist with the cleanup after the meal—clean off the table, clean dishes, or dry utensils placed in his lap (Fig. 14.27).

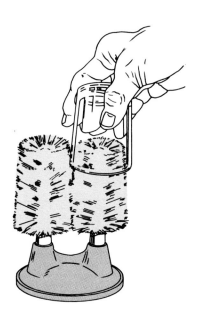
FIGURE 14.27 A glass brush with suction cups can help a client clean up after meals.

# *Feeding*

The person who has difficulty feeding himself, drops utensils, spills food, or chokes and drools when swallowing often gets discouraged. He may refuse to feed himself or to eat as much as he should. He becomes dependent and loses his sense of self-esteem.

Plan mealtimes so that the client can use his available resources and feed himself successfully. He will eat more and feel better emotionally and physically. He will gain many of the motor skills needed to perform other daily living skills.

### HELPING A CLIENT AT MEALTIME

Set up the table or tray so it is convenient and attractive. Give the client utensils and dishes he can handle with a minimum of effort. Use cups and glasses light enough for him to lift and silverware he can grasp securely.

If the client's dominant side is involved and he is still trying to eat with that hand, he may lack sensation and the ability to grasp. You can enlarge the fork or spoon handle by wrapping it with paper towels to about an inch in diameter and tape the paper in place. Or slip a foam rubber curler pad over the handle. Either way will enlarge the gripping surface so the client can hold and lift it more easily. The paper towel is temporary and cannot be washed, but the curler can be removed, washed, squeezed dry, and reused on any utensil. Enlarging the handle also makes it easier to use the nondominant hand. If a person has never used his left or right hand to feed himself, he may need the enlarged handle when he first tries.

A rigid plastic cup may be easier and safer for the client to handle than a breakable glass. If the cup has a large hand opening, it will enable the client to put his fingers or hand around the cup for security (Fig. 14.28).

**FIGURE 14.28**

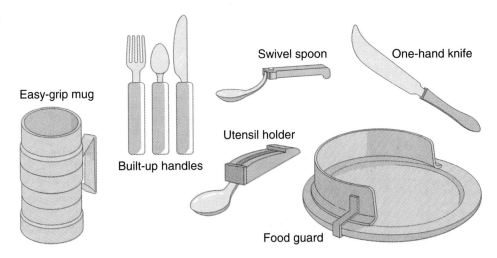

Easy-grip mug

Built-up handles

Swivel spoon

One-hand knife

Utensil holder

Food guard

Some clients have visual problems. They may be totally or partly blind. Objects placed to the far right or far left may not be visible to them. With these clients, you may have to remind them to "look to your left (right)" when they are eating.

Other clients may have sensory deficits that affect eating. If they lack sensation and the facial muscles are weak on one side, these clients will have difficulty with eating. They cannot swallow easily and they tend to "pocket" food between their cheeks and teeth on the involved side of their face. This can cause them to gag and choke as food builds up. You may have to remind this person to move his tongue to that side of the mouth to dislodge the food.

Place a shaving mirror in front of your client and encourage him to glance at it several times during a meal. This will enable him to use his eyes to make him aware of what occurs when he eats. He may begin to automatically wipe his mouth or to search with his tongue to dislodge stored food or food that remains on his lips.

A plate guard is a plastic ring that slips over the edge of a plate and creates a bumper for the client to push food against when eating. As food is pushed against an elevated surface, it piles up and spills onto the client's fork or spoon and enables him to get enough on the utensil to feed himself. Plates, bowls, forks, knives, and spoons with specially built-up handles make it easier for the client to grasp and hold onto while eating. If a client's grasp is too weak to hold a fork or spoon without dropping it, a feeding cuff may help. It fits over the client's hand. The spoon or fork slips into the pocket and allows the client to lift the utensil without having to grasp it tightly. Cups and glasses with handles open at the bottom can "clip" onto the client's hand, reducing his need to hold tightly while lifting the cup.

## Leisure Activities

These skills are given little space in this chapter because you, the homemaker/home health aide, have other responsibilities. Often only the physical part of care is stressed, but if you can incorporate some pleasurable activities into your daily routine, you will contribute to the client's recovery. The client who used to crochet or knit or sew may wish to relearn these skills. The OTR will instruct the client to do these things again in spite of the disability.

Perhaps a client has a perceptual deficit and does not "see" things as they really are. He may not be able to follow the printed lines in a newspaper or read a book because his eyes cannot see the last few words on every line. The OTR works with this client to help him improve his reading ability.

If these pleasurable pastimes are used as tools during therapy, you may be asked to follow through with the program. Of course, you will be told exactly how to help in any activity of this kind.

On your own, if you have time to play a simple card game with a client, read aloud to him, or turn on the record player for him, it will take his mind off his physical problems and bring him pleasure. Any extra activity that expands the area of interest for a client is both pleasurable and beneficial.

## Topics for Discussion

1. Read a few case studies and review the different therapies represented and the aide's role in each case.
2. What would you say to a family when they complain that their relative is not getting better quickly enough?
3. What will you say when a client asks you: "Will I be like I was before this happened to me?"

# Chapter 15

# Measuring and Recording Client Vital Signs

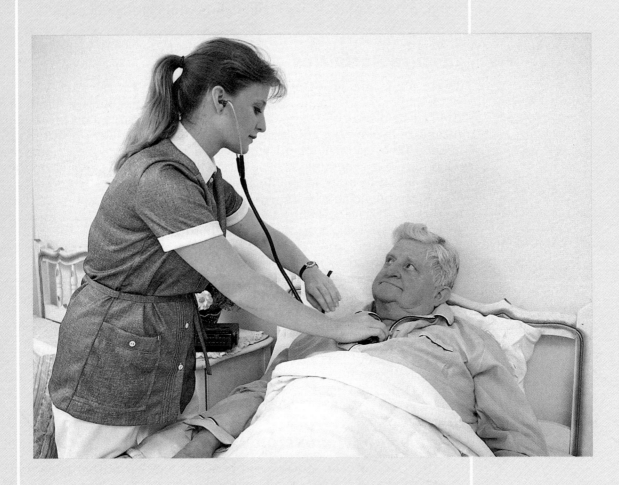

## Objectives: What You Will Learn to Do

- Explain the term *vital signs*.
- State the average adult normal rate for vital signs.
- Explain when vital signs are measured.

### *Introduction: Vital Signs*

**vital signs** temperature, pulse, respiration, and blood pressure

**Vital signs** are those bodily functions that reflect the state of health of the body and that are easily measurable. The term *vital signs* refers to body temperature, pulse rate, respiratory rate, and blood pressure. It is often written as TPR&BP (Fig.15.1).

FIGURE 15.1

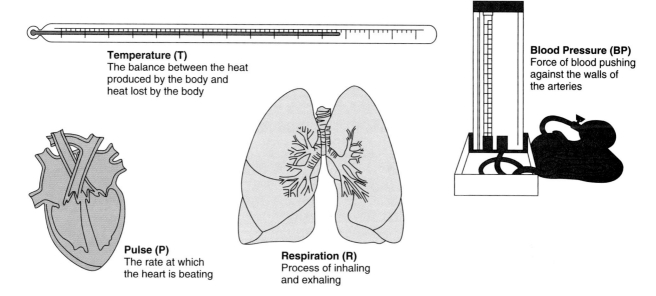

**Temperature (T)**
The balance between the heat produced by the body and heat lost by the body

**Blood Pressure (BP)**
Force of blood pushing against the walls of the arteries

**Pulse (P)**
The rate at which the heart is beating

**Respiration (R)**
Process of inhaling and exhaling

When the body is not functioning normally, the measurable rates of vital signs change. Everyone who measures and records client's vital signs must be very careful and accurate. When you record the reading, write carefully. Be sure your handwriting is clear and easy to read. If you are not sure of your reading, mention this when you report the reading to your supervisor.

### WHEN ARE VITAL SIGNS CHECKED?

Your supervisor will tell you when and how often to check your client's vital signs. This decision will be based on the client's present condition, his past history, and his prognosis. Vital signs are not always checked in the home as often as they are in the hospital because home care clients are often in a more stable condition.

You should check the vital signs if you observe any change in your client or after a fall. Then when you call your supervisor to report the change, report these vital signs. This information will assist her in making a decision over the telephone. Be sure to record all signs when you take them. If you don't, you will forget.

### Average Normal Adult Rates

- Temperature: 98.6°F or 37°C
- Pulse: 60–80 regular beats per minute
- Respiration: 16–20 regular breaths per minute
- Blood pressure: Infants: 50/40 to 80/58 mm of mercury
- Under eighteen years old: below 120/80 mm of mercury
- Eighteen to fifty years old: below 140/90 mm of mercury

These rates are given to you as a guide. A person can have a reading that varies from these figures and be very healthy. But if you took thousands and thousands of TPR&BP, you would have average readings as indicated. On an individual basis, it is more correct to compare several of your client's readings than to compare his with the average rates.

### Reporting Vital Signs

When you are given the assignment of taking a client's vital signs, your supervisor will tell you when you should call her with the readings. In the home, you may often take vital signs without reporting them each time. It is most important, however, for you to know when to report your findings. *Ask* for guidance. If you are in doubt, report. It is far better to report an unnecessary reading than not to report one that is necessary.

### Telling a Client His Vital Signs

There was a time when hospitals and doctors did not share information with clients. This time has passed. Especially in a person's home, you will be expected to share the vital sign readings with your client. Please do so promptly. If you do not, the client may think you are hiding something from him. Remember, it is his body you are caring for and he has the right to know how it is working. There are clients who do not wish to know their vital signs. Do not force the information upon them. You will also work in some homes where, for one reason or another, the client will not be told. Your supervisor will tell you how to handle this situation. Remember, you must abide by the wishes of the family and the physician's decision, even if you do not agree with them!

## Section 2  Measuring Temperature

**Objectives:**
**What You Will**
**Learn to Do**

- Read a thermometer accurately.
- Demonstrate the procedure for measuring oral temperatures.
- Demonstrate the procedure for measuring rectal temperatures.
- Demonstrate the procedure for measuring axillary temperatures.

# Introduction: Body Temperature

Body temperature is a measurement of the amount of heat in the body. The balance between the heat produced and the heat lost is the body temperature. The normal adult body temperature is 98.6°F or 37°C. There is a normal range in which a person's body temperature may vary and still be considered normal (Fig. 15.2).

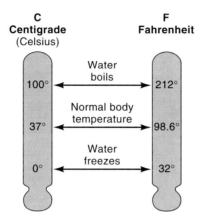

**FIGURE 15.2** The two major scales used for measuring temperature.

temperature measurement of the amount of heat in the body at a given time. The normal body temperature is 98.6°F (37°C)

## NORMAL RANGES OF BODY TEMPERATURE

- Oral: 97.6 to 99°F (36.4 to 37.2°C)
- Rectal: 98.6 to 100°F (37.0 to 37.8°C)
- Axillary: 96.6 to 98°C (35.9 to 36.7°C)

For recording the client's **temperature,** three symbols are used:

1. degrees
2. F **Fahrenheit**
3. C **Centigrade** or Celsius

You will record the client's temperatures according to the method used by your agency.

Fahrenheit temperature can be written in two ways:

98.6°F or 98°F

If you are using a centigrade (Celsius) thermometer, the temperature would be written

37°C or 37.3°C

Write an R with the temperature reading if a rectal temperature was taken. Write an A beside the temperature reading if an axillary temperature was taken.

thermometer instrument used for measuring temperature

The body temperature is measured with an instrument called a **thermometer.** This is a delicate, hollow, glass tube with a liquid metal called mercury sealed inside it. Mercury is an element that is very sensitive to temperature. It expands when the temperature rises and contracts when the temperature goes down. Even if the temperature rises only slightly, the mercury will expand and travel up the tube, indicating the change. The outside of the glass thermometer is marked with lines, or calibrations, and numbers. These markings make it possible to measure exactly the change in the mercury. By knowing the change, you will be able to know the body temperature.

## TYPES OF THERMOMETERS

There are several different types of thermometers. They are:

- Glass
- Battery-operated electronic (Fig. 15.3)
- Chemically-treated paper

*FIGURE 15.3*

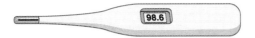

Each battery operated and chemical thermometer is slightly altered. Read the instructions carefully before using them.

This section is concerned only with the standard glass thermometer. This is the most common type of thermometer found in the home. There are three types of glass thermometers (Fig. 15.4). They are:

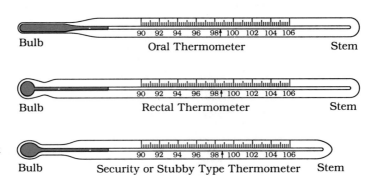

*FIGURE 15.4* Use the correct thermometer for the correct purpose.

1. *Oral.* This type is used to measure the client's temperature by mouth and is also used in measuring the axillary temperature (under the client's arm, in his armpit area). The bulb is long and thin so as to be exposed to as much of the lining of the mouth as possible.
2. *Rectal.* This type is used to measure the client's temperature by inserting the thermometer into the rectum. The bulb is small and round. This type of bulb prevents the thermometer from injuring the rectum.
3. *Security.* This type has a very strong construction. It is used for taking an infant's rectal temperature. Many agencies use the security or stubby type with a red knob at the stem for rectal temperatures and the one with a green knob at the stem for oral temperatures.

---

## ■■■ Guidelines: Safety Considerations While Using Thermometers

- Do not expect a client to talk with a thermometer in his mouth.
- Glass thermometers break and shatter easily. Handle them with care. Be especially careful to avoid breaking a thermometer while it is in a client's mouth or rectum.
- The liquid metal (mercury) inside the thermometer is a poison; that is, it may be harmful if it is swallowed or if it comes in contact with the skin for a prolonged period of time.

- Keep all thermometers in a case. Do not leave them loose in a pocket, drawer, or dresser.
- Never clean a glass thermometer with hot water. The mercury will expand so much that the thermometer will explode.
- If the client feels that he may be about to sneeze, he should remove the thermometer.

## Procedure 43: Shaking Down a Glass Thermometer

1. Assemble your equipment:
   Thermometer in a container
2. Wash your hands.
3. Before using the thermometer, check to make sure that it is not cracked or that the bulb is not chipped.
4. Hold the thermometer firmly between your fingers and your thumb at the stem end farthest from the bulb. The bulb is the end that is inserted into the client's body.
5. Stand clear of any hard surfaces such as counters and tables to avoid striking and breaking the thermometer while you are shaking it. For practice, you might stand with your arm over a pillow or mattress in case you accidentally drop the thermometer.
6. When you are sure that you have a good hold on the thermometer, shake your hand loosely from the wrist. Do it as if you were shaking water from your fingers.
7. Snap your wrist again and again. This will shake down the mercury to the lowest possible point. This should be below the numbers and lines (calibrations).
8. Always do this before and after using a thermometer.

## Procedure 44: Reading a Fahrenheit Thermometer

1. With your thumb and first two fingers, hold the thermometer at the stem.
2. Hold the thermometer at eye level. Turn the thermometer back and forth between your fingers until you can clearly see the column of mercury.
3. Notice the scale or calibrations. Each long line stands for one degree.
4. There are four short lines between each of the long lines. Each short line stands for two tenths (0.2) of a degree.
5. Between the long lines that represent 98° and 99°, look for a longer line with an arrow directly beneath it. This special line points out normal body temperature.
6. Look at the end of the mercury. Notice the line or number where the mercury ends. If it is one of the short lines, notice the previous longer line toward the silver tip that

Accuracy is
Extremely Important.

Look at the Mercury Carefully
When Reading a
Thermometer

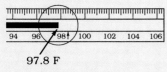

97.8 F

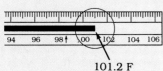

101.2 F

goes into the client's mouth. The temperature reading is the degree marked by that long line plus two, four, six, or eight tenths of a degree. Example: If the mercury ends after the 97 line, on the fourth short line, the temperature is 97.8 (Fig. 15.5a). If the mercury ends between two lines, use the closer line.

7. Write down the client's temperature right away, using the figure you read on the thermometer. Some agencies will write 97.8°F. Others will write 97°F. Follow the method used by your agency.

# Procedure 45: Reading a Centigrade (Celsius) Thermometer

FIGURE 15.5b

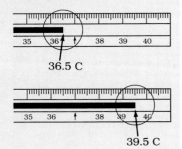

36.5 C

39.5 C

1. With your thumb and first two fingers, hold the thermometer at the stem.

2. Hold it at eye level. Turn the thermometer back and forth between your fingers until you can clearly see the column of mercury.

3. Notice the scale or calibration. Each long line shows one degree.

4. There are nine short lines between each number. These short lines are one, two, three, four, five, six, seven, eight, and nine tenths of a degree. If the mercury ended after the 36° and on the third short line, the temperature would read 36.5°C (Fig. 15.5b). If the mercury ended after the long line 37° and on the eighth short line, the temperature would read 37.8°C. If the mercury ends after line 37° on the fifth short line, the temperature would be 37.5°C.

5. Write down the client's temperature right away. Some agencies write 37°C. Others will write 37C. Follow the method used by your agency.

# Procedure 46: Cleaning a Thermometer

1. Assemble your equipment:
Thermometer
Tissue and/or cotton balls
Soap
Cool running water

2. Wipe the thermometer off from the stem to the bulb. Throw away the tissue (Fig 15.6).

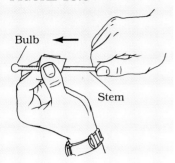

FIGURE 15.6

Bulb ←

Stem

3. Soap a tissue.
4. Holding the thermometer, rotate the soapy tissue around the thermometer from the stem to the bulb.
5. Holding the thermometer under cool running water, repeat the process.
6. Discard the tissue.
7. Dry the thermometer with a dry tissue.
8. Put the thermometer into a case, bulb first.
9. Wash your hands.

## Procedure 47: Measuring an Oral Temperature

1. Assemble your equipment:
   Clean oral thermometer in a case
   Tissue or paper towel
   Pad and pencil
   Watch
2. Wash your hands.
3. Tell the client that you are going to take his temperature orally.
4. Ask the client if he has recently had hot or cold liquids or if he has smoked. If the answer is yes, wait 10 minutes before taking his temperature.
5. The client should be in bed or sitting in a chair. Do not take a temperature while the client is walking.
6. Take the thermometer out of the container, and inspect it for cracks or chips. Do not use it if you see any.
7. Shake the mercury down until it is below the calibrations.
8. Run the thermometer under cool water. This will make the thermometer more pleasant in the client's mouth.
9. Ask the client to lift up his tongue. Place the bulb end of the thermometer under his tongue. Ask him to keep his lips gently around the thermometer without biting it (Fig 15.7). (If the client cannot close his mouth, take the temperature by another method.)

FIGURE 15.7

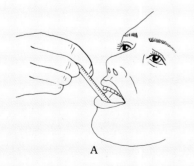
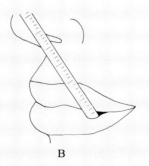
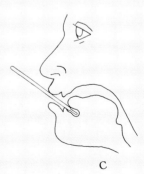

A B C

10. Leave the thermometer in place for 8 minutes. (The latest research shows that oral temperature is more accurate when the thermometer remains in the mouth for 8 minutes. However, if it is the policy of your agency to let the thermometer stay only 3 to 4 minutes, follow the policy of your agency.)

11. Stay with your client if you feel that he cannot keep his mouth closed.

12. Take the thermometer out of the client's mouth. Hold the stem end and wipe the thermometer with a tissue from the stem toward the bulb.

13. Read the thermometer.

14. Record the temperature and your observations concerning the client during this procedure.

15. Shake down the mercury.

16. Clean the thermometer.

17. Make the client comfortable.

18. Wash your hands.

## MEASURING RECTAL TEMPERATURE

Always use a rectal thermometer for taking rectal temperatures. Under the following conditions you would automatically take a rectal temperature:

- When the client is an infant or a child who cannot safely use an oral thermometer
- When the client is having warm or cold applications on his face or neck
- When the client cannot keep his mouth closed around the thermometer
- When the client finds it hard to breathe through his nose
- When the client's mouth is dry or inflamed
- When the client is restless, delirious, unconscious, or confused
- When the client is getting oxygen by cannula, catheter, or face mask
- When the client has had major surgery in the areas of his face or neck
- When the client's face is partially paralyzed, as from a stroke

## Procedure 48: Measuring a Rectal Temperature

1. Assemble your equipment:
   Rectal thermometer in a case
   Tissue or paper towel
   Lubricating jelly
   Pad and pencil
   Watch

2. Wash your hands.

3. Ask visitors to leave the room if appropriate.

4. Tell the client you are going to measure his temperature rectally.

5. Lower the backrest on the bed.

6. Take the thermometer out of its container. Hold the stem.

7. Inspect the thermometer for cracks or chips. Do not use if you see any.

8. Shake down the mercury until it is below the calibrations.

9. Put a small amount of lubricating jelly on a piece of tissue. Lubricate the bulb of the thermometer with the jelly. This makes the insertion easier and also makes it more comfortable for the client.

10. Ask the client to turn on his side. If he is unable to turn, position him on his side. Turn back the top covers just enough so that you can see the client's buttocks. Avoid overexposing him.

11. With one hand, raise the upper buttock until you see the anus. With the other hand, gently insert the bulb 1 inch through the anus into the rectum (Fig 15.8).

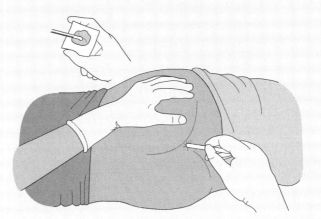

*FIGURE 15.8*

12. If the client is an infant, remove the diaper. Lay the baby on his back. Raise his legs with one hand. Insert the thermometer with the other hand, 1/2 inch into the rectum. Always hold the thermometer while it is in the child's rectum.

13. Hold the thermometer in place for 3 minutes. Do not leave a client with a rectal thermometer in the rectum, no matter what his condition.

14. Remove the thermometer from the client's rectum. Holding the stem end of the thermometer, wipe it with a tissue from stem to bulb to remove particles of feces.

15. Read the thermometer.

16. Record the temperature and your observations concerning the client during this procedure. (Note this is a rectal temperature by writing *R* next to the reading.)

17. Make the client comfortable.

18. Clean the thermometer.

19. Shake the mercury down until it is below the calibrations.

20. Replace the thermometer in its container.

21. Wash your hands.

# Procedure 49: Measuring an Axillary Temperature

1. Assemble your equipment:
   Oral thermometer in a container
   Tissue or paper towel
   Pad and pencil
   Watch
2. Wash your hands.
3. Ask visitors to leave the room if appropriate.
4. Tell the client that you are going to take his temperature by placing a thermometer under his arm.
5. Remove the thermometer from its case and shake down the mercury so that it is below the calibrations.
6. Inspect the thermometer for cracks or chips. Do not use it if you see any.
7. Remove the client's arm from the sleeve. If the axillary region is moist with perspiration, pat it dry with a towel.
8. Place the bulb of the oral thermometer in the center of the armpit in an upright position.
9. Put the client's arm across his chest or abdomen (Fig. 15.9).
10. If the client is unconscious or too weak to help, you will have to hold the arm in place.
11. Leave the thermometer in place 10 minutes. Stay with the client.
12. Remove the thermometer. Wipe it off with a tissue from the stem to the bulb.
13. Read the thermometer.
14. Record the temperature and your observations concerning the client during this procedure. (Note that this is an axillary temperature by placing an *A* next to the reading.)
15. Shake the mercury down until it is below the calibrations.
16. Clean the thermometer.
17. Replace the thermometer in its case.
18. Make the client comfortable.
19. Wash your hands.

FIGURE 15.9

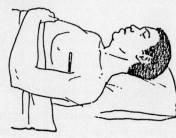

## ■ Using a Plastic Sheath over a Thermometer

Plastic thermometer covers, or sheaths, are used to protect the thermometer from the client's secretions and to aid in the cleanup of the thermometer and the reading of the thermometer. The use of a sheath does not mean that you do not have to wash the thermometer after each use; it only makes the washing easier. Be sure to read the directions for each type of sheath as they differ slightly from manufacturer to manufacturer. Also, remember that sheaths for rectal and oral thermometers are different and should not be used interchangeably.

## Procedure 50: Using a Thermometer Sheath

FIGURE 15.10

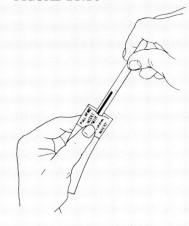

1. Assemble your equipment:
   Thermometer
   Thermometer sheath
   Trash bag
   Tissues
2. Wash your hands.
3. Shake down the thermometer.
4. Hold the sheath so that you can insert the thermometer into the plastic between the paper covering (Fig. 15.10).
5. Withdraw the thermometer, now covered with the clear plastic sheath. Be sure the sheath is covering the entire thermometer and is not hanging off the end (Fig. 15.11).

FIGURE 15.11

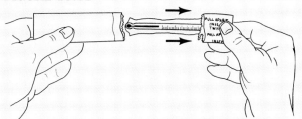

6. Take the client's temperature using the standard procedure (Lubricating the rectal thermometer may be unnecessary as the rectal sheaths usually come prelubricated.)
7. Remove the thermometer from the client.
   a. Remove the sheath with a tissue and discard it in the trash (Fig. 15.12). Or
   b. Insert the sheath back into the package outer sleeve. Remove the thermometer, leaving the contaminated sheath in the sleeve. Discard it in the trash.

FIGURE 15.12

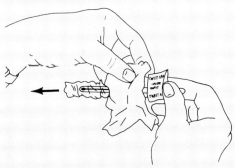

8. Read the thermometer and record the temperature.
9. Wash and store the thermometer according to the standard procedure.
10. Wash your hands.

**Objectives: What You Will Learn to Do**

■ Count the pulse.
■ Report the rate and rhythm of the pulse accurately.

### Introduction: The Pulse

Each time the heart beats, it pumps a certain amount of blood into the arteries. This causes the arteries to expand. Between heart-beats, the arteries contract and return to their normal size. The heart pumps the blood in a steady rhythm. The rhythmic expansion and contraction of the arteries, which can be measured to show how fast the heart is beating, is called the **pulse**. Measuring the pulse is one method of observing how the circulatory system is functioning.

**pulse** rhythmic expansion and contractions of the arteries caused by the beating of the heart

The pulse measures how fast the heart is beating. At certain places on the body, the pulse can be felt easily under a person's fingers (Fig. 15.13). One of the easiest places to feel the pulse is at the wrist. This is called a radial pulse because you are feeling the radial artery (Fig 15.14). When taking the pulse, you must be able to report accurately the following:

■ *Rate:* the number of pulse beats per minute
■ *Rhythm:* the regularity of the pulse beats, that is, whether the length of time between the beats is steady and regular
■ *Force:* the strength of the beat (weak or bounding)

**apical** refers to the apex of the heart

You will use a stethoscope to listen to the **apical** pulse. The apical pulse is the pulse measured at the apex of the heart. The **stethoscope**

**stethoscope** instrument that allows one to listen to various sounds in the human body

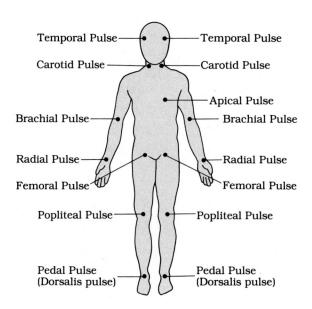

Temporal Pulse — Temporal Pulse
Carotid Pulse — Carotid Pulse
Apical Pulse
Brachial Pulse — Brachial Pulse
Radial Pulse — Radial Pulse
Femoral Pulse — Femoral Pulse
Popliteal Pulse — Popliteal Pulse
Pedal Pulse (Dorsalis pulse) — Pedal Pulse (Dorsalis pulse)

**FIGURE 15.13** Pulses can be felt at many places on the body.

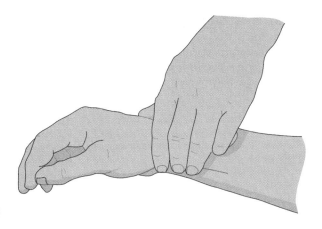

FIGURE 15.14

## Procedure 51: Measuring the Radial Pulse

1. Assemble your equipment:
   Watch with a second hand
   Pad and pencil
2. Wash your hands.
3. Tell the client that you are going to take his pulse.
4. If the client is standing, ask him to sit down. Or have him lying in a comfortable position in bed for 5 minutes before you measure the pulse.
5. The client's hand and arm should be well supported and resting comfortably.
6. Find the pulse by placing the tips of your middle three fingers on the palm side of the client's wrist in a line with his thumb directly next to the bone. Press lightly until you feel the beat. (If you press too hard, you may stop the flow of blood and then you will not be able to feel a pulse. Never use your thumb. Your thumb has its own pulse and you would be counting it instead of the client's.) When you have found the pulse, notice the rhythm. Note if the beat is steady or irregular. Notice the force of the beat.
7. Look at the position of the second hand on your watch. Start counting the pulse beats (what you feel) until the second hand comes back to the same number on the clock.
   a. Method A: Count the pulse beats for 1 full minute and report the full-minute count. This is always done if the client has an irregular beat.
   b. Method B: Count for 30 seconds, until the second hand is opposite its position when you started. Then multiply the number of beats by 2. This answer is the number you record. For example, if the count for 30 seconds is 35, the count for 60 seconds is 70 beats.
8. Record the pulse rate, rhythm, and force immediately.
9. Make the client comfortable.
10. Wash your hands.

is an instrument that makes it possible to listen to various sounds in a client's body. The stethoscope is a tube with one end that picks up sound when it is placed against a part of the body. This end is either bell-shaped and called a **bell**, or it is round and flat and is called a **diaphragm** (Fig. 15.15).

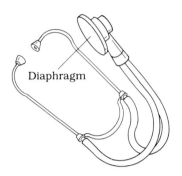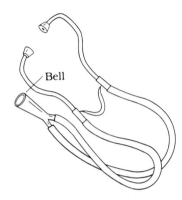

Diaphragm

Bell

*FIGURE 15.15*

## Procedure 52: Measuring the Apical Pulse

1. Assemble your equipment:
   Stethoscope and antiseptic swabs
   Watch with a second hand
   Pad and pencil
2. Wash your hands.
3. Ask visitors to leave the room if appropriate.
4. Explain to the client that you are going to take his apical pulse.
5. Clean the earplugs of the stethoscope with antiseptic solution. Put the earplugs in your ears facing forward.
6. Uncover the left side of the client's chest. Avoid overexposing the client.
7. Locate the apex of the client's heart by placing the bell or diaphragm of the stethoscope under the client's left breast. Be sure this is the place you hear the heart beating the loudest.
8. Count the heart sounds for a full minute (Fig. 15.16).

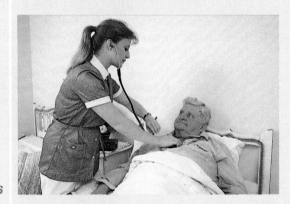

*FIGURE 15.16*

9. Write the full-minute count on the note paper. Also record the rhythm and the quality of the sounds and your observations concerning the client during this procedure.
10. Cover the client and make him comfortable.
11. Clean the earplugs of the stethoscope. Return the equipment to its proper place.
12. Wash your hands.

The apical-radial deficit is the difference between the pulse count at the apex of the heart and the radial artery. This is one way to see if the circulatory system is working properly.

## Procedure 53: Measuring the Apical-Radial Deficit

1. Assemble your equipment:
   Stethoscope and antiseptic swabs
   Watch with a second hand
   Pad and pencil
2. Wash your hands.
3. Ask visitors to leave the room if appropriate.
4. Explain to the client that you are going to take his pulse both apically and radially.
5. There are two methods of taking the apical pulse deficit: Method A. Two people do this procedure together at the same time. One counts the radial pulse. The other counts the apical pulse for 1 full minute (Fig. 15.17). The difference between the two pulses is known as the apical-radial deficit. Method B. The homemaker/home health aide first takes the apical pulse, then the radial pulse. The difference between the two pulses is known as the apical-radial deficit. However, because the readings are not taken at the same time, it is not considered as accurate as the first method.

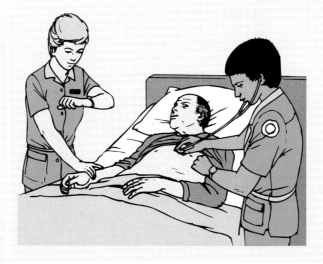

FIGURE 15.17

6. Count the apical pulse and the radial pulse for a full minute, and record both figures.
7. Record the figure for the pulse deficit and your observations concerning the client during this procedure.
8. Make the client comfortable.
9. Clean the equipment and return it to its proper place.
10. Wash your hands.

# Section 4   Measuring Respirations

## Objectives: What You Will Learn to Do

■ Count a client's respirations accurately.
■ Determine if the client's breathing is labored or noisy.

 ### Introduction: Measuring Respirations

The human body must have a steady supply of air. When you breathe in, air is drawn into the lungs. The waste products from this process are removed from the body as we exhale.

**respiration** process of breathing; inhaling and exhaling air

**Respiration** is the process of inhaling and exhaling. One respiration includes breathing in once and breathing out once. When a person breathes in, his chest expands. When he breathes out, his chest contracts. When you count respirations, you watch a person's chest rise and fall as he breathes. Or you feel his chest rise and fall with your hand. Either way, you should count respirations without the client knowing it. If he thinks his breathing is being counted, he will not breathe naturally. What you want to count is his natural breathing. Besides counting respirations, you will be noticing whether the client seems to breathe easily or seems to be working hard to get his breath. When a person is working hard to get his breath, it is called **labored** respiration. You must also notice whether his breathing is noisy.

**labored** difficult

Normally adults breathe at a rate of from 10 to 20 times a minute. Children breathe more rapidly. The elderly breathe more slowly. Exercise, digestion, emotional stress, disease conditions, some drugs, stimulants, heat, and cold can all affect the number of times a person breathes per minute.

### ABNORMAL RESPIRATION

While you are counting the client's respirations, it is important to observe and make note of anything about his breathing that appears to be abnormal. Different types of abnormal respiration that you should be familiar with are:

■ *Stertorous respiration.* The client makes abnormal noises like snoring sounds when he is breathing.

- *Abdominal respiration.* The client breathes using mostly his abdominal muscles.
- *Shallow respiration.* The client breathes using only the upper part of the lungs.
- *Irregular respiration.* The depth of breathing changes and the rate of the rise and fall of the chest is not steady.
- ***Cheyne-Stokes respiration.*** At first the breathing is slow and shallow; then the respiration becomes faster and deeper until it reaches a kind of peak. The respiration then slows down and becomes shallow again. The breathing may then stop completely for 10 seconds and then begin the pattern again. This type of respiration may be caused by certain cerebral (brain), cardiac (heart), or pulmonary (chest) diseases or conditions. It frequently occurs before death.

**Cheyne-Stokes respiration** a type of noisy breathing alternating with periods of no breathing; usually precedes death

# Procedure 54: Measuring Respirations

1. Assemble your equipment:
   Watch with a second hand
   Pad and pencil
2. Wash your hands.
3. Ask visitors to leave the room if appropriate.
4. Hold the client's wrist just as if you were taking his pulse. This way he will not know you are watching his breathing. Count the client's respirations, without his knowing it, immediately after counting his pulse rate (Fig. 15.18).
5. If the client is a child who has been crying or is restless, wait until he is quiet before counting respirations. If a child is asleep, count his respirations before he wakes up. Always count a child's pulse and respirations before you

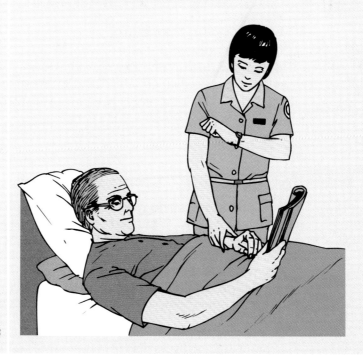

*FIGURE 15.18*

measure the temperature. (Most children get upset when you measure their temperature.)

6. One rise and one fall of the client's chest count as one respiration.

7. If you cannot clearly see the chest rise and fall, fold the client's arms across his chest. Then you can feel his breathing as you hold his wrist.

8. Check the position of the second hand on the watch. Count "one" when you see the client's chest rising as he breathes in. The next time his chest rises, count "two." Keep doing this for a full minute. Report the number of respirations you count.

9. You may be permitted to count for 30 seconds. Count the respirations for 30 seconds and then multiply the number you counted by 2. For example, if you count 8 respirations in 30 seconds (a half-minute), your number for a full minute is 16.

10. If the client's breathing rhythm is irregular, always count for a full minute. Observe the depth of the breathing while counting the respirations.

11. Immediately write down the number you counted.

12. Note whether the respirations were noisy or labored and your observations concerning the client during this procedure.

13. Make the client comfortable.

14. Wash your hands.

# Section 5  Measuring Blood Pressure

## Objectives: What You Will Learn to Do

- Explain systolic pressure.
- Explain diastolic pressure.
- Demonstrate the use of aneroid and mercury types of blood pressure equipment accurately and efficiently.
- Measure a client's blood pressure accurately.

### *Introduction: Blood Pressure*

**blood pressure** force of blood on the inner walls of blood vessels as it flows through them

**Blood pressure** is the force of the blood pushing against the walls of the blood vessels. When you take a client's blood pressure, you are measuring the force of the blood flowing through the arteries.

There is always a certain amount of pressure in the arteries. This is because the heart, by pumping, is constantly forcing blood to circulate. The amount of pressure in the arteries depends on two things: the rate of heartbeat, and how easily the blood flows through the blood vessels.

The heart contracts as it pumps the blood into the arteries. When the heart is contracting, the pressure is highest. This pressure is

**systolic pressure** force with which blood is pumped when the heart contracts

**diastolic pressure** the pressure in the blood vessels measured when the heart is relaxed

called the **systolic pressure**. As the heart relaxes between each contraction, the pressure goes down. When the heart is most relaxed, the pressure is lowest. This pressure is called the **diastolic pressure**. When you take a client's blood pressure, you are measuring these two pressures.

In young healthy adults below forty years old the normal blood pressure range is below 140 millimeters (mm) mercury (Hg) systolic pressure and below 90 millimeters (mm) mercury (Hg) diastolic pressure. These figures are written:

$$140/90 \text{ or } \frac{140}{90} \begin{array}{l} = \text{systolic} \\ = \text{diastolic} \end{array}$$

In adults over forty years old, 160/90 or less is considered normal.

**hypertension** high blood pressure

**hypotension** low blood pressure

When a person's blood pressure is higher than the normal range for his age and condition, it is referred to as high blood pressure or **hypertension**. When a client's blood pressure is lower than the normal range for his age and condition, it is referred to as low blood pressure or **hypotension**. One reading of high blood pressure does not mean that a person has hypertension. This diagnosis can only be made by a physician after a complete medical evaluation.

### INSTRUMENTS FOR MEASURING BLOOD PRESSURE

**sphygmomanometer** apparatus for measuring blood pressure of which there are two types, mercury or aneroid; blood pressure cuff.

When you take a client's blood pressure, you will be using an instrument called a **sphygmomanometer**. Sphygmomanometer is a combination of three Greek words:

1. *Sphygmo*, meaning pulse
2. *Mano*, meaning pressure
3. *Meter*, meaning measure

This instrument, however, is usually called simply the **blood pressure cuff**. The four main parts of this instrument are the manometer, valve, cuff, and bulb (Fig. 15.19).

Two kinds of instruments are used for taking blood pressure. One is the **mercury** type. The other is called the **aneroid** (dial) type. Both kinds have an inflatable cloth-covered rubber bag or cuff. The cuff is wrapped around the client's arm. Both kinds also have a rubber bulb for pumping air into the cuff. The procedure for measuring blood pressure is the same, except for reading the measurement. When you use the mercury type, you will be watching the level of a column of mercury on a measuring scale. When you use the dial or aneroid type, you will be watching a pointer on a dial.

When you take a client's blood pressure, you will be doing two things at the same time. You will be listening to the brachial pulse as it sounds in the brachial artery in the client's arm. You will also be watching an indicator (either a column of mercury or a dial) in order to take a reading (Fig. 15.20).

You will use a stethoscope to listen to the brachial pulse. It is important to note the first tapping sound you hear and the last sound you hear. Sometimes you will hear a tapping sound, then silence, then a tapping sound again. The *true* reading is the *first* sound you hear. Often the first sound is missed by improper techniques and only the second sound is heard and recorded. By following the procedure in this book carefully, you will not miss the first sound and will record an accurate and truthful blood pressure.

## MERCURY SPHYGMOMANOMETER

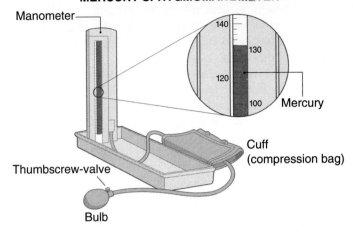

Manometer

140
130
120
100

Mercury

Cuff
(compression bag)

Thumbscrew-valve

Bulb

## ANEROID SPHYGMOMANOMETER

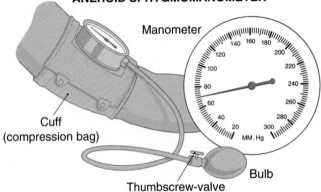

Manometer

Cuff
(compression bag)

Thumbscrew-valve

Bulb

**FIGURE 5.19** Sphygmomano-
meters may look different, but
they all measure blood pressure
accurately.

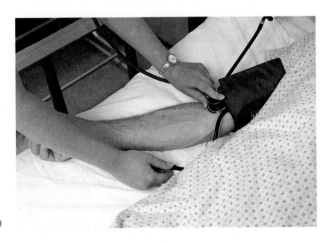

**FIGURE 15.20**

If you should hear the tapping noise all the way to the "O" on your
indicator, try and listen for a change in the sound and record the
client's blood pressure reading as follows:

142/72/0

142  systolic reading—first tapping sound heard

72  diastolic reading—change in sound

0  last sound heard

# Procedure 55: Measuring Blood Pressure

(This procedure is based on the article, "Hypertension—What Can Go Wrong When You Measure Blood Pressure," *American Journal of Nursing* 8, no. 5 (1980): 942–945.)

1. Assemble your equipment:
   Sphygmomanometer (blood pressure cuff)
   Stethoscope
   Antiseptic pad to clean earpieces of stethoscope
   Pad and pencil

2. Wash your hands.

3. Tell the client that you are going to take his blood pressure.

4. Wipe the earplugs of the stethoscope with the antiseptic pad.

5. Have the client resting quietly. He should be either lying down or sitting in a chair.

6. If you are using the mercury apparatus, the measuring scale should be level with your eyes.

7. The client's arm should be bare up to the shoulder, or the client's sleeve should be well above the elbow.

8. The client's arm from the elbow down should be resting fully extended on the bed. Or it might be resting on the arm of the chair or your hip, well supported, with the palm upward.

9. Unroll the cuff, and loosen the valve on the bulb. Then squeeze the compression bag to deflate it completely.

10. Wrap the cuff snugly and smoothly around the client's arm above the elbow. But do not wrap it so tightly that the client is uncomfortable from the pressure.

11. Leave the area clear where you will place the bell or diaphragm of the stethoscope.

12. Be sure the manometer is in position so you can read the numbers easily.

13. With your fingertips, find the client's brachial pulse at the inner side of the arm above the elbow. Hold your fingers there and inflate the cuff until the pulse disappears. Note the reading on the indicator. Quickly deflate the cuff. This is the approximation of the client's systolic reading and is called the palpated systolic pressure (Fig. 15.21).

14. Put the ear pieces of the stethoscope into your ears and place the bell or diaphragm of the stethoscope on the brachial pulse. Hold it snugly but not too tightly. Do not let the stethoscope touch the blood pressure cuff.

15. Tighten the thumbscrew of the valve to close it. Turn it clockwise. Be careful not to turn it too tightly. If you do, you will have trouble opening it.

16. Hold the stethoscope in place. Inflate the cuff until the dial points to 30 mm above the palpated systolic pressure.

**FIGURE 15.21**

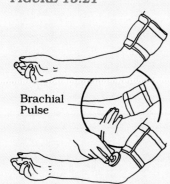

Brachial Pulse

17. Open the valve counterclockwise. This allows the air to escape. Let it out slowly until the sound of the pulse comes back. A few seconds must go by without sounds. If you do hear pulse sounds immediately, you must stop the procedure. Then completely deflate the cuff. Wait a few seconds. Then inflate the cuff to a much higher calibration above 200. Again, loosen the thumbscrew to let the air out. Listen for a repeated pulse sound. At the same time, watch the indicator.

18. Note the calibration that the pointer passes as you hear the first sound. This point indicates the systolic pressure (or the top number) (Fig 15.22).

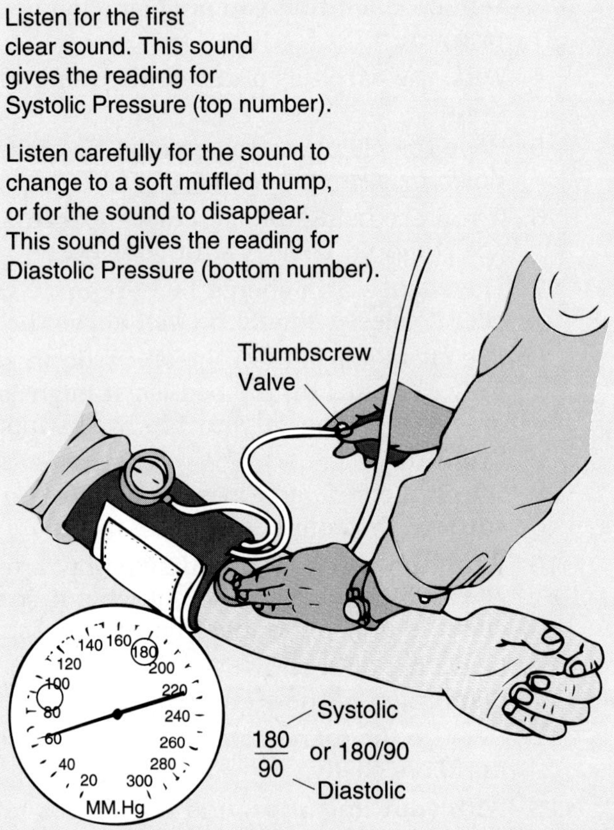

Listen for the first clear sound. This sound gives the reading for Systolic Pressure (top number).

Listen carefully for the sound to change to a soft muffled thump, or for the sound to disappear. This sound gives the reading for Diastolic Pressure (bottom number).

FIGURE 15.22

19. Continue releasing the air from the cuff. When the sounds change to a softer and faster thud, or disappear, note the calibration. This is the diastolic pressure (or bottom number).

20. Deflate the cuff completely. Remove it from the client's arm.

21. Record your reading on the client's chart.

22. After using the blood pressure cuff, roll it up over the manometer and replace it in the case.

23. Wipe the earplugs of the stethoscope again with an antiseptic swab. Put the stethoscope back in its proper place.

24. Wash your hands.

25. Record the blood pressure and your observations concerning the client during this procedure.

## Topics for Discussion

1. A client asks you his vital signs, and you tell him your readings. He says, "That's impossible. The other homemaker/home health aide got different readings." What do you say?

2. You have been taking care of the client for several days. Each day his vital signs have been similar. Today they are very different. What do you do?

# Chapter 16

# Intake
# and Output

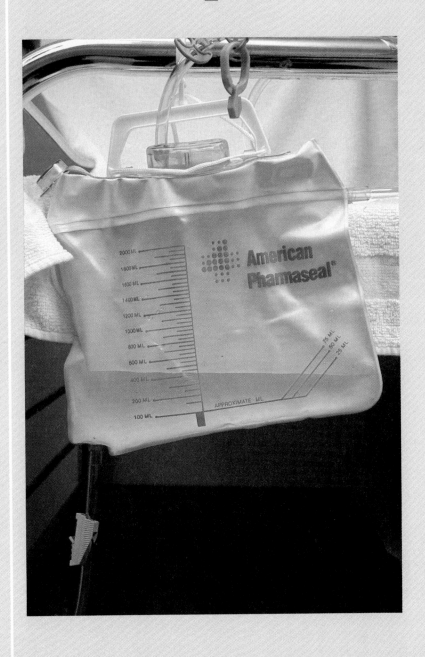

# Section 1  Fluid Balance

## Objectives: What You Will Learn to Do

- Explain fluid balance and imbalance.
- List the factors that affect intake and output.
- List the reasons for keeping accurate records of intake and output.
- Discuss the metric system as it applies to intake and output.
- Demonstrate how to make and use an intake and output record.

### *Introduction: Fluid Balance*

**fluid intake** liquid taken into the body

**fluid output** liquid excreted by the body

**fluid balance** relationship of intake fluid with excreted fluid output

**edema** abnormal swelling of a part of the body caused by fluid collecting in that area

**dehydration** condition in which the body has less than normal amount of fluid

Water is essential to human life. Next to oxygen, water is the most important nutrient the body requires. A person can lose half his body protein and almost half his weight and still live. But losing only one-fifth of his body fluid will result in death.

Through eating and drinking, the average healthy adult will take in about 3½ quarts of fluid every 24 hours. This is called **fluid intake.** The average adult also will eliminate about 3½ quarts of fluid every 24 hours. This is **fluid output.** The human body has several ways of keeping the amount of fluid it eliminates balanced with the amount of fluid it takes in. This balance is what allows the body to continue to function in a healthy state. When this balance is disturbed, the body is said to be in a state of **fluid imbalance** (Fig. 16.1). In some medical conditions, fluid may be held by the body tissues. This causes swelling and is called **edema.** In other conditions much fluid can be lost, and this is called **dehydration.** Fluids can be discharged from the body through:

- The kidneys in the form of urine
- The skin in the form of perspiration
- The lungs during breathing
- The intestinal tract

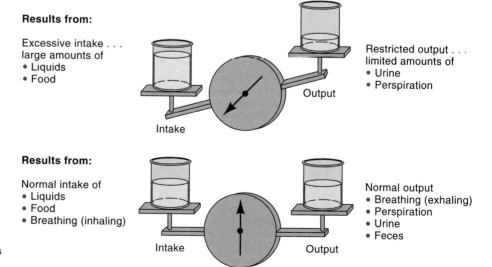

**Results from:**

Excessive intake . . . large amounts of
- Liquids
- Food

Restricted output . . . limited amounts of
- Urine
- Perspiration

Output

Intake

*FIGURE 16.1a*   Intake exceeds output

**Results from:**

Normal intake of
- Liquids
- Food
- Breathing (inhaling)

Normal output
- Breathing (exhaling)
- Perspiration
- Urine
- Feces

Intake

Output

*FIGURE 16.1b*   Intake equals output

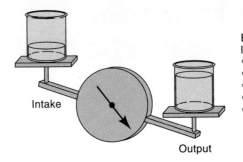

**Results from:**

Restricted intake . . .
limited amounts of
• Liquids
• Food

Excessive output . . .
large amounts of
• Urine
• Vomitus
• Blood
• Drainage
• Perspiration

Intake

Output

*FIGURE 16.1c* Intake is less than output

## REASONS FOR KEEPING RECORDS OF FLUID BALANCE

When a person is healthy, the fluid balancing system works by itself; however, when a person is ill or disabled, this system often does not function to its maximum. By accurately keeping records of an individual's intake and output, a decision can be reached as to the functioning of his fluid balancing system. Many things can affect the fluid balance system:

- Medication
- Emotional stress
- Exercise
- Nourishment
- Weather
- General health

## THE METRIC SYSTEM OF MEASUREMENT

You probably have already noticed that many quantities used in the health care field are measured in cubic centimeters. Because this method of measurement is used more and more, you should understand what it means (Fig. 16.2).

**U.S. CUSTOMARY LIQUID MEASURE WITH EQUIVALENT METRIC MEASUREMENTS**

| | | |
|---|---|---|
| cc | = | cubic centimeter |
| ml | = | milliliter |
| oz | = | ounce |
| 1 cc | = | 1 ml |
| 1/4 teaspoon | = | 1 cc |
| 1 teaspoon | = | 4 cc |
| 30 cc | = | 1 oz |
| 60 cc | = | 2 oz |
| 90 cc | = | 3 oz |
| 120 cc | = | 4 oz |
| 150 cc | = | 5 oz |
| 180 cc | = | 6 oz |
| 210 cc | = | 7 oz |
| 240 cc | = | 8 oz |
| 270 cc | = | 9 oz |
| 300 cc | = | 10 oz |
| 500 cc | = | 1 pint |
| 1000 cc | = | 1 quart |
| 4000 cc | = | 1 gallon |
| pt | = | pint |
| qt | = | quart |
| gal | = | gallon |

*FIGURE 16.2* Liquid measurements must be recorded and reported on the same measurement scale.

**cubic centimeter** a unit of measure used in the metric system

**metric system** a method of measuring temperature, length and volume of fluid which is based on the decimal system

The term *cc* is an abbreviation for **cubic centimeter**, a unit of measurement in the metric system. The **metric system** of measurement is used in many countries of the world. In the United States, we normally use one system for measuring liquids (ounces, pints, quarts) and a different system for measuring lengths (inches, feet, yards, miles). Scientists, engineers, and many health care personnel use the metric system for measuring liquids, lengths, and weight, as well. The basic unit of measurement is the meter, which is a little longer than the yard. A centimeter [one one-hundredth (1/100) of a meter] is about four-tenths (4/10) of an inch long.

A cubic centimeter can be thought of as a square block with each edge of the block 1 centimeter long. If we filled this block with water, we would have a cubic centimeter (1 cc) of water. The list shown here includes liquid amounts with which you are probably familiar. It also gives about the same amounts in cubic centimeters.

## MAKING AN INTAKE AND OUTPUT SHEET

**intake** all substances ingested by the body, sometimes refers only to fluid consumed

**output** material discharged from the body: may refer only to fluids

The amounts of **intake** and **output** (I&O) are written on a special sheet of paper. It is called the intake and output sheet and is usually kept near the client's bed. Some agencies have special forms for this purpose; some do not. The picture will give you a guide as to how to make up an I&O sheet in the client's home (Fig. 16.3). The intake and output sheet is divided into two parts, intake on the left and output on the right. After measuring intake and output, you will record the amount in the proper column. You will also indicate the time and what it was that was drunk or expelled. The amounts in each column are totaled every 24 hours.

| Client's Name_____ | | | Date_____ | | |
|---|---|---|---|---|---|
| INTAKE | | | OUTPUT | | |
| Time | | Amt. | Time | | Amt. |
| | | | *drainage urine* | | |
| | | | *diarrhea* | | *small, medium, large soft, water* |
| | | | *perspiration* | | *small, moderate,* |
| | | | *Diaper* | | *large* |
| | | | *vomitus* | | *" " or saturated* |
| | | | *blood (rectal feces)* | | |
| Total | | | Total | | |

**FIGURE 16.3** Intake and output sheet

### Starting an Intake and Output Record

A 24-hour intake record is started with the first fluids the client drinks in the morning. The first urinary output of the morning, however, is considered to be a part of the previous day's I&O because the fluid that formed the urine was consumed within the previous 24 hours. Therefore, the first urine recorded on the output sheet will actually be the second urination of the day.

### The Responsibility of Keeping I&O

The responsibility for keeping an accurate intake and output (I&O) record is a shared one. Because few clients have a homemaker/home health aide on a 24-hour basis, a family member must be taught to keep the record when you are not in the home. It is most important that all people who write on the sheet use the same procedure, or the total will not be accurate and the sheet will be useless.

Usually, the supervisor of your client's case will teach the family members how to keep a simple I&O record. You will, of course, have to answer any questions they may have and reinforce the teaching. Be sure to report to your supervisor any difficulty the family may have with keeping the records.

# Section 2   Fluid Intake

## Objectives: What You Will Learn to Do

- List the fluids that are considered as intake.
- Measure fluids accurately.
- Demonstrate that you can accurately measure and record intake.

### ■ Introduction: Fluid Intake

Although solid foods also contain liquid, most of the fluids in the body are taken in when a person drinks liquids. A client's intake includes all liquids (Fig 16.4).

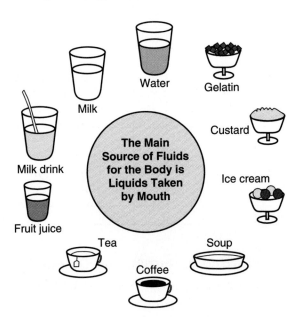

FIGURE 16.4  Fluid intake includes many things. Record all of them.

## How Much Does Each Serving Container Hold?

**calibration** graduations on a measuring instrument

A container or measuring cup is used to measure intake and output. It is marked or **calibrated** with a row of short lines and numbers. These show the amount of liquid in both cubic centimeters and ounces. You can use a regular measuring cup. Another calibrated container may be a baby bottle. Be sure that you use one container to measure intake and a different one for output. Do not mix them up.

For you to record accurately the exact amounts of fluids taken by the client, you will have to measure the amount of liquid contained in each serving container, bowl, glass, and cup that the client uses. It is helpful to make a list of how much each one contains. Then you can refer to it rather than measuring the liquid each time you fill the container.

## Procedure 56: Measuring the Capacity of Serving Containers

1. Assemble your equipment:
   Complete set of dishes, bowls, cups, and glasses used by the client
   Measuring cup
   Water
   Pen and paper
2. Fill the first container with water.
3. Pour this water into the measuring cup.
4. Look at the level of the water and determine the amount in cc (cubic centimeters).
5. Write this information on the paper. For example, carton of milk equals 240 cc.
6. Repeat these steps for each dish, glass, bowl, or cup used by the client.
7. You now have a complete list to use when measuring intake.

### MEASURING FLUID INTAKE

You should tell the client that his intake is being measured. Encourage him to help you as much as he can by asking him to keep track of how much liquid he drinks. This procedure must, of course, be a shared responsibility between you, the client, and the client's family.

Record the fluid intake as soon as the client has consumed the fluids. Do not wait. You will forget. Think about fluid intake every time you remove a tray, glass, or cup.

When measuring fluid intake, you will have to note the difference between the amount the client drinks and the amount he leaves in the serving container.

It is a good idea to list the intake and output in the same unit of measurement. If you keep the output in cc, record the intake in cc, too. If you keep the output in ounces, also record the intake in ounces.

## Procedure 57: Determining the Amounts Consumed

1. Assemble your equipment:
   Measuring cup
   Pen and paper
   Leftover liquids in their serving containers
2. Pour the leftover liquid into the measuring cup.
3. Look at the level and determine the amount in cc.
4. From your list determine the amount in the full serving container.
5. Subtract the leftover amount from the full container amount. This figure is the amount the client actually drank.
6. Immediately report this amount on the intake side of the intake and output sheet.

## Section 3  Fluid Output

### Objectives: What You Will Learn to Do

 List the fluids that are considered output.
 Demonstrate the technique for measuring and recording output.

### Introduction: Measuring Fluid Output

emesis vomitus

vomitus material which is vomited; emesis

Fluid output is the sum total of liquids that come out of the body. Most fluid is discharged from the body as urine. Other terms for this bodily function are "void" or "pass water." Output also includes **emesis (vomitus),** drainage from a wound, loss of blood, and excessive perspiration. Every time your client uses the urinal, emesis basin, or bedpan, the urine and other fluids must be measured.

You should tell a client his output is being measured and ask him to cooperate. All clients must urinate in a bedpan, urinal, or container. Ask the client not to place toilet paper in this container. Provide a plastic bag for this purpose. Then dispose of the tissue into the toilet. If at all possible, ask your client not to move his bowels while urinating.

## Procedure 58: Measuring Urinary Output

1. Assemble your equipment:
   Bedpan and cover or urinal or container for urine
   Measuring container
   Pad and pencil
2. Wash your hands.

3. Pour the urine from the bedpan or urinal into the measuring container.
4. Place the container on a flat surface for accuracy in measurement.
5. At eye level, carefully look at the container to see the number reached by the level of urine. Remember it.
6. Rinse and return the measuring container to its proper place. Pour the urine and the rinse water into the toilet.
7. Rinse and return the urinal or bedpan to its proper place. Pour the rinse water into the toilet.
8. Wash your hands.
9. Record the amount of urine in cc and the character of the urine on the output side of the I&O sheet.

 ## Measuring Output from an Indwelling Catheter

catheter a tube used to remove body fluids from a cavity

Some clients have a **catheter** (tube) inserted into their urinary bladder by the doctor or nurse. This catheter drains all the client's urine into a plastic urine container, which hangs on the bed below the level of the urinary bladder (Fig. 16.5). You will empty this container, measure the urine for amount, and record the amount. This will always be done whenever it is full and always before the end of your working shift. The measurement is not taken from the soft, expandable, plastic urine container. A hard plastic container is always used, as it is more accurate.

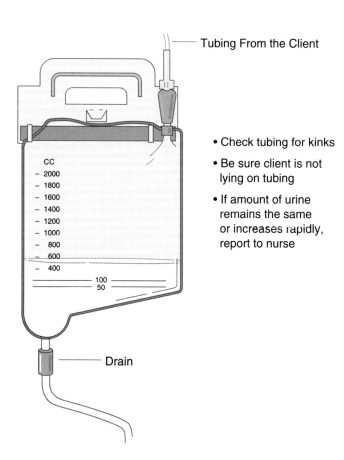

Tubing From the Client

cc
- 2000
- 1800
- 1600
- 1400
- 1200
- 1000
- 800
- 600
- 400

100
50

Drain

• Check tubing for kinks

• Be sure client is not lying on tubing

• If amount of urine remains the same or increases rapidly, report to nurse

FIGURE 16.5 A plastic urine collection container should be hung on the bed frame below the level of the bladder.

## Procedure 59: Emptying a Urinary Collection Bag from an Indwelling Catheter

1. Assemble your equipment:
   Measuring container
   Paper towels
   Pad and pencil
2. Wash your hands.
3. Protect the floor with paper towels.
4. Open the drain at the bottom of the plastic urine container and let the urine run into the measuring cup. Then close the drain. Be sure the urine does not touch the floor. Be sure the tubing from the catheter bag does not touch the floor.
5. Place the measuring container on a flat surface for accuracy in measurement.
6. At eye level, carefully look at the container to see the level of urine. Remember it.
7. Rinse the measuring container, and put it in its proper place. Put the urine and rinse water into the toilet.
8. Wash your hands.
9. Record the time, amount in cc, and anything unusual concerning the urine on the output side of the I&O sheet.

### FLUID OUTPUT FROM THE INCONTINENT CLIENT

**incontinence** the inability to control one's bowel movements or urination

If the client is **incontinent** (cannot control elimination or urine), record this on the output side of the I&O sheet each time the bed is wet. Even though the urine cannot be measured, it will be obvious that the client's kidneys are functioning.

#### Measuring Fluids Other than Urine

Vomitus and diarrhea are also measured according to the procedure for measuring urinary output. Be sure to indicate on the I&O sheet what fluid you are recording.

If a client bleeds a great deal, has wound discharge, or perspires heavily, indicate this on the I&O sheet. Include in your recording:

■ What was wet
■ How wet (damp, dripping, etc.)
■ The size of the area that was wet
■ The time this occurred

## Section 4   Forcing and Restricting Fluids

**Objectives: What You Will Learn to Do**

■ Explain the terms *force fluids* and *restrict fluids*.
■ Demonstrate the homemaker/home health aide's role when a client is to be on restricted fluids.
■ Demonstrate the homemaker/home health aide's role when a client is to force fluids.

# Introduction: Balancing Fluid Intake

force fluids extra fluids taken in according to doctor's orders

Clients who need to have more fluids added to their normal intake are told to **force fluids.** FF is the abbreviation for force fluids. A client who is to force fluids often needs encouragement to drink. Be sure you know how much fluid the client is to have within a 24-hour period. Some ways you can assist the client to drink the amount of fluids are by:

- Showing enthusiasm and being cheerful
- Providing different kinds of liquids that the client prefers, as permitted
- Offering liquids without being asked
- Offering hot and cold drinks
- Offering liquids in divided amounts. For example, 800 cc every eight hours means the client ought to drink 100 cc an hour.

Record the amount taken in by the client in cc and on the intake side of the I&O. Report to your supervisor if the client is unable to drink the amount required.

Some clients must **restrict** their fluid intake. This means that fluids are to be limited to a certain amount. Be sure you know what that amount is. Follow orders, and measure accurately. Your calm and reassuring attitude can make a big difference in how the client feels and reacts.

- Alternate different fluids as permitted.
- Record the amount of intake on the intake side of the I&O sheet.
- Frequent oral hygiene is often necessary.
- Discuss with your supervisor the client's reaction to this restriction.
- If the restriction is severe, the client may be permitted to suck on ice chips or candy. Check with your supervisor before you start any of these practices.

# Topics for Discussion

1. If the client is all alone and has no family assistance, what are some of the things you would do to ensure an accurate I&O?
2. What are some of the characteristics of urine that you would record on the intake and output sheet? Color, sediment, and so on.
3. If a client refused to use a urinal or bedpan, can you keep an accurate I&O?

# Chapter 17

# Specimen Collection

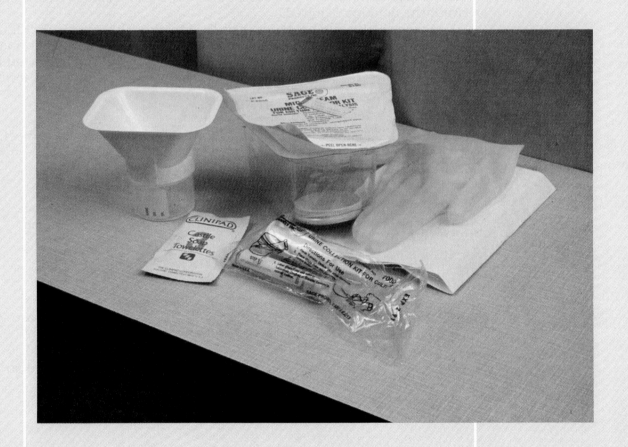

# Section 1 ■ Specimen Collection

---

## Objectives: What You Will Learn to Do

■ Explain what specimens are.
■ Collect specimens correctly.

---

### ■ *Introduction: Specimen Collection*

As one of its natural functions, the human body regularly gets rid of various waste materials. Most of the wastes are discharged in the form of urine and feces. The body also discharges waste in sputum, which is coughed up from the lungs.

When bodily wastes are tested in the laboratory, changes in the body function can be detected. This information is used by the doctor to decide on an appropriate treatment for the client. Specimens are samples of bodily waste products that are collected and sent to the laboratory for examination.

When you are collecting a specimen, you must be accurate in following the procedure and labeling the specimen. You have to collect the specimen at exactly the right time. The name of the client, his address, the date, and the time of specimen collection should be printed on the label in clear letters. This label must be attached securely to the specimen container. Unlabeled specimens will be thrown away by all laboratories. If this happens, another one will have to be collected, resulting in extra time and cost for the client.

Many specimens must be stored in the home for a short period before they are taken to the laboratory. It is your responsibility to be sure of the correct storage procedure for a specimen.

Urine specimens must be free of fecal matter. They must also be free of menstrual blood. If your client is menstruating, a vaginal tampon must be in place while the urine specimen is collected. Before you suggest this, however, discuss it with your supervisor.

#### OBTAINING A SPECIMEN

Few of us can urinate on demand, but if we know we will be expected to give a urine specimen, we will cooperate. Tell your client that a specimen will be needed some time before you actually try to collect it.

Some clients are embarrassed by the procedures involved in obtaining some types of specimens. Your client will be calm and cooperative if you show understanding and assist him when necessary. If your client understands the procedure, he should obtain the specimen himself.

Human waste material has many names. Street language uses one set of terms. Many cultures use other sets of terms. Many people do not know the correct English words for human waste material. It is usually a good idea to try to use the words that the client and his family use (this is especially true of children). If these words are offensive to you, discuss this situation with your supervisor.

*Need for Accuracy*

Be sure you follow all the "rights" listed here:

- *The right client:* from whom the specimen is to be collected.
- *The right specimen:* as ordered by the doctor.
- *The right time:* when the specimen should be collected.
- *The right amount:* amount needed for the laboratory to test.
- *The right container:* the cup that is correct for each specimen.
- *The right label:* filled out properly and neatly.
- *The right method:* procedure by which you collect the specimen.
- *The right asepsis:* washing your hands before and after collecting the specimen.
- *The right attitude:* how you approach and speak to the client.

*Asepsis in Specimen Collection*

As you learned from Chapter 8 on infection control, asepsis means "free of disease-causing organisms." When collecting specimens, it is very important to use good medical aseptic technique to prevent contamination. Wash your hands carefully before and after collecting each specimen. Handwashing before you collect the specimen prevents contamination of the specimen by anything that may be on your hands. Handwashing after you collect the specimen prevents microorganisms from the specimen from remaining on your hands.

# Section 2 Collecting Urine for a Specimen

## Objectives: What You Will Learn to Do

- Define a routine urine specimen.
- Demonstrate the correct procedure for collecting a routine urine specimen.
- Demonstrate the correct procedure for collecting a urine specimen from a client who has a Foley catheter.
- Demonstrate the correct procedure for collecting a urine specimen from an infant.
- Define a clean-catch urine specimen.
- Demonstrate the correct procedure for collecting a clean-catch urine specimen.
- Demonstrate the correct procedure for collecting a 24-hour urine specimen.

 ### Introduction: Routine Urine Specimen

**specimen** sample of urine obtained at any time during the day in a clean container

This is a single sample of urine taken from the client as he voids the usual way. No special precautions are taken. At times you will be told to take a **specimen** of the first urine of the day, but if you are not given time instructions, this specimen may be taken when convenient.

## Procedure 60: Collecting a Routine Urine Specimen

1. Assemble your equipment:
   Bedpan or urinal
   Measuring container for measuring output
   Urine specimen container and lid
   Paper or plastic bag for toilet tissue
   Label
   Wet washcloth and towel for the client

2. Prepare the label. Write clearly the client's name, address, date, and time. Also write what type of specimen this is: Routine Urine.

3. Wash your hands.

4. Ask visitors to leave the room if appropriate.

5. Tell the client a urine specimen is needed. Explain the procedure to him. If he is able to collect the specimen himself, he should do so.

6. If the client is able, he can urinate directly into the container. If he is not, ask the client to urinate into the bedpan or urinal. Remind the client not to put toilet tissue into the bedpan but to use a paper bag or a plastic bag. You will discard the tissue in the toilet.

7. Offer the client a washcloth and towel to wash his hands.

8. Make the client comfortable.

9. Take the bedpan or urinal into the bathroom.

10. If the client is on I&O, pour the urine into a clean measuring container and note the amount of urine on the I&O sheet.

11. Pour the urine into the specimen container. Fill it 3/4 full.

12. Put the lid on the container. Wipe off the outside of the container. Secure the label to the container.

13. Pour the urine remaining in the bedpan, urinal, or measuring container into the toilet.

14. Clean and rinse the bedpan, urinal, or measuring container. Put them in their proper place.

15. Wash your hands.

16. Make a notation on the client's chart that you collected the specimen, the time, and anything you observed about the client during this procedure.

17. Store the specimen in the correct place before it is taken to the laboratory.

### Collecting a Urine Specimen from a Client with a Foley Catheter

A urine specimen from a client with a Foley catheter in place takes time to collect. Be sure the client has had some fluid to drink before you attempt this. Tell the client what you will be doing because he will be unable to see the procedure or take an active part in it. It is imperative that the specimen be labeled properly. Include the fact that the specimen was obtained from a catheter.

## Procedure 61: Obtaining a Urine Specimen from a Client with a Foley Catheter

1. Assemble your equipment:
   Specimen container and lid
   Measuring container
   Label
   Disposable gloves
   Padding to protect the bed
   Protective cap for drainage tubing or sterile gauze pads
2. Prepare the label. Write clearly the client's name, address, date, and time. Write what type of specimen it is and how it was obtained.
3. Wash your hands.
4. Ask visitors to leave the room if appropriate.
5. Tell the client a urine specimen is needed. Explain the procedure to him.
6. Place the client in a comfortable position, usually on his back.
7. Spread bed protectors on the bed between the client's legs.
8. Disconnect the catheter from the tubing going to the collection bag. Protect the drainage tubing to prevent contamination of it.
9. Hold the end of the catheter over the specimen bottle and allow the urine to drip in. This may take time so do not be impatient. Do not allow the catheter to drop into the bottle.
10. Fill the specimen bottle at least half full, if at all possible.
11. If the client is on I&O, allow the urine to drip from the catheter into a measuring container, and then transfer it to the specimen bottle. Be sure to note on the I&O sheet the amount of urine obtained.
12. Reattach the catheter to the collection bag tubing.
13. Wash your hands.
14. Make the client comfortable.
15. Put the lid on the collection container. Wipe off the outside of the container. Secure the label to the container.
16. If you used a measuring container to measure urine, wash it and replace it in the proper place.
17. Wash your hands.
18. Make a notation on the client's chart that you collected the specimen, the time, and anything observed about the client during this procedure.
19. Store the specimen in the correct place before it is taken to the laboratory.

## Midstream Clean-Catch Urine Specimen

A special method is used to collect a client's urine when the specimen must be totally free from contamination. This special type of specimen is called a midstream clean-catch urine specimen. **Clean-catch** refers to the fact that the urine is not contaminated by anything outside the client's body. The procedure requires careful washing of the genital area. Midstream means catching the urine specimen between the time the client begins to void and time he stops.

clean-catch urine specimen obtained, following the careful cleansing of the urinary meatus and surrounding area, into a sterile container

All the equipment and supplies necessary for this specimen are usually found in a special kit the laboratory sends to the client. If you are unable to get such a kit, sterilize a jar. Wash the genital area with a nonirritating sterile cleansing solution and sterile gauze. Be sure all soap is off the area before collecting the specimen.

## Procedure 62: Collecting a Midstream Clean-Catch Urine Specimen

1. Assemble your equipment:
   Clean-catch kit or sterilized jar, sterile cleansing solution, sterile gauze, and sterile gloves
   Bedpan or urinal if the client is unable to go to the bathroom
   Wet washcloth and towel
   Waste bag

2. Prepare the label if it is outside the kit. If not, wait until the end of the procedure. Write clearly the client's name, address, date, and time. Write what type of specimen it is and how it was obtained.

3. Wash your hands.

4. Ask visitors to leave the room if appropriate. You may want to explain this procedure to a family member.

5. Tell the client you need a midstream clean-catch urine specimen.

6. Explain the procedure. If the client is able, he may collect the specimen himself.

7. If the client is not able to collect the specimen, assist him with the procedure.

8. Open the disposable kit.

9. Put on the gloves. Remove the towelettes and the urine specimen container. Do not put your hand inside the container or lid.

10. For female clients:
    a. Separate the folds of the labia and wipe with one towelette from the front to the back along one labia. Throw away the towelette. The labia must be separated during cleansing and collection of the specimen.
    b. Wipe the opposite labia with the second towelette. Throw it away.
    c. Wipe down the middle using the third towelette. Throw it away.

11. For male clients:
    a. If the male is not circumcised, pull the foreskin of the penis back before cleansing the penis. Hold it back during urination.
    b. Use a circular motion to clean the head of the penis. Use all three towelettes. Throw each one away after you use it.
12. Ask the client to start urinating into the bedpan or the toilet. Then ask him to stop. Place the sterile urine container under the stream of urine and ask the client to start urinating again. Fill the container 1/2 to 3/4 full. The remaining urine may be discarded.
13. If the client is on I&O, all the urine must first be voided into a sterile measuring container and measured, then put into the sterile specimen container provided. Be sure to note on the I&O sheet the amount of urine that was sent as a specimen.
14. Cover the urine container with the proper lid. Be sure not to touch the inside of the lid or the container. Wipe off the outside of the container.
15. Take off your gloves.
16. Wash your hands.
17. Make the client comfortable. Offer the client a wet wash-cloth and towel to wash his hands.
18. Clean all the equipment, and replace it.
19. Wash your hands.
20. Make a notation on the client's chart that you collected the specimen, the time, and anything observed about the client during this procedure.
21. Store the specimen in the correct place before it is taken to the laboratory.

## 24-Hour Urine Specimen

A 24-hour urine specimen is a collection of all urine voided by a client over a 24-hour period. All the urine is collected for 24 hours, usually from 7 A.M. on the first day to 7 A.M. the following day (Fig. 17.1).

When you are to obtain a 24-hour urine specimen, it is necessary to ask the client to void and discard this voided urine at 7 A.M. This is done because this urine has been in the bladder an unknown length of time. The test should begin with the bladder empty. For the next 24 hours, save all the urine voided by the client. On the following day at 7 A.M. ask the client to void and add this specimen to the previous collection. This way the doctor can be sure that all of the urine for the test came into the urinary bladder during the 24 hours of the test period.

It is very important that the client and his family understand the importance of collecting *all* the urine voided within the 24 hours. If one urination is accidentally thrown away, the test is not accurate and will have to be repeated.

It is your responsibility to be sure of the correct placement of the 24-hour urine collection bottle. Some specimens must be kept on ice and others not. Ask!

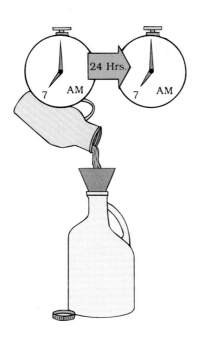

*FIGURE 17.1* Write down the 24 hours in which you are collecting the urine.

## Procedure 63: Collecting a 24-Hour Urine Specimen

1. Assemble your equipment:
   Large container, usually a 1-gal bottle (the laboratory usually supplies this)
   Bedpan or urinal
   Funnel if the neck of the bottle is small
   Measuring container used for measuring output if the client is on I&O
   Label for the container
   Wet washcloth and towel
2. Fill out the label. Clearly write the client's name, address, date, and time the collection started.
3. Wash your hands.
4. Ask visitors to leave the room, if appropriate.
5. Tell the client that a 24-hour specimen is needed. Explain the procedure to him and his family. Discuss the placement and care of the gallon container of urine.
6. You may be instructed to refrigerate the urine. If so, one way is to keep it in a bucket of ice. This ice will have to be changed as it melts. It may, of course, be kept in the refrigerator if that is acceptable to the client and his family.
7. During the collection of the specimen, ask the client to use the bedpan or urinal each time he voids. Remind him not to throw toilet tissue into the bedpan or urinal and to try to urinate without moving his bowels at the same time. Provide a waste bag for the toilet tissue, and then discard it promptly in the toilet.
8. If the client is on I&O, measure all urine each time the client urinates and write it on the I&O sheet.

9. When the collection starts, have the client urinate. *Throw away this first urine.* This is to be sure that the bladder is completely empty as the collection starts. If this urine is discarded at 7 A.M., the collection will continue until 7 A.M. the following morning.

10. For the next 24 hours save all the client's urine. At the end of the collection, write the time the collection stopped on the label. Store the bottle in the proper place until it is sent to the laboratory.

11. Offer the client a washcloth and towel to wash his hands each time he voids.

12. Be sure to clean all equipment *after each urination.* Note in your charting that the collection was done and your observations about the client during this procedure.

## Collecting Urine from an Infant

It is often difficult to collect urine from an infant because they are unable to cooperate and void when we ask them. Therefore, it is very important to gather the specimen in the correct manner the first time so that the procedure need not be repeated. The procedure may appear to be uncomfortable to the child, but it does not hurt him. Reassure the child's parent or guardian that you are not hurting the child and that the information the doctor will have after the laboratory examination of the urine will help in the child's care. Be kind, efficient, and thoughtful of both child and parents.

## Procedure 64: Collecting a Urine Specimen from an Infant

1. Assemble your equipment:
   Urine specimen bottle or container
   Plastic disposable infant urine collector

2. Prepare a label. Write the client's name, address, date, and type of specimen. Fill in the time when the actual specimen has been obtained.

3. Wash your hands.

4. Ask visitors to leave, except the parent or guardian of the child.

5. Explain to the child and his parent that you want to collect a urine specimen. Children who are not yet toilet trained can understand language and are more likely to cooperate if they know what is expected of them. Use language the children understand and are familiar with.

6. Take off the child's diaper.

7. Clean the genital area. Be sure it is dry or the collector bag will not stick.

8. Remove the outside piece that surrounds the opening of the plastic urine collector. Be sure the skin is not folded under the sticky part as you apply it. Place the opening of the bag

FIGURE 17.2

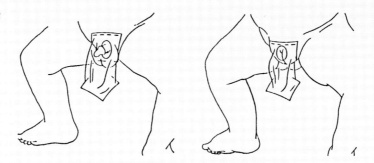

around a male penis or a female meatus (Fig. 17.2). Do not cover the rectum. The specimen is useless if it is contaminated with fecal matter.

9. Put the child's diaper on as usual.

10. Check every half hour to see if the infant has voided. You cannot feel the diaper. You must look inside the diaper.

11. When the infant has voided, remove the urine collector gently. Do not spill the urine. Pour the urine into a specimen container.

12. Wash off any excess sticky material on the genitalia. Make the baby comfortable.

13. Wash your hands.

14. Make a notation on the client's chart that you collected the specimen, the time, and anything you observed about the client during the procedure.

15. Store the specimen in the correct place before it is taken to the laboratory.

# Section 3 Collection of a Stool Specimen

## Objectives: What You Will Learn to Do

■ Define stool specimen.

■ Demonstrate the correct procedure for collecting a stool specimen.

### Introduction: Stool Specimen

**stool** solid waste material discharged from the body through the rectum and anus. Other names include feces, excreta, excrement, bowel movement, and fecal matter

The solid waste from a person's body has many names—**feces, stool, B.M., bowel movement.** They all mean the same thing. The doctor sometimes requires a sample of the client's feces to assist him in diagnosing the client's illness or in monitoring the client's progress. A sample of feces is a stool specimen. There are certain tests that must be performed only on a warm stool. You will be told whether the specimen is to be warm or cold.

## Procedure 65: Collecting a Stool Specimen

1. Assemble your equipment:
   Bedpan
   Stool container
   Label
   Wooden tongue depressor
   Plastic bag for warm specimen if used by your agency
   Washcloth and towel for the client

2. Fill in the label with the client's name, address, date, and type of specimen. Fill in the time when the actual specimen has been obtained.

3. Wash your hands.

4. Ask visitors to leave the room.

5. Tell the client that a stool specimen is needed. Explain that he is to call you whenever he can move his bowels.

6. Have the client move his bowels in the bedpan. If the client is unable to use the bedpan, place several layers of toilet tissue in the bottom of the toilet and have the client move his bowels on the paper (Fig. 17.3). This way you will be able to take a specimen easily.

FIGURE 17.3

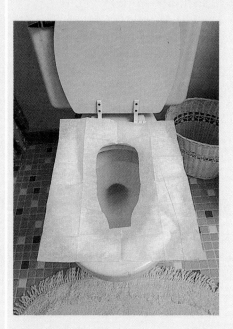

7. Ask the client not to urinate into the bedpan and not to put toilet tissue into the bedpan. Provide him with a plastic or paper bag to dispose of the tissue temporarily. Then discard it in the toilet.

8. After the client has had a bowel movement, take the bedpan into the bathroom.

9. Wash your hands.

10. Offer the client a washcloth and towel for his hands.

11. Make the client comfortable.

FIGURE 17.4

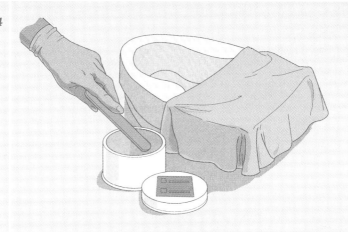

12. Using the wooden tongue depressor, take 1 to 2 tablespoons of stool from the bedpan and place it into the stool specimen container (Fig. 17.4).

13. Cover the container. Do not touch the inside of the container or the top of it.

14. Wrap the depressor in a piece of toilet tissue and discard it into a plastic or paper bag.

15. Empty the remaining feces into the toilet.

16. Clean the bedpan and return it to its proper place.

17. Wash your hands.

18. Make a notation on the client's chart that you collected the specimen, the time, and anything you observed about the client during this procedure.

19. Store the specimen in the correct place before it is taken to the laboratory.

# Section 4  Collection of a Sputum Specimen

## Objectives: What You Will Learn to Do

■ Define *sputum.*

■ Demonstrate the correct procedure for collecting a sputum specimen.

### *Introduction: Sputum Collection*

**Sputum** is a substance collected from a client's lungs. It contains saliva, mucus, and sometimes blood or pus. It is usually clear in color but can be gray, yellow, green, or red. The best time to collect a sputum specimen is in the morning, right after the client awakens.

## Procedure 66: Collecting a Sputum Specimen

1. Assemble your equipment:
   Sputum container with lid
   Tissues
2. Label the container with the client's name, address, date, and type of specimen. Fill in the time when the actual specimen is obtained.
3. Wash your hands.
4. Ask visitors to leave the room if appropriate.
5. Tell the client a sputum specimen is needed.
6. If the client has eaten recently, have him rinse out his mouth. If he wants oral hygiene at this time, help him as necessary.
7. Give him the sputum container. Ask him to take three consecutive deep breaths. On the third breath, ask him to exhale deeply and cough. He should be able to bring up sputum from within the lungs. Explain to him that saliva is not adequate for this test.
8. Have the client spit the sputum directly into the specimen container.
9. Cover the container immediately. Be careful not to touch the inside of either the container or the cover.
10. Offer the client oral hygiene.
11. Make the client comfortable.
12. Wash your hands.
13. Make a notation on the client's chart that you collected the specimen, the time, and anything you observed about the client during this procedure.
14. Store the specimen in the correct place before it is taken to the laboratory.

## Topics for Discussion

1. Your client has several specimens that are required. What are the factors you must consider in order to get the specimens with the least amount of discomfort to the client?
2. Review the sterilization procedures in the home. If you contaminate a bottle or are unable to get a specimen bottle from the laboratory, how will you prepare one?

# Chapter 18

# Special Procedures

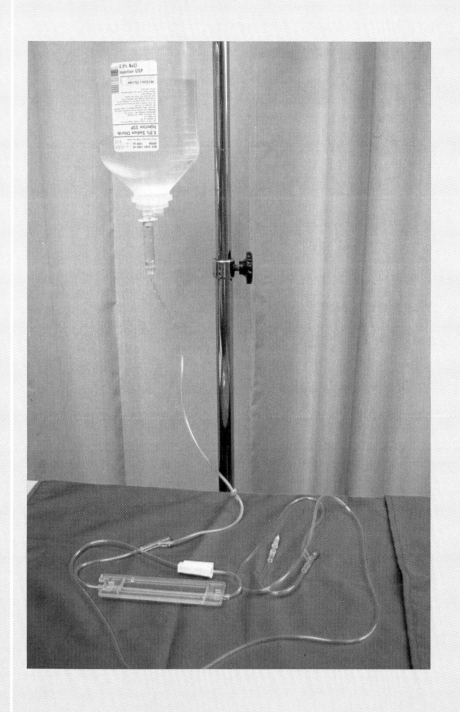

## Objectives: What You Will Learn to Do

- Discuss the difference between administering medication and assisting with medication.
- Define the role of the homemaker/home health aide in relation to medication.
- Demonstrate the proper techniques for assisting clients with various types of medication.
- Discuss methods of medication storage and disposal.
- Define the role of the homemaker/home aide when there is oxygen in the home.

### Introduction: Assisting with Medications

**medication** substance or preparation used in treating a disease

**administer** to give a client medication without his assistance

**Medication** is prescribed by a physician, dispensed by a pharmacist, and **administered,** or given without client assistance, by a nurse. All these professionals are licensed by the state to perform their duties. These duties are very specific. Failure to stay within the state guidelines can result in a legal action ending in a fine, the revoking of a license to practice the profession, and possibly jail. In addition, these people are paid for their services. As a homemaker/home health aide, you are *not* licensed to administer medication, nor are you paid to do so. You are, however, expected to assist your clients as they take their own medication. When you administer you take all responsibility that goes along with giving medication. When you assist a client, he shares the responsibility. If you ever have a question about a situation with your client, ask your supervisor.

Prescription drugs are prescribed by a physician and cannot be bought without a prescription. Over-the-counter drugs can be bought without a prescription. As a homemaker/home health aide, you will not administer either type of drug and will assist the client only with those drugs about which you have specifically been instructed.

### Your Role as a Homemaker/Home Health Aide

As a homemaker/home health aide, you probably will spend more time with the client than any other member of the health care team. During this time you will often be assigned to assist the client with his medication. To do this correctly, you will have to have certain information. Without this information, an accident could happen. Accidents involving medication are very serious because they can cause the client pain, delay his recovery, and sometimes even cause death.

Your supervisor will find out all information about your client's medication. She will then make a medication plan for the client and review it with the client, the family, and you. Your supervisor will tell you your specific duties about the client's medication. You must be sure you have all the information you need to perform your duties to the best of your ability.

To perform your duties well, you must know the Five Rights of medication (Fig. 18.1).

| | |
|---|---|
| The Right Client | Is this medication for the client? |
| The Right Medication | Is this the correct medication? |
| The Right Time | Is this the prescribed time to take it? |
| The Right Route | How to take it? By mouth, apply to the skin, swallow it, suck on it? |
| The Right Amount | Is this the prescribed quantity? |

FIGURE 18.1 The five rights of medication must be completed every time a client takes medication.

You should also know the side effects of the medication, how to store the medication, and how it reacts with food.

As you spend time in your client's house, there are many things you will observe. Here are a few of the observations you should report to your supervisor immediately:

■ If your client is not taking the medication exactly as it has been prescribed (Fig. 18.2).

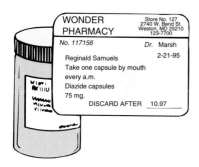

FIGURE 18.2 The label on the medication bottle must be checked every time the client takes the medication.

WONDER PHARMACY
Store No. 127
2740 W. Bend St.
Weston, MD 25210
123-7700
No. 117156
Dr. Marsh
2-21-95
Reginald Samuels
Take one capsule by mouth
every a.m.
Diazide capsules
75 mg.
DISCARD AFTER  10.97

■ If your client is taking medication (prescription or over-the-counter) of which your supervisor is not aware.

■ If your client does not know why he is taking his drugs.

■ If your client has nausea, vomiting, diarrhea, itching, difficult breathing, a rash, or hives soon after he takes his medication.

■ If his orientation, concentration, memory, or mood changes soon after he takes his medication.

■ If your client is confusing his medications.

## Procedure 67: Assisting a Client with Medication

1. Assemble your equipment:
   Medication
   Spoon
   Water or juice
   Dressings if medication is applied to the skin
   Tissues or cotton balls

2. Wash your hands.

3. Ask visitors to leave the room if appropriate.

4. Remind the client it is time for his medication.

5. Check the five rights of medication.

6. Place the medication within reach of the client. Loosen the tops of bottles or tubes.

7. Assist the client as necessary:
   a. Oral medication. Hold client's hand, assist him with liquid.
   b. Ointments. Assist him as needed with medication and dressing.
   c. Eyedrops. Guide his hand, wipe excess liquid or ointment from under eye from nose to outer area.
8. Make the client comfortable.
9. Put the medication in its proper place. Dispose of the used equipment.
10. Wash your hands.
11. Make a notation on the client's chart that he took his medication, the time, and how he took it. Also note your observations of the client during this procedure.

## MEDICATION STORAGE

Each year there are many accidents resulting from the improper storage of medication. As you make your first tour around your client's house, observe how he keeps his medication. If it is poorly stored, you will want to correct this. If you are unable to discuss the problem with your client directly, discuss it with your supervisor and together you will make a plan to correct the situation.

- Clients save medication, but some of it changes its chemical makeup as it stands. Clients save medication so if they have symptoms they can medicate themselves. But the same symptoms are often caused by different physical problems. This practice is most dangerous. Old medication should be disposed of with the client's permission.
- Many medications have similar names and look alike. Store these separately.
- Do not assist a client with a medication from an unlabeled container.
- Do not change the place your client stores his medication without his permission. People do not always read labels but take medications from the place they expect to find them.
- Keep medications out of reach of children and confused, forgetful clients.
- Keep medication away from extreme heat, cold, or light.
- Dispose of medication by flushing it down a toilet or pouring it down a drain. Dispose of old medication so that no one else can make use of it or eat it by mistake.

### Assisting a Client with Oxygen Therapy

**oxygen** a colorless, odorless gas making up about one-fifth of the air we breathe. It is essential for life.

**Oxygen** is considered a medication. All the rules and responsibilities that apply to you while you are assisting a client with medication apply to you while you are assisting a client with oxygen. Oxygen is prescribed by a physician. It is delivered to the home in a tank by a special company. The tank may look like a vacuum cleaner canister or a piece of furniture. It may also look like the tanks in the hospital. The oxygen can be delivered by a concentrator, a tank, or a liquid oxygen system. The company is responsible for refilling the tank, servicing the equipment, and teaching the client and his family how to use the equipment. If this is not the case, report it to your supervisor.

Oxygen is dispensed from the tank to the client through a rubber tube connected to a nasal cannula or catheter. Oxygen is very drying, so a nebulizer filled with water or medication is usually attached to the tank. The oxygen passes through the water and takes on moisture before it goes to the client (Fig. 18.3).

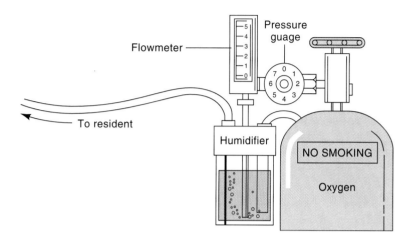

FIGURE 18.3 Although some oxygen delivery systems look different, they all have the same parts and function.

**Nasal Catheter:** This catheter is a piece of tubing that is longer than a cannula. It is inserted through the client's nostril into the back of his mouth. The nasal catheter is used when the client must have additional oxygen at all times. The nasal catheter is fastened to the client's forehead or cheek with a piece of tape that holds it steady (Fig. 18.4).

**Nasal Cannulas:** Nasal cannulas, or tubes, are used to give oxygen to a client. The cannulas are inserted into the client's nostrils. The plastic cannula is a half-circle length of tubing with two openings in the center. It fits about 1/2 inch into the client's nostrils. Nasal cannulas are held in place by an elastic band around the client's head and are connected to the source of oxygen by a length of plastic tubing (Fig. 18.5).

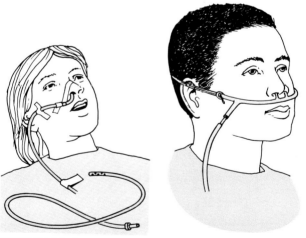

FIGURE 18.4 The nasal catheter should be securely taped to the client's face to decrease possible irritation.

FIGURE 18.5 Nasal cannulas move easily, so check their placement frequently.

**Face Mask:**  This is a piece of plastic shaped like a cup which covers the client's nose and mouth. It has holes in it. A tube connects the mask to the oxygen tank, and a piece of elastic holds the mask securely to the client's face. This mask is used when the client requires more oxygen than can be given by cannula or catheter. This mask must be removed for the client to eat. Some clients can say a few words with the mask in place, but most remove it to speak (Fig. 18.6).

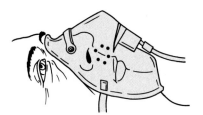

*FIGURE 18.6*  Clients cannot talk with a face mask in place. Be sure the client can signal for assistance.

## HOMEMAKER/HOME HEALTH AIDE RESPONSIBILITIES

- Put up a "No Smoking" sign in the room where the client uses the oxygen. *Enforce this rule.*
- Report to your supervisor if the client does not use the oxygen as it was prescribed.
- Use cotton bed clothes to decrease static electricity.
- Do not use electric shavers or hair dryers while the oxygen is running. Keep the electric plugs out of the walls while the oxygen is running. If an electric plug is pulled from the outlet while the oxygen is running, a spark could cause an explosion.
- Do not use candles or open flames in the room.
- Avoid combing a client's hair while he is receiving oxygen. A spark of electricity from his hair could set off an explosion.
- Ask for careful instructions as to which valve turns the oxygen on and off.
- Do not change the setting on any oxygen equipment. The setting has been chosen by the physician. Too much or too little oxygen can cause the client to change his breathing pattern, his heart rate, and his speech pattern.
- Call your supervisor immediately if you notice any of these signs. *Do not change the oxygen setting.*

Too much oxygen:

- Sleepiness or difficulty waking up
- Headache
- Difficulty speaking
- Slow, shallow breathing

Too little oxygen:

- Tiredness
- Blue fingernails and/or lips
- Anxiety, restlessness
- Irritability
- Confusion

## Objectives: What You Will Learn to Do

- List the types of dressing a homemaker/home health aide may change.
- Demonstrate the correct technique for changing a nonsterile dressing.

### *Introduction: Nonsterile Dressings*

**dressing** bandage for an external wound

**nonsterile** not subjected to the sterilizing process and therefore possibly having pathogens

**drainage** discharge from a sore, wound, or body part

Some of your clients will have wounds or areas of their bodies that will have to be covered by a bandage or **dressing**. Those dressings that do not require you to use sterile technique or to apply medication to the wound will often be assigned to your care. These are called **nonsterile**. When you change a dressing, always note the color, odor, amount, and consistency of the **drainage** (discharge) on the old dressing. Also note how big the wound is and the condition of the skin surrounding the wound. Note any change in the wound since you last saw it. If the nurse is scheduled to visit, save the old dressing for her to see. Each dressing is somewhat different, but the following procedure is a general rule for changing all nonsterile dressings.

#### EXAMPLE OF CHARTING FOLLOWING A DRESSING CHANGE

7/3/90 Dressing changed on Mrs. C's right thigh at 10 A.M. Old dressing has light red drainage, 25-cent size, no odor, wound 5-cent size. Surrounding skin had several small red raised areas. Clean dressing applied. Tape not applied to red areas. Called supervisor to report this. Mary Jones H/HHA.

## *Procedure 68: Changing a Nonsterile Dressing*

1. Assemble your equipment:
   Clean dressing and tape
   Cleansing solution
   Paper bag or plastic bag for old dressings
   Medication the client will apply
2. Wash your hands.
3. Ask visitors to leave the room if appropriate.
4. Tell the client you are going to change his dressing.
5. Open the paper bag.
6. Open the clean dressings without touching the center of them. Prepare the tape in a convenient place.
7. Position the client so that the wound is exposed.

8. Remove the old dressing. Note the drainage for amount, color, odor, and consistency. Note the size of the wound and the condition of the surrounding skin.

9. Cleanse the wound and the skin as you have been instructed. Use circular motions, and clean from the clean areas to the dirty. The wound is considered clean and the skin dirty.

10. Allow the client to assist you as much as possible.

11. If a medication is to be applied to the wound, assist the client with the application as needed.

12. Apply clean dressings. Hold all dressings by the corners as you apply them. Do not contaminate the center of the bandages. Tape the dressing in place, leaving the edges free. Do not put tape completely around the edges of the bandage (Fig. 18.7).

13. Make the client comfortable.

14. Discard the dressing in a covered container. Clean the equipment.

15. Wash your hands.

16. Make a notation on the client's chart that you changed the client's dressing. Also note your observations of the client during this procedure.

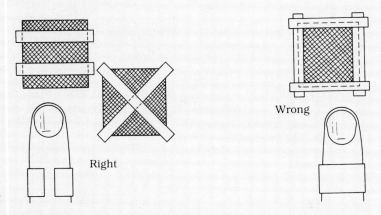

Right          Wrong

*FIGURE 18.7*

# Section 3  Care of the Indwelling Catheter

**Objectives: What You Will Learn to Do**

- Understand what an indwelling catheter is and when it is used.
- List your responsibilities as a homemaker/home health aide in caring for an indwelling catheter.
- Demonstrate the proper technique for giving catheter care.
- Demonstrate the proper technique of changing the catheter from a straight drainage bag to a leg drainage bag.

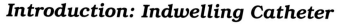

## *Introduction: Indwelling Catheter*

**catheter** a tube used to remove body fluids from a cavity

The urinary catheter is the most common kind of **catheter** used for taking fluids out of the body. This catheter is made of plastic or rubber and is inserted by a nurse or physician through the client's urethra into his bladder. A catheter may be used when a client is unable to urinate naturally, or it may be used to measure the amount of urine left in the bladder after a client has urinated naturally. It may also be used to help keep an incontinent client dry. An incontinent client is one who cannot control his urine or feces.

Sometimes a urinary catheter is used for only one withdrawal of urine. Sometimes, however, it is kept in place in the bladder for a number of days or even weeks. This type of catheter is called an indwelling catheter or Foley catheter (Fig. 18.8). This catheter is specially made so that it will stay in the bladder. It is two tubes, one inside the other. The inside tube is connected at one end to a balloon. After the catheter has been inserted, the balloon is filled with water or air so the catheter will not pass out through the urethra. Urine drains out of the bladder through the outer tube. The urine collects into a container. The container is attached to the bed frame lower than the client's urinary bladder. This is always a closed system, which means it is never opened except when emptying the urine collecting bag.

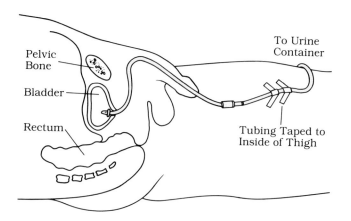

**FIGURE 18.8** A catheter is a possible source of irritation and infection. Care for it carefully and according to the plan of care.

Sometimes, in male clients, the catheter is secured to the abdomen. This reduces the pressure on the catheter and provides the straightest route for the urine drain.

**straight drainage** method of collecting urine from a Foley catheter into a closed container

**Straight Drainage:** Urinary indwelling catheters drain by **straight drainage** from the client into a bag. This type of drainage gets its name from the fact that the tubing from the bed to the bag must be kept straight and all other tubing must be kept above this. When the tubing is in its proper position, the urine will drain freely into the bag. If the tubing is not in the proper position, the urine could back up into the bladder or the kidneys (Fig. 18.9).

## *Guidelines: Indwelling Urinary Catheter*

*It is normal for urine to change from light yellow to dark yellow, depending on the concentration and the amount of fluid the client has consumed.*

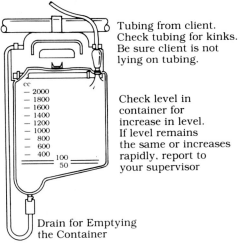

Plastic Urine
Container
Hung on Bedframe

Tubing from client.
Check tubing for kinks.
Be sure client is not
lying on tubing.

cc
— 2000
— 1800
— 1600
— 1400
— 1200
— 1000
— 800
— 600
— 400    100
          50

Check level in
container for
increase in level.
If level remains
the same or increases
rapidly, report to
your supervisor

Drain for Emptying
the Container

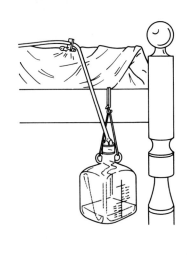

**FIGURE 18.9** Check the tubing from the client to the drainage bag frequently to be sure it is free of kinks.

■ Check from time to time to make sure the level of urine has increased. If the level stays the same, report this to your supervisor.

■ If the client says he feels that his bladder is full, or that he needs to urinate, report this to your supervisor.

■ If the client is allowed to get out of bed for short periods, the bag goes with him. It must always be held lower than the client's urinary bladder, to prevent the urine in the tubing and bag from draining back in the urinary bladder.

■ Check to make sure there are no kinks in the catheter and tubing.

■ Be sure the client is not lying on the catheter or the tubing. This would stop the flow of urine.

■ Be sure the tubing from the bed to the bag is always straight.

■ The catheter should be secured at all times to the client's inner thigh or in the case of male clients, the abdomen. This keeps it from being pulled on or being pulled out of the bladder. Tape can be used, or special straps are made for this purpose (Fig. 18.10).

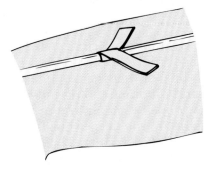

**FIGURE 18.10** Taping the tubing to the client decreases irritation.

■ Most clients with urinary drainage through a catheter are on intake and output measurement.

■ If urine leaks around a catheter, report this to your supervisor.

■ A male client may have an erection while the catheter is in place. This is a natural occurrence. Assure him there is nothing the matter with him, and maintain a concerned attitude. Discuss this with your supervisor for additional information.

▨ Empty the collection bag frequently and from the correct port. Protect the floor from spillage. There are many types of collection bags. If you find one that is new to you, ask for assistance.

▨ Clean the collection tubing and the bag as instructed by your agency. Some agencies discard collection equipment after a specified amount of time. Some agencies use a cleansing procedure.

▨ Keep the client's urinary opening clean. Even though he is not urinating, mucus and perspiration collect in the area.

▨ Be sure the catheter is free of fecal matter and mucus.

▨ Cover the exposed ends of tubing only with sterile covers.

▨ Notify your supervisor if you see sediment or blood in the tubing or collection bag.

## Procedure 69: Catheter Care

*Note:* This procedure may be incorporated into the morning bath routine. Be sure you use clean water for this procedure.

1. Assemble your equipment:
   Basin of water and mild soap or cleaning solution
   Washcloth or gauze pads
   Paper or plastic bag for waste
   Disposable gloves
2. Wash your hands.
3. Ask visitors to leave the room if appropriate.
4. Tell the client you are going to give him catheter care.
5. Position the client on his back so the catheter and urinary meatus are exposed. Put on your gloves.
6. Wash the area gently. Do not pull on the catheter, but hold it with one hand while wiping it with the other.
7. Observe the meatus for redness, swelling, or discharge.
8. Wipe away from the meatus. Wipe from the meatus to the anus.
9. Wipe one way and not back and forth.
10. Remove your gloves.
11. Dry the area.
12. Apply lotion to the thighs or cornstarch or powder in small quantities. Ask your supervisor if this area should be kept dry or moist.
13. Make the client comfortable.
14. Dispose of the dirty water into the toilet. Clean your equipment, and put it in its proper place.
15. Wash your hands.
16. Make a notation on the client's chart that you have completed this procedure. Also make a note of your observations of the client during this procedure.

## Leg Bag

A leg bag is a small plastic bag worn on the client's leg. This apparatus allows the client to be more active than when using the traditional straight drainage. It cannot be used when the client is lying down as the drainage is improper in that position (Fig. 18.11).

The same rules of asepsis that apply to changing a straight drainage bag apply to putting on a leg bag. Be sure to put the top of the bag at the top and the bottom at the bottom. Empty the bag immediately after it is removed or when it gets full. If the client is on I&O, record the amount of urine collected. Clean the bag as you have been taught by your supervisor.

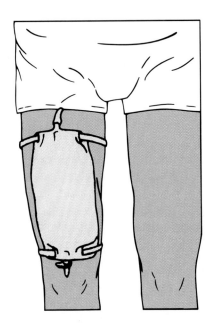

**FIGURE 18.11** The use of a leg bag increases the client's mobility but must be emptied frequently.

**Procedure 70: Changing a Catheter from a Straight Drainage Bag to a Leg Bag**

1. Assemble your equipment:
   Leg bag with straps
   Alcohol wipes or antiseptic solution
   Sterile cover for straight drainage tubing or sterile 4 x 4
   bed protector
2. Wash your hands.
3. Ask visitors to leave the room if appropriate.
4. Tell the client you are going to put on his leg bag.
5. Expose the end of the catheter and the drainage tubing.
   Put a bed protector under this area.
6. Disconnect the drainage tubing from the catheter and allow
   it to drain. Put a sterile cover on the end, and place it out
   of the way, but *not* on the floor. Do not put the catheter on
   the bed.
7. Wipe the attachment tube of the leg bag with an alcohol
   swab, and insert it into the catheter.
8. Secure the leg bag to the client's thigh.

9. Make the client comfortable.
10. Empty the drainage bag. Measure the urine, and note it on the chart.
11. Wash your hands.
12. Make a notation on the client's chart that you have completed this procedure. Also make a note of your observations of the client during this procedure.

# Section 4 Care of External Urinary Drainage

**Objectives: What You Will Learn to Do**

 List the reasons a male client may have an external urinary drainage system.

 *Introduction: Uses of External Urinary Drainage Systems*

When a male client is incontinent of urine, the nurse may suggest the use of an external drainage system that will collect the urine and keep the client dry. One end of the catheter is kept in place at the end of the penis and one end is connected to straight drainage (Fig. 18.12).

This device should not be left on for more than 24 hours at a time and must be removed at least that often so that the penis may be

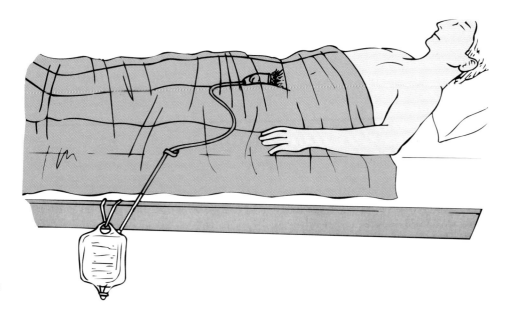

*FIGURE 18.12* Check the placement of external drainage frequently and change it at least every 24 hours.

washed and inspected. If there is any change in the skin and the client complains of pain or discomfort or the catheter does not drain, remove the entire device, discard it, and call your supervisor. Observe the client shortly after you put on the catheter and then frequently when you are with him.

The cleaning of the bag and the catheter should be discussed with your supervisor.

## Procedure 71: External Urinary Drainage

1. Assemble your equipment:
   External urinary system, consisting of a condom, a catheter, and a straight drainage system
   Material to secure condom to penis: tape, strap, or adhesive foam
   Soap and water
   Towel
2. Wash your hands.
3. Ask visitors to leave the room if appropriate.
4. Tell the client you are going to put on an external urinary collection device.
5. Position the client on his back so that the penis is exposed. Cover the client so he is not exposed.
6. Wash the entire penis and dry thoroughly. Observe the penis for any discharge or redness.
7. Roll the condom onto the entire length of the penis.
8. Secure the condom. Be sure the strap is tight enough to hold the condom in place but not so tight as to hurt the client.
9. Attach the catheter to the condom and to the straight drainage. Secure the collection bag on a bed or chair.
10. Make the client comfortable.
11. Dispose of the dirty water into the toilet. Clean your equipment and put it in its proper place.
12. Wash your hands.
13. Make a notation on the client's chart that you have completed this procedure. Also make note of your observations of the client during this procedure.

## Section 5   Intravenous Therapy: Peripheral or Central

## Objectives: What You Will Learn to Do

■ Define the difference between peripheral and central intravenous therapy.
■ List two reasons for intravenous therapy.
■ Discuss the role of the homemaker/home health aid in caring for a client receiving intravenous therapy.

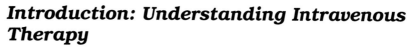

# Introduction: Understanding Intravenous Therapy

**intravenous therapy** giving of fluids or medication directly into the vein

**Intravenous therapy** (IV) is prescribed by a physician and administered by a registered nurse. During this procedure, the nurse inserts a needle into the client's veins to provide a way to give fluids or medication. The medication or fluids are either given by single injection, continuous drip slowly from a bottle or bag, or by a pump which regulates the flow of the medication or nourishment through a tube secured to the needle and the tubing (Fig. 18.13).

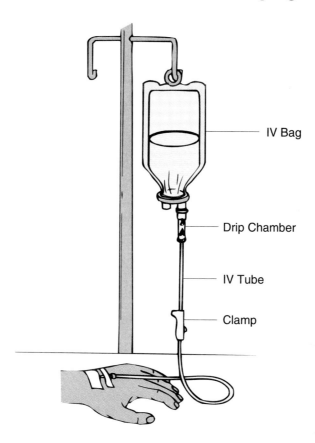

IV Bag

Drip Chamber

IV Tube

Clamp

**FIGURE 18.13** Clients with IVs do not have to be in bed, but they must be in a relaxed environment.

**continuous infusion** uninterrupted: without a stop

**intermittent infusion** alternating, stopping and beginning again

**peripheral line** intravenous lines in place in the upper extremities

**central venous lines** intravenous lines in place, surgically, in large veins of the body

■ **Continuous infusion:** fluid and/or medication is always running. This type of therapy is most often prescribed for clients who have a family member or friend who is able to assume responsibility for the insertion site and care of the bottles or bags.

■ **Intermittent infusion:** small amounts of fluid or medication are given over short periods of time. Each time a dose is needed, the IV must be started again.

There are three types of intravenous therapy:

■ **Peripheral lines:** the use of veins usually of the upper extremities.

■ **Central venous lines:** the use of a catheter that has been surgically implanted into one of the large veins. The end of the catheter used for medication administration is visible on the chest area.

■ **Peripherally inserted central venous catheters (PICC):** which are inserted at the bedside by a specially trained nurse or physician.

## Your Role as a Homemaker/Home Health Aide

Be observant and supportive. Support the client and the family as they learn to care for the equipment. If the client has a continuous infusion, he may walk around as long as the bottle of fluid is above the insertion site and does not pull on the tubing. Remind the client not to sit or lean on the tubing.

You will not be responsible for the care or dressing change of the IV site. Central lines will be covered by a dressing when they are not in use. Sometimes, a peripheral line will have a cap on it when it is not in use. This cap is usually covered by a dressing. Do not disturb these dressings. You will be asked to keep the dressing dry and clean. Check the dressing at least every eight hours to be sure it is secure. You should also be alert to changes in the site and report them immediately. Report if:

- The client complains of pain in the area.
- The area is red, hot, and/or swollen.
- You notice blood or any drainage from the area.
- The client removes the needle or tubing or it falls out.
- The tubing has blood in it.
- The level of fluid in the bag or bottle does not decrease.
- The bag or bottle breaks.

Be sure to document when you check the dressing. Write down that you checked the area and the condition of the dressing and the skin.

> Example: Jan. 28, 1995 2:00 P.M. IV site on left arm checked. Client did not complain of discomfort. Skin intact. No drainage noted on dressing which was secure and dry. Mary Cummings, H/HHA

## Section 6 Cast Care

## Objectives: What You Will Learn to Do

- List the reasons for plaster casts.
- Describe the role of the homemaker/home health aide in caring for clients with plaster casts.

## Introduction: Casts

cast rigid dressing molded to the body to give support and proper alignment

Clients who have broken a bone or sprained or strained a muscle may have a **cast** or splint placed on the body part to immobilize it. The procedure provides support to the injured part and prevents deformity by keeping it in the correct body alignment. Splints and casts are temporary. Permanent support to the bones in the form of pins, plates, and replacement of joints may also be necessary.

Plaster casts are, in reality, a form of a bandage. They are used as a support to hold injured bones in alignment while they are healing. Casts are wet when applied, then allowed to dry. Once it is hardened, the cast should not be allowed to get wet. Plastic or fiberglass casts perform the same task but are lighter, cleaner, and easier to use and remove.

While a plaster cast is drying, the client's position must be maintained and the cast left uncovered. It is normal for the cast to feel hot to the touch and to the client as it is drying. Pillows can be placed to support the cast so it will not move while it is still soft.

- Casts should not restrict circulation to the part.
- Casts should not cause pain. The pain should be only from the healing bone or muscle.
- The skin under casts frequently itches. Do not put anything into the cast. This might cause a scratch and lead to a skin infection.

## Your Role as a Homemaker/Home Health Aide

Casts should be kept clean and dry. They should be protected while a client is using the bedpan or toilet. Do not wash a plaster cast, as it will crumble.

There are casts that can be wet and allowed to air dry. Check with the client and your supervisor as to how to care for each cast. Just because casts look alike, they are not all cared for in the same way.

Encourage your client to take an active part in his care. Some people feel restricted in a cast and do not use the part as much as they are able. This unnecessary restriction of activity leads to a feeling of uselessness and loss of muscle tone.

Frequent careful checking of the cast and the injured part will help prevent complications. If you notice any of the following, call your supervisor:

- Numbness or tingling of toes or fingers
- Discoloration of toes or fingers
- Swelling of the limb at the edge of the cast
- Unusual odors coming from the cast
- Rough or cracked edges of the cast
- Loosely fitting cast
- Discolorations on the cast

Clients will often ask you how much movement they will have when the cast is removed. Tell them that you will get an answer for them. Then call your supervisor and discuss what to tell the client. Do not promise the client he will be fine unless that is what the physician has told him. Beware of telling him that everyone who has a broken arm is eventually fine. Everyone heals differently.

## Objectives: What You Will Learn to Do

■ Define ostomy.
■ Demonstrate the proper techniques for assisting with ostomy care.

## Introduction: The Ostomy

**ostomy** artificially created opening through the abdominal wall that provides a way for the intestinal organs to discharge waste products

**stoma** artificially made opening connecting a body passage with the outside

**colostomy** surgical procedure that creates an artificial opening through the abdominal wall into a part of the large bowel through which feces can leave the body. Can be temporary or permanent

**ileostomy** surgical procedure that makes an artificial opening through the abdominal wall into the ileum, through which waste material is discharged

**ureterostomy** an incision through the abdominal wall into the ureters resulting in drainage to the outside of the body

The creation of an ostomy is a surgical procedure. An **ostomy** is a new opening in the abdomen for the release of wastes from the body. The opening is called a **stoma**. This operation is necessary when the colon or urinary system is diseased or injured. Ostomies are created for many reasons—not only because a client has cancer. Sometimes the surgery is done to permit the colon to heal following an injury. Some ostomies are temporary, while others are permanent. The word *ostomy* means "opening into." A **colostomy** is an opening into the colon. An **ileostomy** is an opening into the ileum. A **ureterostomy** is an opening into the ureter. The opening is from the abdominal wall to the affected organ. The part you see, the stoma, will look like a pink rosebud (Fig. 18.14).

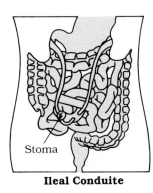

**Ileal Conduite**

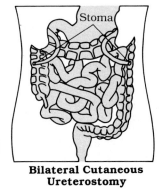

**Bilateral Cutaneous Ureterostomy**

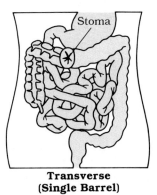

**Transverse (Single Barrel)**

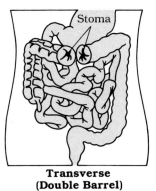

**Transverse (Double Barrel)**

*FIGURE 18.14* The placement and type of ostomy is the decision of the physician before surgery.

There are several types of colostomies. The type of colostomy takes its name from the placement of the stoma. It can be in the ascending, descending, or transverse colon. It can have one opening (single barrel) or two openings side by side (double barrel). The surgeon decides which type of colostomy is made.

A person with an ostomy must wear an appliance to collect the matter released through the stoma (Fig. 18.15). This collecting bag is held over the stoma by special paste, adhesive, and/or a belt. Some ostomy appliances are permanent. This means that they are reused after they are cleaned and dried. Some bags are disposable and used only once (Fig. 18.16).

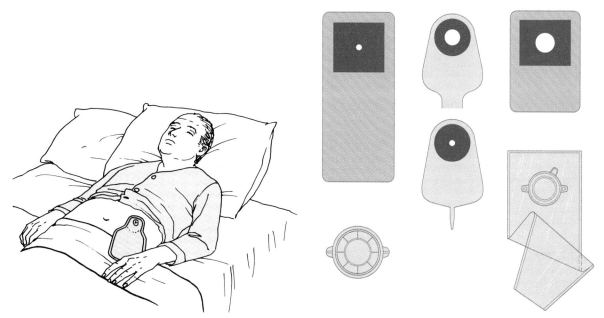

**FIGURE 18.15** The choice of a collection device is a personal one.

**FIGURE 18.16** There are various types of ostomy applicances.

##  *Your Role as a Homemaker/Home Health Aide*

When you receive your assignment, your supervisor will tell you the reasons the client had an ostomy. You will be told exactly for how much of the client's care you will be responsible. You will also be told what the client knows about his operation.

Your client's goal is to be as self-sufficient as possible. If the client will be unable to assume his total care, you will assist the client and his family as they establish a routine that they can maintain when you are no longer in the home.

Clients and families may want to discuss this operation with you. They will ask you questions. Do not lie to them. If they ask you questions that you cannot answer, assure them you will get the answers and call your supervisor. If the client asks you questions about death, recovery, and the future and you are uncomfortable, discuss this with your supervisor. Frequently, a client or family member will ask you the same question many times. This is a way of confirming that the first answer you gave was the real one. Report this to your supervisor. Your supervisor can then help you plan your care to meet this client's need.

All ostomy care is based on several considerations. They are:

■ Aseptic technique (rules of cleanliness)
■ Client and family reaction to the procedure

- Client prognosis
- Frequent changing of the collection bag

A collection bag must be changed when it is full or when the adhering seal is broken. Some clients will be well enough to sit in the bathroom on the toilet to do this procedure. Also, many clients will be learning to do this procedure independently, in which case you will assist them less and less.

**irrigate** cleanse or wash with water or fluid

Some clients will have to **irrigate** their colostomy as part of their routine. Irrigating a colostomy is like giving an enema into the ostomy. You may, after you have been instructed, assist the client as he carries out this procedure.

## Procedure 72: Assisting with an Ostomy

*Note:* Each client has his own routine for caring for his ostomy. This procedure is a general guide.

1. Assemble your equipment:
   Bedpan
   Disposable bed protector
   Bath blanket
   Clean ostomy belt (ostomy appliance), adjustable
   Toilet tissue
   Basin of water
   Soap or cleanser
   Washcloth
   Disposable gloves (optional)
   Towels
   Lubricant or skin cream, as ordered
   Plastic waste bag
2. Wash your hands.
3. Ask any visitors to leave the room if appropriate.
4. Tell the client that you are going to assist him with changing his ostomy appliance.
5. Cover the client with the bath blanket. Ask the client to hold the top edge of the blanket. Without exposing him, fanfold the top sheet and bedspread to the foot of the bed under the blanket.
6. Place the disposable bed protector under the client's hips. This is to keep the bed from getting wet or dirty.
7. Place the bedpan within easy reach.
8. Put the wash basin, soap, washcloth, and bath towels near the bed.
9. Open the belt. Protect it if it is clean and can be used again. If the belt is dirty, remove it. It must be replaced with a clean one.
10. Remove the soiled plastic stoma bag from the belt carefully.
11. Put the soiled plastic bag into the bedpan. Wipe the area around the ostomy with toilet tissue. This is to remove any loose feces. Place the dirty tissue in the plastic bag. Flush the tissues down the toilet later.
12. Wet and soap the washcloth. Wash the entire ostomy area with a gentle circular motion.

13. Dry the area gently with a bath towel.

14. Apply a small amount of lubricant or protective cream (if ordered) around the area of the ostomy. The lubricant is to prevent irritation to the skin around the ostomy. Wipe off all excess lubricant so that the ostomy device will adhere to the skin. If using a wafer, secure it around the stoma. Be sure the size is correct (Fig. 18.17).

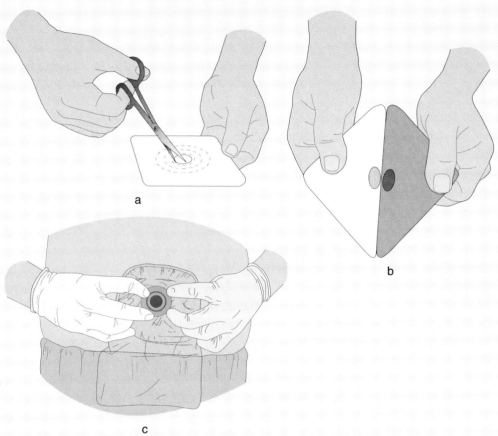

**FIGURE 18.17** (a) Cut the hole in the center of the wafer 1/8 inch larger than the stoma. (b) Peel the backing from the wafer. (c) Place the wafer around the stoma and attach a clean bag.

15. Put a clean adjustable belt, if the client wears one, on the client. Place a clean stoma bag in place through the loop.

16. Remove the disposable bed protector. Change any damp linen.

17. Replace the top sheet and bedspread, and remove the bath blanket.

18. Make the client comfortable.

19. Remove all used equipment. Dispose of waste material into the toilet. Do not throw the plastic collection bag down the toilet but into the plastic liner in the wastebasket.

20. Clean the bedpan, and put it in its proper place.

21. Empty the wash basin into the toilet. Wash it thoroughly with soap and water. Rinse and dry it, and return it to its proper place.

22. Wash your hands.

23. Make a notation on the client's chart that you have completed this procedure. Also make a note of your observations about the client during this procedure.

As a homemaker/home health aide, you will be assisting clients and their families in many phases of ostomy care. Clients are often afraid or disgusted by this procedure. Be patient and understanding. Let the client and his family express their feelings. Listen. Although most ostomy clients are encouraged to assume their own care, each one does so at a different pace. Respect the client's feelings and his individual wishes. Discuss your client's reactions and your feelings and activities in this house when you see your supervisor. In this way you will gain a better understanding of your client and yourself.

## Gastrostomy, Duodenostomy, and Jejunostomy

These ostomies are surgical openings directly into various parts of the upper gastrointestinal tract. These incisions are kept open by the presence of a tube or a screw cap. The client will receive part or all of his nourishment through this opening. He may also take his medication through this opening (Fig. 18.18).

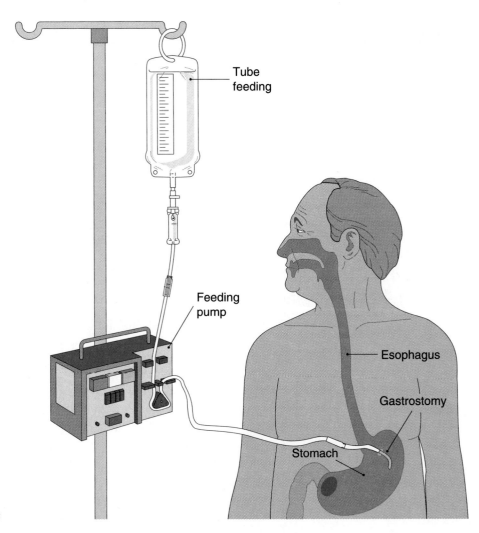

*FIGURE 18.18*

## Your Role as a Homemaker/Home Health Aide

Your role in working with a client who has one of these openings is to assist him in feedings and in the care of the area. You will not be given complete responsibility for the procedure as it is very important that a family member be able to assist the client when you are not there.

Cleanliness is an important part of the care. Be sure that the client's or family member's hands are clean before he cares for the site and before he starts the feeding.

Assist the client in making the feeding or in preparing commercially prepared feeding. Be sure to read directions and to follow them closely. When mixing the solution, date the container with important information. It is wise to discard any feeding that is more than 24 hours old. Warm the solution to room temperature. Observe the client as to how he tolerates the feeding. Report to your supervisor your observations.

Note the time of the feeding, how long it lasts, and how the client tolerates it. Also note if he complains of any nausea, vomiting, diarrhea, cramps, or sweating after the feeding.

# Section 8   Assisting a Client Having a Seizure

## Objectives: What You Will Learn to Do

- Describe a grand mal seizure.
- Describe a petit mal seizure.
- Demonstrate safety measures for the client having a seizure.

### Introduction: Creating a Safe Environment for a Client Having a Seizure

**seizure** convulsions or involuntary muscular contractions and relaxations

A **seizure** is caused by an abnormality within the central nervous system. This abnormality is thought to be an electrical problem in the nerve cells. Seizures can occur from the time of birth or may be the result of a head injury or disease. Often the cause of seizures is unknown. Seizures are often controlled by medication.

As a homemaker/home health aide, you may be present when a client has a seizure. Therefore, it is important for you to know what the warning signals of a seizure are and what to do if one occurs.

**aura** sensation before an epileptic seizure

Some clients know they are going to have a seizure. This is called an **aura.** An aura may be a smell or sensation that always occurs before the client has a seizure. There are two types of seizures. One type is known as grand mal. The other type is a partial body seizure known as a petit mal. In the **grand mal seizure,** there may be stiffness of the total body followed by a jerking action of the muscles. Usually, the client becomes unconscious. Sometimes the client bites his tongue. Sometimes he becomes incontinent. These seizures can last for several minutes.

**grand mal seizure** type of epileptic seizure

**petite mal seizure** type of epileptic seizure

In the **petit mal seizure,** the client may appear to be daydreaming. His eyes may roll back, and there may be some quivering of the body muscles. The petit mal seizure usually lasts less than 30 seconds. The client usually has no memory of the seizure. Clients who have been diagnosed as having epilepsy, or who have seizures due to other diseases, often lead normal productive lives. Ignorance about seizures is their biggest enemy.

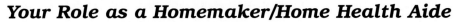

### Your Role as a Homemaker/Home Health Aide

Your role as a homemaker/home health aide in caring for a client having a seizure is to prevent the client from injuring himself. If you are present at the beginning of a seizure, you may place a padded tongue depressor or tongue blade, or a belt, in the client's mouth, if this is the policy of your health care agency. Some health care agencies prefer that you simply turn the client's head to the side. If the client's jaw is already tight or he has his teeth clenched, *do not try to pry his teeth apart to insert a tongue depressor.* Help the client to lie down on the floor. Loosen his clothing, and move any furniture that he might hit as he moves. Place a pillow or something soft under his head. *Turn his head to the side to promote drainage of saliva or vomitus. Never try to move or restrain the client.* Protect the client from people who may stare at him. Protect him from embarrassment.

Comfort the client after the seizure. Clean him of any saliva, urine, or fecal matter. Assist him with mouth care and care of his body after the seizure. After the client is comfortable and safe, chart the client's actions and your actions during this occurrence. Notify your supervisor of the entire incident.

## Section 9 Testing Urine for Sugar and Acetone

### Objectives: What You Will Learn to Do

- Discuss the reasons for testing a client's urine for sugar and acetone.
- Demonstrate the proper technique for testing urine for sugar and acetone.

### Introduction: Testing Urine for Sugar and Acetone

The testing of a client's urine provides an accurate and easy method of checking the client's metabolism of carbohydrates. This procedure is usually done with diabetic clients but may be done with other clients.

**glucose** sugar

**acetone** a chemical found in urine

**ketones** chemical compounds sometimes found in urine

**reagent** a substance used to measure or detect another substance

The Clinitest and Clinistix tests determine the amount of **glucose** (sugar) in the client's urine. The Acetest or Ketostix reagent strip determines the amount of **acetone** or **ketones** in the urine.

These tests are usually done four times a day: 1/2 hour before breakfast, lunch, supper, and at bedtime.

For each test you will be using either a reagent strip or a reagent tablet. A **reagent** is a substance used in a chemical reaction to determine the presence of another substance. The names of these tablets or strips vary greatly according to geographical area and the pharmaceutical company that makes them. When testing for sugar (doing the Clinitest), you will use Clinitest tablets, Tes-tape, Clinistix, or Uristix. When testing for acetone (doing the Acetest), you will use Ketostix, Tes-tape, Acetone, Uristix, or Labstix. Instructions for these tests are on the package of reagent strips or reagent tablets. All tablets and strips used for these tests are poisonous. Always put equipment in a safe place where children cannot reach it. Be sure to wash and dry all equipment between tests and keep bottles tightly closed. Heat is generated during the Clinitest. Do not touch the bottom of the glass test tube while doing the tests as it will be hot and you could burn yourself. Be sure to pay attention to the time. Many incorrect readings are made because of incorrect timing.

Some readings are recorded as percentages and some as "plus" (++, etc.). Be sure you ask how the client reports his readings.

Each client will decide with his physician which tests he will do at home depending on client need, cost, and availability of alternative tests, such as glucometer equipment. This is an accurate blood test that often replaces the need for frequent urine testing.

## FRESH FRACTIONAL SPECIMENS

A fresh specimen is needed for each testing. However, since the sugar test and the acetone test are done at the same time, only one specimen is needed. The word *fresh* is used to refer to urine that has accumulated recently in the client's urinary bladder. To obtain fresh urine, it is necessary to discard the first urine voided because this urine has remained in the urinary bladder for an unknown length of time. One-half hour after discarding the urine, collect a fresh urine specimen for the test. This will be urine recently accumulated in the urinary bladder. The word *fractional* is used to refer to a small portion of the urine voided. Only a very small amount of urine is needed for these tests.

*Note:* There are two Clinitest methods. One is the older 5-drop method. The newer method is the 2-drop method. *Special notes about the 2-drop method:*

- It gives expanded readings up to 5% sugar in the urine.
- It requires a special chart to read it, not a different tablet.
- It requires careful watching.
- If the urine contains more than 5% sugar, the color will "pass through" the bright orange color (5%) and become greenish orange. This indicates that the sugar is higher than 5%.

## Procedure 73: The Clinitest

1. Assemble your equipment:
   Fresh urine specimen
   Clean and dry test tube
   Color chart
   Medicine dropper
   Clinitest reagent tablets
   Paper cup of water for rinsing dropper
   Paper cup of clean water for test
   Paper towel
   Disposable gloves (optional)
2. Wash your hands.
3. Place the paper towel on the countertop that will be your working area.

4. Rinse the dropper in the paper cup of water that is used for rinsing only.

5. With the dropper in the upright position, place 5 drops of urine in the center of the test tube.

6. Rinse the dropper.

7. Place 10 drops of clean water in the center of the test tube.

8. Place one Clinitest tablet in the test tube by dropping the tablet into the cover of the bottle and then dropping the tablet into the test tube from the cover. Never touch the tablet with your hands. (If your hands are wet and you touch the tablet, the moisture will activate the reaction and you will be burned.) Then cap the bottle immediately. If the tablets are individually wrapped, open the foil carefully and drop the tablet into the test tube without touching the tablet.

9. Wait 15 seconds after the reaction (boiling) has stopped. Then shake the test tube.

10. Compare the test tube contents with the color chart.

11. Match the color of the liquid in the test tube to the nearest matching color on the chart. Be sure to use the color chart that goes with the tablets you have used for the test.

12. Read the number inside the matching color box. For example, if the color is bright orange, it will say 2% or 4 ++++ inside the orange-colored box.

13. Throw away used disposable equipment. Wash the test tube with cold water. Replace it upside down so that any remaining water will drain out. The test tube will then be ready for the next test. Rinse the medicine dropper with cold water. Put it in a safe place.

14. Wash your hands.

15. Note on the client's chart that you have completed this procedure and what the test result was. Also make a note of your observations of the client during this procedure. If you are to call your supervisor now, do so and note this on the chart.

## Procedure 74: The Acetest

1. Assemble your equipment:
   Fresh urine specimen
   Color chart
   Medicine dropper
   Acetest reagent tablets
   Paper cup of water for rinsing dropper
   Paper towel
   Disposable gloves (optional)

2. Wash your hands.

3. Place the paper towel on the countertop that will be your working area.
4. Place one acetone tablet on the paper towel.
5. Never touch the tablet, but drop it into the cover of its container. Then place it on the paper towel from the cover.
6. Rinse the medicine dropper with water from the paper cup.
7. Place 1 drop of urine on the tablet. Wait 30 seconds.
8. Compare it to the color chart.
9. Match the color of the tablet to the nearest matching color on the chart.
10. Read the results from the chart. For example, if the color is dark purple, it will say "Large Quantity."
11. Throw away used disposable equipment.
12. Wash your hands.
13. Note on the client's chart that you have completed this procedure and what the result was. Also make a note of your observations of the client during this procedure. If you are to call your supervisor now, do so and note this on the chart.

## Procedure 75: The Clinistix Test

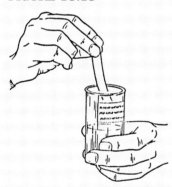

FIGURE 18.19

1. Assemble your equipment:
   Fresh urine specimen
   Clinistix reagent strips
   Disposable gloves (optional)
2. Wash your hands.
3. Dip the reagent strip into the urine in the specimen container (Fig. 18.19).
4. Remove it immediately.
5. Tap the edge of the strip against the side of the urine container to remove excess urine.
6. Hold the strip in a horizontal position to prevent mixing of the chemical from the adjacent reagent area.
7. Clinistix reagent strips are used for the glucose level. Therefore, read the results 10 seconds after removing the strip from the urine. The color chart is on the Clinistix bottle label.
8. Read the results from the color chart, matching the color carefully.
9. Discard disposable equipment.
10. Wash your hands.
11. Note on the client's chart that you have completed this procedure and what the result was. Also make a note of your observations of the client during this procedure. If you are to call your supervisor now, do so and note this on the chart.

## Procedure 76: The Ketostix Reagent Strip Test

1. Assemble your equipment:
   Fresh urine specimen
   Ketostix reagent strips
   Disposable gloves (optional)
2. Wash your hands.
3. Dip the Ketostix strip into the urine in the container.
4. Remove it immediately.
5. Tap the edge of the strip against the side of the urine container to remove excess urine.
6. Hold the strip in a horizontal position to prevent possible mixing of the chemical from the adjacent reagent area.
7. The ketone test is read 15 seconds after removing the strip from the urine.
8. Read the results from the color chart in good lighting, matching the color carefully. The color chart is on the bottle label that holds the Ketostix strips.
9. Throw away disposable equipment.
10. Wash your hands.
11. Note on the client's chart that you have completed this procedure and what the result was. Also make a note of your observations of the client during this procedure. If you are to call your supervisor now, do so and note this on the chart.

# Section 10  Deep-Breathing Exercises

## Objectives: What You Will Learn to Do

- State the reasons for shallow breathing. State your role in assisting clients with deep-breathing exercises.
- Demonstrate the correct technique for assisting clients with deep-breathing exercises.

### Introduction: Deep Breathing

Shallow breathing takes place in the upper lobes of the lungs, which are surrounded by bony areas on all sides. The lungs cannot expand very much in the bony enclosure, so they cannot take in much oxygen or exhale much carbon dioxide. People who have had lung disease for a long time have "barrel chests." The chest cavity has taken on this shape in an attempt to have the lungs inhale more oxygen.

Deep breathing helps people inhale more air with less effort than their usual type of breathing. When people breathe deeply, the lower lobes of the lungs push the soft tissue of the abdomen out of the way and expand to take in more air.

People who have lung disease continue to breathe with shallow breaths because of fear and misinformation about how their bodies are built. You will be able to help clients trust deep breathing by explaining how their lungs work. Your supervisor will do this, too, but it will be your responsibility to answer questions. If you do not know the answer, tell the client that you will get the information and ask your supervisor.

### Your Role as a Homemaker/Home Health Aide

Clients who are learning to deep breathe are often frightened. Have patience and be gentle. Praise the client, and point out small successes. Continue to reinforce the reasons why deep breathing is important.

When the client takes a deep breath, his shoulders and chest should *not* move. His abdomen should expand. When he exhales his abdomen should get *flat*. If the client is confused about how to do this, tell him to cough. The squeezing of the abdominal area will make him aware of where the muscular activity should take place.

Coughing is forced expiration. Deep breathing sometimes produces a coughing response. This is true especially if the lungs are congested. Keep a basin, tissue, or specimen container (if ordered) near the client. Collect any mucus he may bring up. Encourage him to spit it out. Note the color, amount, and odor.

Protect the client from visitors and friends when he is coughing. Deep breathing is frequently unpleasant, although it is very important. Because it also makes some people cough and bring up mucus, plan this exercise between mealtimes. By doing this, you will not cause vomiting or loss of appetite.

The physical therapist will instruct you as to how often this exercise is to be done. She may also give you some special instructions for your client. Remember, all clients are different and though the exercise may look the same for two people, the reasons it is done may be different. The physical therapist will also tell you if there are any special observations you are to make while you are helping the client.

Even though you are able to do these exercises, do not start them until you have been instructed to do so. The aim of teaching clients deep breathing, or abdominal breathing as it is also called, is to change their breathing habits permanently.

## Procedure 77: Helping a Client with Deep-Breathing Exercises

1. Assemble your equipment:
   Equipment for mouth care following this procedure
   Tissues and basin or specimen container
   Plastic bag for waste
2. Wash your hands.
3. Ask visitors to leave the room if appropriate.
4. Tell the client you are going to help him with deep-breathing exercises.
5. Direct the client to breathe in deeply through his nose.

6. Direct the client to blow out through his mouth with his lips "pursed" (as though he were blowing out a match) (Fig. 18.20).
7. This should be repeated 10 times.
8. Offer the client mouth care.
9. Dispose of the tissues into a plastic bag.
10. Make the client comfortable.
11. Make a notation on the chart that you have completed this procedure. Also note anything you observed about the client while doing this procedure.

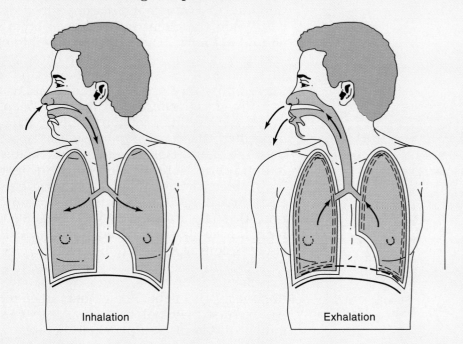

*FIGURE 18.20*

Inhalation      Exhalation

## Section 11   Making Normal Saline

**Objectives: What You Will Learn to Do**

▮ Describe some uses of normal saline.
▮ Demonstrate the procedure to make normal saline.

### *Introduction: Making Normal Saline*

Normal saline is a solution of salt and water that has many uses. Its chemical makeup is very close to the fluids in the body. It is usually used to wash open areas or to clean very sore bony prominences or bedsores. It may also be used by a nurse to irrigate a Foley catheter.

## Procedure 78: Making Normal Saline

1. Assemble your equipment:
   Large pot
   Sterilized 1-qt jar and lid
   2 tsp of salt
   1 qt of water
   Source of heat (stove, Sterno, fire)
2. Wash your hands.
3. Measure 1 qt of water into pot. Add 2 tsp of salt. Boil covered for 10 minutes (Fig. 18.21a).
4. Pour into sterilized jar, and replace cover. Allow solution to cool (Fig. 18.21b).
5. May be used up to 48 hours after making the solution.

FIGURE 18.21a

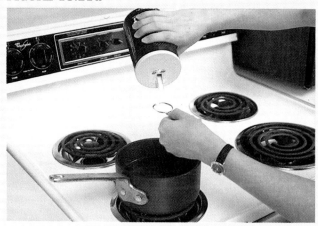

FIGURE 18.21b

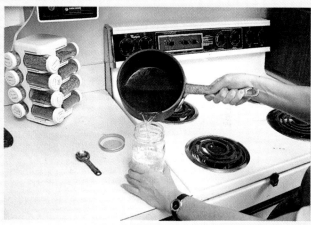

# Section 12  Sitz Bath

## Objectives: What You Will Learn to Do

- List three reasons a client may have to take a sitz bath.
- Describe the safety precautions you will take when assisting a client with a sitz bath.
- Demonstrate what you will report to your supervisor after your client has taken a sitz bath.

###  Introduction: The Sitz Bath

**sitz bath** bath in which the client sits in a specially designed chair or tub with his hips and buttocks in water

The term **sitz bath** means seat bath or a bath that is given while sitting. The area that is bathed is the perineal area. Such a procedure may be ordered to promote healing of the area, to decrease pain following surgery or a procedure, and to increase relaxation of the muscles in the perineal area.

A sitz bath can be taken by the client either in a specially designed bath that fits into the toilet or commode or in a bathtub that has had a covered rubber ring placed in it so that the perineal area is suspended off the tub floor (Fig. 18.22).

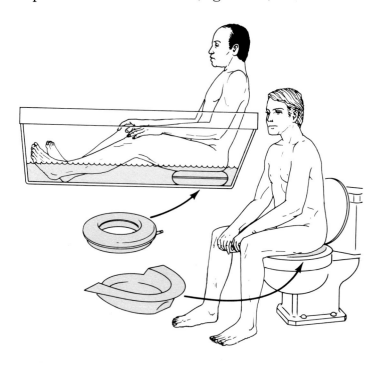

FIGURE 18.22 Provide a safe and private place for the client during a sitz bath. Be sure he can signal for assistance.

**Safety Considerations:** Be sure the water is the correct temperature. It should be comfortable to the touch and measure between 95 and 110°F or 35 to 43°C. Water that is too hot will burn the client, and water that is too cold will cause the muscles to tighten up rather than relax.

Help the client start and finish the procedure. Safely getting on and off the commode or in and out of the tub should be done slowly and at the client's speed. Protect the client from slipping and falling on towels, clothes, or dressings.

Maintain the water temperature by adding warm water when necessary.

Help the client keep track of the time. The usual length of time for a sitz bath is between 10 and 15 minutes. You will be told how long and how often your client should have a sitz bath. Check on your client frequently, and tell him how long he has yet to go. Ask your client how he feels, and observe him, too.

### ■ *Your Role as a Homemaker/Home Health Aide*

Your role is to assist the client take his sitz bath as it has been ordered. If you find the client deviates from the order, report that to your supervisor.

You will also be responsible for cleaning the sitz bath or the bath tub following the procedure. Be sure that the bath area is clean and dry and ready for the next time the client must bathe. Assist the client with dressings that he may have to apply and dispose of old soiled dressings in plastic bags in the outside trash.

Following the procedure, when the client is comfortable and the area is clean, you will chart your activities. These are the elements to include:

- The length of time the client remained in the bath
- The client's reaction to the bath
- A description of any drainage from the wounds
- How the client finished the procedure—new dressing, returned to bed, and so on

# Section 13   Hyperalimentation

## Objectives: What You Will Learn to Do

- Recognize the reasons that a client would receive hyperalimentation.
- Discuss the role of the homemaker/home health aide as an observer during the feeding.
- List at least five occurrences when you would call your supervisor.

## *Introduction: Working with Hyperalimentation*

**hyperalimentation** process of giving nutrients directly into the blood stream

Clients who are severely malnourished and who are unable to eat often receive their nutritional requirements by means of **hyperalimentation.** For long term administration a catheter is surgically placed in a large vein and the nutrition is administered directly into the blood stream. A physician orders the exact dose of the supplement, and it must be mixed by a special pharmacy. The pharmacy has the responsibility for delivering the correct bottles to the client every 24 hours. The catheter that is used for the feeding is not used for any other purpose. Some bottles or bags must be kept refrigerated. Some must be at room temperature. If the delivery does not arrive on time or you notice that the feedings are not stored properly, call your supervisor. Do not discard any unused feedings. Return them to the pharmacy.

Clients may receive this treatment for a short amount of time or for several years. Some clients receive their feeding in the evening and work during the day. Others receive feeding over a 24-hour period. Clients who receive this treatment must be able to assume the responsibility for the feedings or have a responsible family member who can do it. This teaching takes place in the hospital and will be reinforced in the home. Usually, there is an emergency telephone number that can be called with questions. The professionals from the supply company will take responsibility for checking the pump and the catheter insertion site. If the family has any questions between visits, they should be encouraged to contact the supplier via the emergency telephone number.

You will not be asked to administer the feedings or change the dressings on the catheter, but you will be responsible for assisting with preparation of the bottles. Allow the bottles to stand at room temperature at least one hour before use.

## Your Role as a Homemaker/Home Health Aide

You will be caring for the client's personal needs during the administration of the hyperalimentation. Be observant for any changes in the client. Report them immediately. If you are to keep a record of intake and output, vital signs, and weights, do so accurately.

■ Report any shortness of breath, tingling in arms or feet, or weakness or temperature.

■ Report any irritation or drainage near the catheter site.

■ Report any change in the client.

■ Help the client maintain a comfortable position during the feeding. The tubes should be straight and not under the client.

## Topics for Discussion

1. Review actual homemaker/home health aide assignments and make a plan as to when you would do all the procedures. Discuss different routines and the things that you would take into consideration as you made up each plan.

2. How do you feel about all the procedures that you learned in this section? Are there some you do not feel comfortable with? Why?

# Chapter 19

# Common Diseases
You Will See

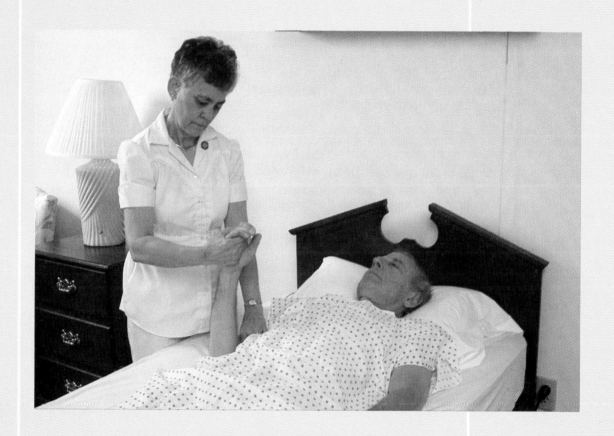

## Objectives: What You Will Learn to Do

- Discuss the most common signs and symptoms of hypertension.
- Discuss your role in caring for clients with hypertension.

 *Introduction: Hypertension*

hypertension high blood pressure

**Hypertension,** or high blood pressure, is a treatable chronic disease. People who have hypertension have more stress placed on their circulatory systems than people without high blood pressure. Latest estimates are that over 35 million Americans suffer from hypertension. Hypertension contributes to death from heart disease and kidney disease. Treatment for hypertension is available, but must be kept up forever. Once blood pressure has been brought to an acceptable level, it does not mean the disease has gone away. It only means that the disease has been brought under control, and this control must be continued.

### HOW DO PEOPLE KNOW THEY HAVE HYPERTENSION?

Hypertension has been called "the silent killer" because it gives no warning. In the early stages of this disease, there often are no symptoms. As the disease develops, people may complain of headaches, vision changes, or problems with their urinary output. If they would consult a physician at this point in their disease, permanent damage to a vital organ could be avoided. Some people with high blood pressure do not seek help until they have severe problems. By this time there is often permanent damage to their vital organs. It is important to find those people who have hypertension before they suffer permanent damage.

Certain people are more apt to have hypertension than others. You have a higher risk of hypertension if you:

- Have a family history of hypertension, heart disease, or kidney disease.
- Smoke cigarettes.
- Are overweight.
- Use a lot of salt in your diet.
- Are black.
- Eat a large amount of saturated fats.

### CAUSES AND TREATMENT OF HYPERTENSION

Many conditions seem to cause hypertension, and some of the causes are still unknown. Research scientists are investigating diet, heredity, birth control pills, kidney infections, and chemicals as possible causes of this chronic disease.

An individualized treatment plan is developed by a physician after a thorough medical examination. Treatment may consist of a combination of diet, medication, and exercise.

 ### *Your Role as a Homemaker/Home Health Aide*

Follow the plan of care for your client. Support your client in complying with his medication plan, diet, and exercise. Report to your supervisor any deviation from the care plan.

Assist the client with incorporating his treatment into his usual daily routine. Because he will always be on some treatment for this disease, it is important that the treatment become a regular part of his day.

Listen to your client. If he has questions about hypertension and/or his treatment, answer him honestly. If you do not know the answer, call your supervisor, but be sure that the client gets his answers.

Be observant for possible side effects from the medication. Depending on the drug and the client, side effects range from a stuffy nose to muscle cramps, weakness, nightmares, and impotence. Careful observations and objective, timely reporting of these and other symptoms will result in a treatment plan the client can live with the rest of his life. If the client starts taking any medications, including nonprescription drugs, report this to your supervisor.

# Section 2  Heart Attack/Myocardial Infarction

## Objectives: What You Will Learn to Do

- Define *myocardial infarction.*
- Define *atherosclerosis.*
- List the common symptoms of a heart attack.
- Discuss three kinds of pacemakers.
- Discuss the role of the homemaker/home health aide in caring for a client recovering from a myocardial infarction.

 ### *Introduction: Myocardial Infarction*

**heart attack** layman's term referring to damage to the heart; a myocardial infarction

**myocardial infarction** death of a part of the heart due to blockage in a blood vessel

**Heart attack** is a general term that describes sudden damage to the heart. There are many medical reasons people have heart attacks, but they all have the same results—a decrease in the blood supply to the heart (Fig. 19.1). This eventually leads to heart muscle damage and possibly permanent tissue death.

The word *infarct* means the death of tissue due to lack of blood. The word *myocardial* refers to heart muscle. So a **myocardial infarction,** or MI, is really the death of part of the heart due to a blockage in a blood vessel. If the blood vessel involved is a small one and only a small amount of heart muscle is affected, this may be called a minor or small heart attack. If the blood vessel involved is a large one and a large portion of the heart is damaged, it is often called a massive heart attack. The ultimate recovery of the injured heart depends on the location of the MI within the heart, age, sex, atherosclerosis, and health history of the individual.

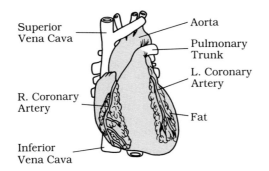

**FIGURE 19.1** All these blood vessels are necessary for the heart to function at an optimum level.

## ARTERIOSCLEROSIS

**Arteriosclerosis** is hardening of arteries and leads to a decrease in the blood supply to body tissue due to a thickening of vessel walls (Fig. 19.2). **Atherosclerosis** is a form of arteriosclerosis that takes place in several well-defined steps:

**arteriosclerosis** "hardening of the arteries" due to thickening of the blood vessel walls

**atherosclerosis** increased formation of fatty deposits and fibrous plaques, resulting in decrease of the lumen of the blood vessel

■ A fatty streak develops in the vessel.
■ A fibrous plaque develops on top of this. Depending on the size of this plaque, the vessel remains open or becomes completely obstructed.
■ Sometimes a clot develops in the same spot as the fibrous plaque.

If atherosclerosis is discovered and treated after the first stage, the condition is reversible. However, once a vessel is completely blocked by plaque, it usually remains that way.

### Signs and Symptoms of Heart Attack

The following signs and symptoms may appear in your client or in a member of the family. Call for emergency help immediately, and keep the client quiet and warm until help arrives.

■ Chest pain that may or may not radiate to the arm or jaw
■ Wet, clammy skin

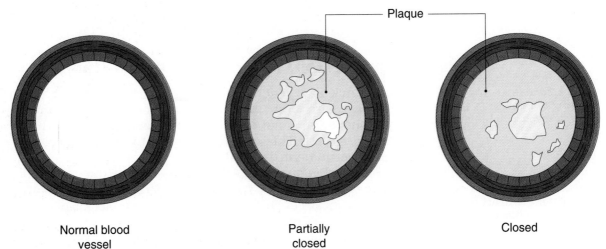

| Normal blood vessel | Partially closed | Closed |

**FIGURE 19.2** The elimination of plaque forming foods from the diet should begin in early childhood.

- Weak and/or rapid pulse rate
- Pale color
- Low blood pressure
- Shortness of breath
- Nausea

## Your Role as a Homemaker/Home Health Aide

After hospitalization, your client will return with an individualized plan of care based on:

- The type of heart attack he had
- His recovery up to that point
- His home situation
- His prognosis

As you assist your client with his daily routine, you will develop a relationship with him. Allow him to have as active a part in his care as his activity level permits. You will get to know him and what he can tolerate.

The plan of care you will receive from your supervisor will include instructions about:

- Activity restrictions
- Diet restrictions
- Medications
- Emotional support

While giving care to a person with a cardiac disability, all caregivers balance the desire to allow the client to be a self-sufficient person and the need to restrict his activity level. Continual discussion with your supervisor as to your client's condition will assist you in making correct decisions.

Many clients are given an exercise regime. Assist your client with the regime as it has been prescribed. If your client is unable to progress with the exercise or tries to advance too quickly, report this to your supervisor.

After a heart attack, many people become "cardiac cripples." They are so afraid of another heart attack that they do not exert themselves at all or take any part in their care. They even remove themselves from family relationships. Everything they do is blamed on their heart attack and their fear of another one.

The opposite of this is a total disregard for one's condition. The client denies any disability. He does not follow any suggestions from his physician, take his medication, nor adhere to his diet. Report this to your supervisor also.

Clients are concerned about how their heart attack will affect their sexual activities. Most clients will return to a full sexual life; however, the discussion is best handled by the client's physician or nurse, who knows what the client has already been told. Do not give the client any opinions or old wives' tales but rather say, "I know you are concerned about this, and I will tell the nurse. She will get you the information you want."

Family members often need help in dealing with the stress of lifestyle changes and fear caused by cardiac disease. Suggest that any family member who expresses these fears seek the assistance of support groups or their physician.

# PACEMAKERS

**pacemaker** electrical device used to stimulate the heart

**Pacemakers** are electrical devices placed in the left upper chest under the skin (Fig. 19.3). The job of this device is to regulate the heart rhythm. A pacemaker can be temporary or permanent. There are three types of pacemakers:

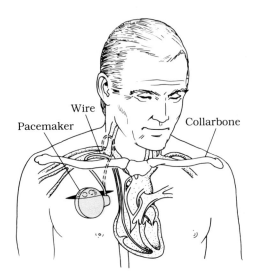

*FIGURE 19.3* Pacemakers permit people to live normal productive lives with only a few restrictions.

1. *Fixed rate:* Stimulation rate is fixed usually between 60 and 70 beats per minute. This is used only if the heart is totally dependent on electrical stimulation.
2. *Synchronous:* Stimulation occurs after a predetermined lack of the heart's own activity.
3. *Demand pacemaker:* When the heartbeat falls below a predetermined rate, the pacemaker takes over. This is the most common type.

### Care of the Pacemaker

It is helpful to know what type of pacemaker your client has. It is also important to know at what rate it is set. There are several guidelines to keep in mind when you have a client with a pacemaker.

- Electrical appliances may be used around pacemakers.
- Microwave ovens should not be used around pacemakers. Some clients have difficulties being around lawn mowers and cellular telephones.
- If your client has hiccups, report this immediately. This could be an indication that the electrical wires are out of place.
- If your client's pulse is below the preset level of the pacemaker, report it immediately.
- Report pain or discoloration near the pacemaker.
- Detecting devices in airports should be avoided.
- Report any complaints of dizziness, **edema** (swelling), shortness of breath, or irregular heart beat.
- Batteries have to be replaced from time to time. The physician decides when this is to be done. It varies from client to client.
- Assist your client with his telephone monitoring procedure. Be sure he understands it so that he can do it when you are no longer in the house.

**edema** abnormal swelling of a part of the body caused by fluid collecting in that area

## Objectives: What You Will Learn to Do

- Define *angina*, and list the major causes and risk factors.
- Discuss some of the treatments for angina.
- Discuss your role as a homemaker/home health aide when caring for a patient with angina.

### *Introduction: Angina*

**angina** brief, temporary chest pain resulting from a decrease in oxygen to the heart

**Angina** is a brief, temporary pain or heaviness in the chest that results from lack of oxygen to the heart. Usually after resting and medication, the discomfort disappears. These episodes may be brought on by stress or physical activity. Angina differs from person to person. Changes in your client's angina signal a change in his cardiac status and should be reported to your supervisor immediately.

#### CAUSES OF ANGINA

Angina is due to the narrowing of the coronary arteries that bring oxygen to the heart. As these vessels narrow, the amount of oxygen decreases, causing pain and discomfort. This is not a heart attack or myocardial infarction because it is a temporary condition. However, if the angina is allowed to continue without treatment, the sufferer could have a heart attack, resulting in permanent damage to the heart.

You have a higher risk of angina if you:

- Have high blood pressure.
- Have high blood cholesterol.
- Smoke cigarettes.
- Are overweight.
- Have high stress levels.

#### TREATMENT

There is no sure cure for angina. Most people, however, learn to live productive and meaningful lives with the disease. The aim of all treatment is to increase the flow of blood and oxygen to the heart. This is accomplished in one of several ways.

- *Medication.* The physician will prescribe a regime of medication that will help the client and decrease his pain. The medication will be individualized for his particular condition and should not be altered without consulting the doctor.
- *Control of risk factors.* The patient may be put on a weight-reducing diet, told to decrease his use of cigarettes, and advised to decrease his stress. These alterations in lifestyle are very difficult, and the patient and his family will need a great deal of encouragement and support to reach the goal.
- *Surgery.* If this treatment has been recommended by a physician and your client or his family have questions, report this to your

supervisor immediately so that answers to the questions can be provided.

## Your Role as a Homemaker/Home Health Aide

Your role is to help the client and his family maintain the regime set up for him. Remember, activity levels, diets, and medications are individualized and should not be compared to other clients or changed without medical consultation.

By providing support to your client and his family as he tries to alter his lifestyle and decrease his risk factors, you will be giving him the care he needs. Point out the achievements he has made and the progress he hopes to make in the near future. Do not dwell on his failures. It is usual for a client who is trying to make changes in his lifestyle to slip back into old patterns from time to time. Do not be judgmental, but rather encourage him to return to the more healthy activity.

Be alert to stress in the family. Sometimes when there is change in the family function, the other members, not the patient, will exhibit stress. If you notice such family discord, report it to your supervisor.

# Section 4   Diabetes

## Objectives: What You Will Learn to Do

■ Define *diabetes*.
■ Recognize the signs and symptoms of diabetes.
■ Recognize the signs and symptoms of too much insulin and not enough insulin.
■ Discuss the role of the homemaker/home health aide in caring for a diabetic client.

## Introduction: Diabetes

**carbohydrate** one of the basic food elements necessary for the body to function properly; includes all sugars and starches

**insulin** hormone produced by the pancreas that is needed for the metabolism of sugars and starches

**diabetes mellitus** condition that develops when the body cannot change sugar into energy

When the body cannot change **carbohydrates** (sugars and starches) into energy because of an imbalance of **insulin**, the result is the chronic disease known as **diabetes mellitus**. The pancreas usually produces insulin on a feedback mechanism. When the body needs insulin following a meal or when extra energy is needed, the pancreas is alerted and it pumps extra insulin into the bloodstream. If, however, the body needs insulin and none is produced, starches and sugars cannot be converted into energy and absorbed by the cells. Sugar remains in the bloodstream and is eventually excreted in the urine as waste.

### SIGNS AND SYMPTOMS OF DIABETES MELLITUS

■ Fatigue, tiredness
■ Loss of weight
■ Sores heal poorly and slowly
■ High blood sugar
■ Sugar in the urine

- Frequent and large amounts of urine
- Excessive thirst
- Poor vision
- Inflammation of the vagina

There are two types of diabetes. Type I results in the person having to take insulin. In Type II diabetes the pancreas produces some insulin but not enough for normal body function. In this type of diabetes the person may take oral medications or just regulate his diet. Because diabetics have a regulated amount of insulin in their bodies, their food intake must be regulated also. If the amount of food is greater than the amount of insulin available, there will be too much unmetabolized sugar left in the blood. If the amount of insulin is greater than the amount of food available, there will not be any carbohydrates for the insulin to metabolize, and this will cause other problems.

Diabetes can be controlled, but never cured. A diabetic must maintain a special diet and must sometimes take medication by mouth or insulin by injection forever. People with diabetes can live full and productive lives if they keep to a diet and a medication schedule. Diagnosis of this disease can be made only by a physician following laboratory tests.

## SIGNS AND SYMPTOMS OF DIABETIC COMA (HYPERGLYCEMIA/HIGH BLOOD SUGAR-DIABETIC KETOACIDOSIS)

**diabetic acidosis or coma**
hyperglycemia: an excess of circulating sugar in the blood

**insulin reaction or shock**
hypoglycemia due to too much insulin in the blood

**ketoacidosis** a condition characterized by a large amount of ketone bodies in the urine

Be alert for signs and symptoms of **diabetic coma** or **insulin shock** or **insulin reaction,** and follow the emergency procedure for your client.

Diabetic coma (**ketoacidosis**) occurs when there is too much carbohydrate and not enough insulin to metabolize it. The symptoms include:

- Air hunger; heavy, labored breathing; increased respiration
- Loss of appetite
- Dulled senses
- Nausea and/or vomiting
- Weakness
- Abdominal pains or discomfort
- Generalized aches
- Increased thirst and parched tongue
- Sweet or fruity odor of the breath
- Flushed dry skin
- Increased urination
- Soft eyeballs
- Upon examination: large amounts of sugar and ketones in the urine and high blood sugar

## SIGNS AND SYMPTOMS OF INSULIN SHOCK (HYPOGLYCEMIA/LOW BLOOD SUGAR-INSULIN REACTION)

Insulin shock occurs when a person has more insulin than the amount of carbohydrate available for metabolism. The symptoms include:

- Excessive sweating, perspiration
- Faintness, dizziness, weakness
- Hunger

- Irritability, personality change, nervousness
- Numbness of tongue and lips
- Not able to awaken, coma, unconsciousness, stupor
- Headache
- Tremors, trembling
- Blurred or impaired vision
- Upon examination: low blood sugar and no sugar in the urine

## *Your Role as a Homemaker/Home Health Aide*

Your role is to help the client and his family learn to live with this disease and the routine of medication and diet. Point out the positive aspects of the client's situation. Help the family adapt the prescribed diet to the family lifestyle. If this diet seems to be difficult, report to your supervisor. She will get in touch with the nutritionist, who will try to adapt the diet to the family's individualized needs.

Assist your client with his medication, but never give him an injection or oral medication. Insulin is always taken by injection, not by mouth. Insulin should be kept in a cool place, away from heat and strong light. Notify your supervisor if the client does not keep to his medication schedule or has any reaction to his medication.

You may be asked to test the client's urine for sugar and acetone. Be sure that you ask your supervisor when to call her with the results. If possible, the client may do this procedure under your supervision.

Many diabetics have difficulty with their feet. Observe nails and toes for infection or pressure areas. Report these immediately. Do not cut toenails or fingernails. This is a procedure that should be done by a podiatrist or a family member who has been specially trained.

As you care for the client, notice the condition of his skin. Is it dry, is it flaky, are there bruises, are the bruises healing? Because diabetics have a harder time healing than nondiabetics, it is important to prevent bruises and pressure areas. If the skin is dry, lubricate it. Dry skin often itches, and clients who scratch themselves could injure the skin, causing bruises or infection.

# Section 5   Cerebrovascular Accident

**Objectives:
What You Will
Learn to Do**

- Describe a CVA.
- List several causes of a CVA.
- Discuss your role as a homemaker/home health aide when caring for a client who has had a CVA.

## *Introduction: Cerebrovascular Accident*

**cerebrovascular accident** a blockage of blood vessel within the brain leading to death of brain tissue

The term **cerebrovascular accident** (CVA) has three important parts:

1. *Cerebro:* having to do with the brain
2. *Vascular:* having to do with the blood vessels
3. *Accident:* something unpredictable and unexpected

**stroke** cerebrovascular accident

A CVA (or **stroke**) occurs when the blood supply to a part of the brain is stopped due to a blocked blood vessel. When blood flow is stopped, the tissue dies. Because each part of the brain controls a different function, the result of a CVA depends on which blood vessel is blocked and which brain center is destroyed.

It is important to remember that the results of the CVA may be paralysis, loss of speech or vision, but that the cause of the problem is disruption of nerve impulse transmission due to brain tissue damage.

**collateral circulation** circulation taken over by smaller blood vessels after obstruction of the larger ones has occurred

In some brains, when a blood vessel is blocked, the surrounding blood vessels take over to supply the injured part of the brain. This is called **collateral circulation**. In this case, the damage may not be as great as if there were no collateral circulation.

The speech center of the brain is on the left side, so if the CVA occurs on that side, speech may be affected. If the CVA occurs on the right side, varying degrees of muscle weakness may be the result (Fig. 19.4).

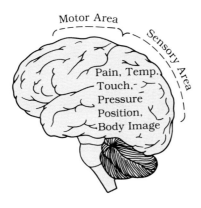

*FIGURE 19.4* Every part of the brain governs a specific function.

**clot** semisolid mass of blood

**embolus** a clot carried by the circulatory system from its place of formation to another site usually causing an obstruction

**thrombus** blood clot which remains at its site of formation

**plaque** fatty deposits within the blood vessels attached to the vessel walls

**hemorrhage** excessive bleeding

## CAUSES OF CVA

There are four main causes of a CVA:

1. A blood **clot** can form elsewhere in the body, travel to the brain, and lodge in a small vessel. This is called an **embolus** (Fig. 19.5a).
2. A blood clot can form in the brain itself and remain there. This is called a **thrombus.**
3. **Plaque** can accumulate in the blood vessels and eventually close them.
4. A blood vessel can burst, causing a **hemorrhage.** This is most common in people who have hypertension (Fig. 19.5b).

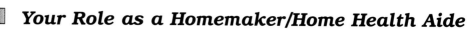

## *Your Role as a Homemaker/Home Health Aide*

It is important to remember that when you meet the client, he will be in a stable condition. However, his condition may change, so be alert. Caring for a person recovering from a CVA is a team effort. You are the team member who will spend the most time with the client. Your careful, objective observations of the client are important to his eventual recovery.

It is impossible to predict when the function of a body part will return following a CVA. Do not try! Do not promise! Do not compare one client with another! People who have suffered a CVA resulting in severe speech and/or motor loss have been known to live thirty or forty years with tender care from their families.

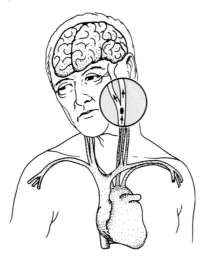

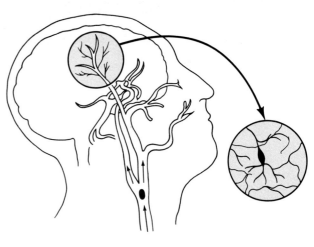

**FIGURE 19.5a** An embolus can form anywhere and travel to the brain.

**FIGURE 19.5b** A hemorrhage can take place in any part of the brain.

Follow the principles of good personal care and the instructions of the physical, occupational, and speech therapists. These therapists will plan an individualized program for your client. You will play an important part in seeing that he and the family follow this routine. The care will be planned with the following in mind:

- Prevention of complications due to decreased mobility
- The need for proper nutrition
- Safety
- Emotional aspects of the chronic condition for both the client and his family

After you have received the care plan of the therapists, it will be your responsibility to make these plans part of the client's daily routine. Arrange them throughout the day so that the client does not get tired. There will be many things for him to relearn, which is emotionally painful and at times frustrating. Just think how you would feel if you had to relearn the alphabet or how to walk.

- Always encourage the client. Point out the positive aspects of his progress.
- Use simple instructions in words that are familiar to the client and his family.
- Always show patience and understanding.
- Do only the exercises you have been told to do. If you have a question, call the appropriate therapist.
- Assist the client with his medication. Some clients cannot remember if they took their medication. Work out a system with your supervisor so that the client and his family can keep track of which medication has been taken.
- If visitors tire your client, tactfully suggest that they leave so that your client can rest.
- Listen to the client and his family. Discuss your conversations with your supervisor. Clients and their families may benefit from a mental health clinician or psychiatric nurse to help them cope with the changes in their family.

# Section 6  Arthritis

## Objectives: What You Will Learn to Do

- Define *arthritis*, and tell how it affects people.
- List the four most common types of arthritis.
- Discuss your role as a homemaker/home health aide in caring for clients with arthritis.

 ## *Introduction: Arthritis*

**arthritis** disease characterized by inflammation and destruction of the joints

**Arthritis** means inflammation and destruction of joints. At times there may be other symptoms also. The shoulders, ankles, elbows, wrists, fingers, and toes are the most common joints affected by this disease. Arthritis or inflammation can be due to an allergy, an injury, or an infection. The cause of some arthritis cannot be determined—it just appears. Everyone seems to have a different reaction to this disease.

There are over 100 types of arthritis, but we will only discuss the 4 most common ones.

**osteoarthritis** the most common type of arthritis

**Osteoarthritis:** This is the most common type. It is thought that after continual use, the joints and their linings just wear out and become very thin (Fig. 19.6). The bony surfaces become thick and develop little spurs. This combination causes pain every time the joint moves. Then the bones rub against each other, causing pain and inflammation. This type of arthritis is most common among the elderly.

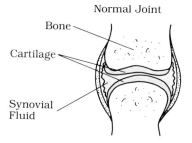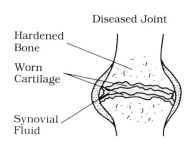

**FIGURE 19.6** Osteoarthritis causes a deterioration in the joints.

**Rheumatoid Arthritis:** This is a crippling, chronic disease. All connective tissue may be affected (Fig. 19.7). If the disease starts in the joints, connective tissue in other organs may eventually be affected. This type of arthritis usually starts in young adulthood or childhood. Three times more women than men have this type of arthritis.

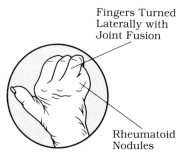

**FIGURE 19.7** Rheumatoid arthritis causes joints to become deformed.

**gout** the buildup of uric acid crystals in the blood and joints

**ankylosing spondylitis** an arthritis-type disease that affects the spine and/or shoulders and hips

**Gout:** This disease is most common among men. Uric acid crystals build up in the blood and lodge in the joints, causing inflammation and pain. This can be sudden and very painful. Any joint can be affected, but the big toe is often the site.

**Ankylosing Spondylitis:** This disease, more common in men than in women, may start in childhood and almost always before the age of thirty-five. It is an arthritic disease that only attacks the spine and/or the shoulders and hips. Following treatment, these people usually remain stiff but are able to function and lead normal lives.

### *Your Role as a Homemaker/Home Health Aide*

Remember, arthritis is a chronic disease. That means the client will have it forever. Help him to establish a routine for daily care that is safe and efficient, and that decreases muscle stress and fatigue.

Exercise and rest are important parts of the client's plan of care. Follow the exercise routine. Do not change it unless you have discussed the change with your supervisor. If you notice that your client's response to the exercises has changed, report it.

Many clients will try unconventional methods of treating their arthritis. Do not assist in these treatments, and make your supervisor aware of them. It is not your role to judge these treatments; just report their existence.

Assist the client with his medication and treatment plan. Each client is treated differently, so do not compare them. Treatment may include diet, weight reduction, rest, and exercise. An occupational therapist and physical therapist may also be involved with this client.

Listen to the client. He may have many feelings about this disease, and he may require emotional counseling from a mental health clinician or psychiatric nurse. Discuss your conversations in the home with your supervisor so that she can make the decision to call these professionals if needed.

## Section 7   Cancer

## Objectives: What You Will Learn to Do

- Define *cancer.*
- Become familiar with possible causes of cancer.
- Become familiar with your role in caring for clients with cancer.

### *Introduction: Cancer*

**malignant** cancerous

Cancer, or a **malignancy**, is a tumor made up of cells that have changed from normal ones to abnormal ones. This change can happen in any organ, at any time, and at any age. As the abnormal cells reproduce and multiply, they destroy the normal tissue and usually form a tumor. The course of the disease depends on many factors:

- Location of the tumor
- Type of tumor
- When the cancer was discovered
- Type of treatment available
- General health of the client

## CAUSES AND SYMPTOMS OF CANCER

There is no definite cause of cancer, but many possible ideas are being investigated (Fig. 19.8). Although a change in the way your body functions may mean many things (not necessarily cancer), there are eight changes, usually called early warning signs of cancer, that should be reported to a doctor immediately (Fig. 19.9).

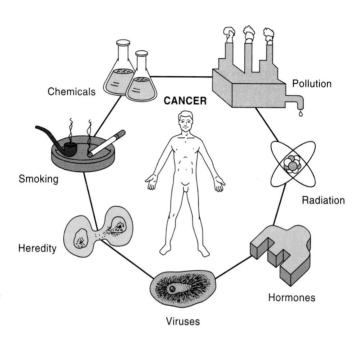

**FIGURE 19.8** Cancer may be caused by a combination of these elements and by elements not yet identified.

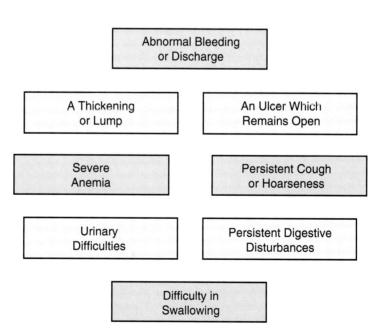

**FIGURE 19.9** Any of the warning signs of cancer should be investigated immediately.

metastasis the spreading of cancer within the body

primary site place of the original cancerous lesion

secondary site place in the body in which cancerous cells are found following the location of the primary site

benign nonmalignant

biopsy examination of tissue taken from the body

The spread of cancer cells from one area to another is called **metastasis.** This does not always occur when there is cancer in the body, but it may. The first site of the cancer is called the **primary site,** and the place it metastasizes to is called the **secondary site.**

The only way a tumor is known to be malignant (cancerous) or **benign** (not malignant) is by taking a small piece of it and examining it under a microscope. This is called a **biopsy.** It is usually done in the operating room in the hospital.

## TREATMENT

Treatment varies from client to client. The client may undergo surgery, radiation, or chemotherapy. He may also undergo a combination of these. The choice of treatment is usually made by the doctor after discussion with the client and his family.

Sometimes a family will choose not to tell the client he has cancer. Even though you may not agree with this decision, you must go along with it. It is not your place to give the client his diagnosis. Discuss this situation with your supervisor so that you will know what to tell the client if he asks you. Do not lie to the client and tell him he will get better unless this is what the family and doctor have decided to tell him.

## *Your Role as a Homemaker/Home Health Aide*

Your role is to give the client the best care you can. This includes both physical and emotional support. Taking care of a client who has cancer is like taking care of any other client. If the client is terminally ill, you and the supervisor will make a plan of care to meet his specific needs. A person is usually said to be terminally ill when there is little or no hope for recovering from the disease.

Cancer is not contagious. Encourage the family members to visit the client and be supportive. Follow the principles of good personal care. Follow the instructions of the therapists within the limits of the client. Discuss with the therapists your responsibilities for exercises. Encourage the client to take part in his care.

Provide an atmosphere of concern. If the client wishes to talk, let him. If he does not seem to be able to talk to you, ask him if you can call the nurse or someone else. Many people live for many years with cancer. Do not give the client false hope, but do not assume he will die unless you have been told this. Help the family deal with this diagnosis by letting them take part in the client's care if they wish. Encourage them to talk to someone who can help them accept this diagnosis.

# Section 8  Alzheimer's Disease

## Objectives: What You Will Learn to Do

■ Define *Alzheimer's disease*.
■ Recognize several of the behaviors exhibited by Alzheimer's sufferers.
■ Discuss the effect of Alzheimer's disease upon the family.
■ Discuss your role in caring for these clients.

## *Introduction: Alzheimer's Disease*

**Alzheimer's disease** a form of irreversible mental deterioration

**Alzheimer's disease** is the major cause of mental deterioration among the over–sixty-five population. It is the diagnosis of more than 50 percent of the nursing home residents of this country. Most of the victims of this disease, however, receive treatment and care in their homes. This disease is chronic, progressive, and ultimately renders the client totally dependent on others. There is no known cure.

There are two known causes of the mental deterioration. One is the inability of the brain to transmit and receive information, and the other is the increasing thickening and intertwining of the brain cells. The thick cells become more and more entangled. When either of these two conditions occur, familiar information cannot be processed by the brain and the client is unable to function. As this condition progresses, the brain actually shrinks in size.

### BEHAVIOR OF CLIENTS WITH ALZHEIMER'S DISEASE

You may see a client in any one of three stages of this disease. If you care for a client for a long time, you will see him progress from one stage to the next.

#### Stage I

At this beginning stage, many people are able to cover up their memory loss, decreased speech, and even their emotional agitation, depression, or apathy. During this stage, many clients sense that something is changing and rather than be embarrassed, they simply withdraw from their familiar activities. Family members may not recognize the pattern of this deterioration, may not admit to it, or may feel all older people are forgetful and withdrawn. Family members may label the client careless or disinterested. This condition, however, gets progressively worse.

#### Stage II

During this period extending over many years, the client's memory progressively worsens. He may stop speaking, wander, and repeat movements in a meaningless way. At this time the client becomes less involved in his care and less and less a contributing member of the family. He may put all types of things in his mouth. His appetite may increase, and his activity may be in the form of continual pacing in small areas.

### Stage III

This is the terminal stage. It is a time when families must give continual supervision to the client. His appetite may decrease, and he must be coaxed to eat and drink. The client may become unresponsive. It is at this point that an exhausted family often seeks to institutionalize the client.

## Your Role as a Homemaker/Home Health Aide

You are an important part of the care of this client and the relief of the family. Follow the care plan carefully. The maintenance of a routine is one way to ease the care of the client. If you find the need to change the plan of care, be sure and discuss it with the family and your supervisor. Your continued support is important for the family of an Alzheimer's victim. Be on time and be conscientious about coming to work. A change of personnel is a disrupting factor in these households.

- Be alert for the safety of the client. Remember, he is unable to remember your instructions, so you must be aware of his activities and movements.
- Provide a quiet, unstressed environment.
- Maintain the personal hygiene of the client. Careful washing of the perineal area will prevent skin breakdown. Frequent cleaning of the teeth will decrease mouth odor and improve general appearance.
- Maintain a toileting routine. If the client is incontinent and can no longer participate in his personal hygiene, discuss with your supervisor the use of various appliances.
- Small nutritious meals should be offered. Frequent sips of water will decrease the chance for dehydration.
- Monitor the client's sleep habits, and report if they are markedly disturbed or they change.
- Be supportive of the family who cares for the client. Encourage them to leave the house when you are there. Encourage them to seek some relief and enjoyment while you are available to care for the client.
- Be alert to family tension. Report this to your supervisor, who will discuss with the family the appropriate counseling or support groups.
- Do not be judgmental or compare the care one family gives to the way another family cares for their relative.
- Be alert to your feelings. If you find you are unable to continue caring for the client, discuss your feelings with your supervisor so that relief can be arranged.

# Section 9 Chronic Obstructive Pulmonary Disease

## Objectives: What You Will Learn to Do

- State what chronic obstructive pulmonary disease is.
- Describe some of the behaviors exhibited by clients who have this disease.
- Describe the effect of this disease on families.
- Discuss your role as a homemaker/home health aide in caring for a client with COPD.

## Introduction: Chronic Obstructive Pulmonary Disease

**chronic obstructive pulmonary disease** refers to diseases that cause permanent damage to lung tissue, including emphysema, asthma, and chronic bronchitis

**Chronic obstructive pulmonary disease (COPD)** is a term that refers to all diseases that cause irreversible damage to the lungs over a period of time. This condition is one of the leading causes of death in the United States. People with a diagnosis of asthma and emphysema are often said to have COPD. This means that their lungs are not able to expand, remove oxygen from the air that is breathed in, or expel the waste products, such as carbon dioxide. These clients also find it difficult to perform activities that require exertion of any kind. Eating and speaking are difficult, and exercise is often impossible. Most of these clients are susceptible to infection, due to the pooling of pulmonary secretions in their lungs. When the levels of carbon dioxide and other gases are not correct, these clients exhibit unusual behavior and are unable to make decisions or be left alone. When the blood gases are corrected, this behavior disappears.

Clients with COPD also suffer from a change in body image. They must learn to live with machines as constant companions because they depend on oxygen equipment and suction equipment to help them breathe. Some clients may have a tracheostomy tube, IVs, or even feeding tubes.

### EFFECTS ON THE FAMILY

As the client demands more and more care, the family function changes. Usually, the spouse cares for the client, but that is not always the case. The caregiver, whoever it is, becomes more and more isolated from friends because the care of the client takes up so much time. Family members become socially isolated, depressed, and often suffer from sensory deprivation. Relationships with friends change because the client often is too tired, or even unable, to speak (Fig. 19.10). Visitors may stop coming, and family members often find themselves without any outside activities.

While all this is occurring, families must often become accustomed to a change in finances and a change in the work status of the client.

## Your Role as a Homemaker/Home Health Aide

Your presence in a home where your client has COPD is a most important one. You will assist the primary caregiver so that there is

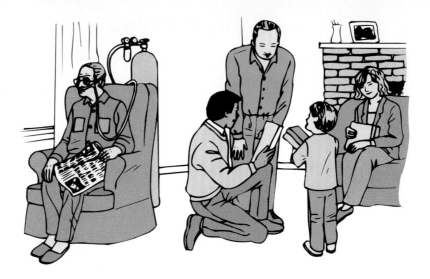

**FIGURE 19.10** Make a special effort to include clients in normal family activities.

a break in his or her routine. Encourage the caregiver to go out and tend to personal needs while you are in the house. Assure both client and family that you will adhere to the routine they have established and will not make changes without discussing them with your supervisor and the client. This respite for the caregiver often enables him or her to continue the care for the rest of the day and possibly into the night.

Encourage the client to adhere to his medication schedule. Report any change in behavior. No change is too small. If you report changes as soon as they occur, your supervisor can change the plan of care to meet the client's changing needs. Often you will be the first person to see a change in behavior, which will mean that the client's blood gases are not correct.

Try to interest the client in eating nutritious, small meals. Because eating is a chore for these people and the taste buds are often not as sensitive as yours, every bit of food should be nutritious and tasty. Fluids may or may not be restricted. Be sure to check. Prepare foods the client likes. This is not the time to introduce new foods.

Expose the client to some activities to occupy his time. If the client does not have any hobbies, discuss with him and his family what type of activities he might enjoy. Then keep on trying each one. Do not be discouraged. The client and the family will appreciate your concern and interest, and you will eventually find an activity that will please the client. For example, if the client liked to play sports but is no longer able to, be sure to have him listen to the radio when ballgames are on, or make him comfortable so he can look at TV. Plan your schedule around these important times in his day.

Many of the clients you care for will be using oxygen therapy in some form. This is not necessarily a problem except that many of the people who have COPD also smoke. Although the client and family are taught that oxygen cannot run when there is an open flame or someone is smoking in the area, these clients often forget. Be firm, but polite. Tell the client and the family that oxygen and smoking is a dangerous combination and that you will have to report this situation. In addition, discuss with your supervisor how she wants you to act. Does she want you to remove the matches and cigarettes?

# Section 10  Neurological Disorders

## Objectives: What You Will Learn to Do

- Discuss the signs and symptoms of Parkinson's disease, multiple sclerosis, and amyotrophic lateral sclerosis.
- Discuss the role of the homemaker/home health aide in caring for clients with neurological disorders.

### *Introduction: Common Neurological Diseases*

Three neurological diseases you will see in the home setting are Parkinson's disease, multiple sclerosis (MS), and amyotrophic lateral sclerosis (ALS). Clients who have these diseases usually remain in the home setting using adaptive aids. Some remain at home until they die. Although the diseases are different, there are many similarities in the care of these clients. All three diseases result in the need for assistance with care, attention to safety, and support for client and family. As these diseases progress, clients require a great deal of personal care and protection. Their ability to respond to changes and slight infections becomes progressively less.

#### *Causes of the Three Diseases*

Parkinson's disease is a progressive disease that affects the part of the brain controlling movement and balance. The first signs are usually tremors of the hands or legs, difficulty walking, and slowness of movement. Other symptoms may be changes in vision, drooling, difficulty swallowing, and inability to control bowel and bladder function. The cause of the disease is unknown, but clients respond to drug therapy that replaces certain chemicals they seem to be lacking. People with this disease often work many years after the diagnosis. Drugs must be carefully and continuously regulated. Side effects from the drugs often occur many years after the therapy has started. Sometimes, a client may appear to be getting better and concludes that he no longer needs the medication or may change his routine. This is a great mistake and should be reported to the physician immediately.

Multiple sclerosis is a progressive disease that affects the transmission of impulses through the central nervous system. The first signs are usually fatigue, emotional changes, and difficulty with speech. This disease affects young adults with young families who are in the first stages of their careers. The people who have this disease are often able to work for many years if they are protected from infection and have a safe environment. There are medications that help some people, but no one medication has been found to be useful for all clients. The cause is unknown, and the course of the disease varies.

Amyotrophic lateral sclerosis is a progressive disease resulting in the degeneration of the neurons. The cause is unknown, and most clients die within the first three years of diagnosis. Many of these clients choose to stay at home. They need assistance with all aspects of personal care and maintenance of a safe environment.

## Your Role as a Homemaker/Home Health Aide

Treatment is prescribed by a physician. Support the client and the family as they follow the regime. Most clients find that it is important to follow the same routine every day. This may seem difficult for people who like variety. But these clients find the same routine to be comforting. They know what to expect. They know how it will affect them. Assist them as they incorporate the regime into their daily lives. If you have suggestions for change, discuss them with the client and the family. Do not change the routine without first telling everyone involved. Areas of concern are:

- *Medication:* must be taken as prescribed and should not be stopped unless the physician is notified. Report client reaction to medication. Be sure to report the slightest changes as that may indicate that a change in dosage is necessary.

- *Regular exercise:* can take the form of active or passive exercise. It could also be walking, swimming, or riding a bike. Exercises should be supervised and done regularly. Report fatigue or pain. Be alert to safety needs during exercise. Clients who tire easily should have several short exercise periods rather than one long one. Do not alter the exercise routine without discussing the change with your supervisor.

- *Nutritional intake:* small meals high in nutrients and fiber are important. Swallowing of liquids may be difficult, so monitor fluid intake. Safety is important. Be sure the foods are at an acceptable temperature and not too hot. Pieces of food should be small enough to chew easily. Report bowel and bladder changes.

- *Support:* encourage the client to be as independent as possible. Encourage the family members to pursue their own interests. There are many local support groups for clients and families. Discuss the possibility of referrals with your supervisor. Allow all family members time to express their feelings. Do not be judgmental. Support the family members in their roles. Be alert to changes in roles. Family members, as well as the client, often need to voice their feelings of frustration, fear, and fatigue. Listen attentively. Offer to put them in touch with a professional counselor if they wish. Discussing feelings can be helpful to both the client and the caregivers.

## Section 11  Tuberculosis

**Objectives: What You Will Learn to Do**

- Describe the causes of tuberculosis.
- Describe three common misconceptions about the disease.
- Describe the most common treatments for this disease.
- Discuss your role as a homemaker/home health aide in caring for a client with tuberculosis.

## Introduction: Tuberculosis

Tuberculosis is a disease caused by a germ. It is spread by people, not animals, when they laugh, cough, sneeze, or speak to one another. Coughing or sneezing into a tissue or a handkerchief is one way to decrease the spread of the disease. The other way is to wash hands frequently and not touch hands to eyes, nose, or mouth.

The disease is known all over the world. It was once thought that the disease was only seen in poor people and was unknown in the United States. This is now known to be untrue. Today the disease is seen in all countries and in people in all living conditions. People are more at risk, however, when living in crowded, poorly ventilated conditions; when malnourished; and when in poor health.

Some people have TB infection. This mean the germ is in their body, but it is inactive and cannot be spread or cause harm. Medication is often prescribed for these people to prevent the germs from becoming active.

## SIGNS AND SYMPTOMS

There are many signs and symptoms of this disease. Any combination of them could mean that a person has active tuberculosis. These should be brought to the attention of a doctor immediately. Some people may be embarrassed to know they have the disease, and this fear prevents them from seeking medical help. Postponing medical help may result in the person getting worse and spreading the disease to many people with whom he comes in contact.

Any of the following symptoms should be brought to the attention of a doctor, clinic, or emergency room immediately.

- Weight loss, loss of appetite
- Feeling sick, weak, or tired
- Fever
- Sweating, especially during the night
- Chest pain
- Coughing
- Coughing up blood
- Unexplained pain in any body part

## HOW IS TUBERCULOSIS DIAGNOSED?

The diagnosis of tuberculosis, active or inactive, can only be made by a physician after a skin test, an X ray, and/or a sputum sample is done. Any hospital, clinic, or health department can assist with finding a place to have these tests done quickly and inexpensively.

Usually once the diagnosis of tuberculosis is made, close contacts of the person are also tested. It is important that all contacts be tested whether they are family members, live in the same house, or are close by.

## TREATMENT FOR TUBERCULOSIS

Medication is always prescribed and is taken for a long time. It is important that the medication be taken exactly as it is prescribed. If not, the disease may not be cured and may return. Often, more than one medication is given. Other activities, such as physical exercise, diet, and breathing exercises, may also be part of the regime.

When the medication is first started, the client is usually hospitalized and isolated to decrease contact with others. As soon as the disease is under control, the client can go home and be around others without fear of infecting them.

## Your Role as a Homemaker/Home Health Aide

You are important in maintaining a routine in the house, in encouraging the client to maintain the regime set up by the physician, and in teaching the family the truth about this disease. A nourishing diet is important. If the medication causes the client to have a decreased appetite, encourage small frequent meals rather than a few large ones. Encourage adequate fluid intake. This should include water, juice, and nourishing soups.

Some family members may be afraid they will catch the client's disease and therefore isolate or ignore him. Explain to them that once the disease is under treatment, the chance of contracting the disease is past. The family may make the client feel guilty or even ashamed he has contracted tuberculosis. If this should happen, contact your supervisor and request written information that you can share with the family.

# Section 12  AIDS  Acquired Immune Deficiency Syndrome

## Objectives: What You Will Learn to Do

■ Describe three common misconceptions about the disease.
■ Describe the most common treatments for this disease.
■ Discuss your role as a homemaker/home health aide in caring for a client with AIDS.

## Introduction: AIDS

AIDS is a virus that is spread through sexual contact between two people and by sharing IV drug equipment when one person is infected with the virus. It cannot be transmitted by holding hands, by giving blood, or by being near someone who has the disease. There is no evidence that AIDS can be spread from sharing the same equipment or bathroom. You will not get sick if you sit next to someone who has any form of AIDS. The virus is not spread by food or sharing a kitchen. It is only transmitted by contact with blood, seminal fluid, or vaginal fluid in the mouth, rectum, vagina, or penis.

There are several forms of this infection. Only a physician can diagnose the disease. Anyone who thinks they have been exposed to AIDS should go to a physician, a hospital, or health department immediately. Although a person may not appear to have the disease, if he is infected in any form, he can transmit it to another person.

### RISK FACTORS

You are at risk of giving, getting, or having AIDS if:

■ You are an IV drug user who shares needles
■ You have received blood or blood products before 1978

- You have several sexual partners and do not use condoms
- You do not know your sexual partners well
- Any of your sexual partners have had "unsafe" sex since 1978

## FORMS OF AIDS

There are three forms of AIDS:

1. *AIDS carrier:* The only sign of the disease to these people may be a positive blood test. Some carriers never show active signs of the disease. Some carriers remain healthy for many years and then gradually show signs and symptoms. There is no way to predict which course the disease will take. The carrier can, however, transmit the disease.

2. *AIDS-related conditions:* Some people may be healthy for years after the first positive blood test and then show related symptoms. Whether or not they have mild symptoms or severe symptoms, they can transmit the disease.

3. *AIDS:* The disease may appear years after the first positive blood test and years after AIDS-related conditions have appeared and been treated. When this happens, the immune system is compromised and the body is no longer able to protect itself against infection. Death eventually occurs.

## *Your Role as a Homemaker/Home Health Aide*

You will be asked to demonstrate universal precautions while caring for the client just as you would when caring for any other client. Use these precautions only when necessary so that neither the client nor the family feel you are afraid of catching the disease. AIDS clients are often very lonely. Family and friends often do not want to spend time with them, touch them, or hold their hands. Your demonstration that this activity is without danger will help decrease needless fears and myths.

AIDS clients often take medication and have set routines to conserve strength and maintain their muscle tone. Assist the client with this and maintain the routine that is comfortable for the family and the client. If the family is unavailable to assist the client when you are not there, discuss with your supervisor the availability of support groups or community volunteers. Make these suggestions carefully so the client knows that you are concerned, but not trying to get somebody else to assume the care.

Report all changes in behavior, pain tolerance, activity tolerance, and skin integrity. Often AIDS clients have difficulty breathing, so be alert to possible changes in their ability to breathe or speak. Protect the client from friends and neighbors who may have slight colds or infections. If you feel a visitor is not 100 percent healthy, suggest he return at another time or speak to the client on the telephone.

Should you have any questions about the disease or the safest way to care for the client, discuss this openly with your supervisor to increase your knowledge and decrease your fears.

## Topics for Discussion

1. Review each disease, and discuss some of the observations you will make while caring for a client with a particular disease.
2. Choose a disease, and discuss how you think you would feel if you had this condition. What changes in your lifestyle would you have to make? How would you feel about that?
3. Choose a disease, and discuss how a family is affected when one of its members contracts this disease. How would you feel if you were faced with a family member who had a chronic disease? a terminal disease?

# Chapter 20

# Emergency Procedures

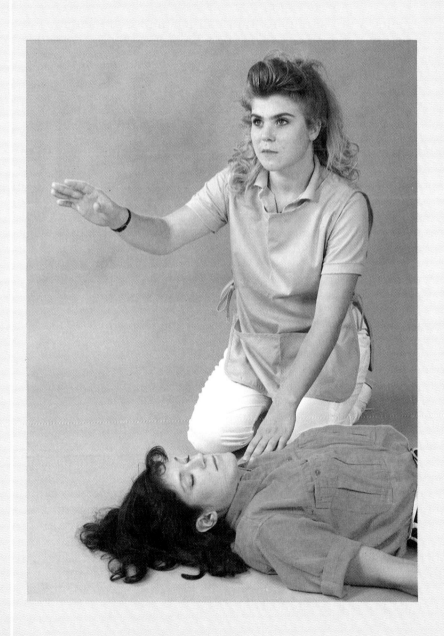

# Section 1   What an Emergency Is

## Objectives: What You Will Learn to Do

- Define emergency.
- Define first aid.
- Discuss the steps to take in an emergency.

 **Introduction: Agency Policies**

*This chapter covers the essentials of emergency procedures in the home. You and your instructor may want to refer to the many other texts on emergency care for further detail.*

**emergency** a sudden unexpected crisis, injury or illness

**first aid** emergency treatment given for injury or illness before regular medical treatment is available

**Emergencies** are situations that call for immediate action. **First aid** is the action taken to assist people who suffer injuries or sudden illnesses until more complete help arrives.

Every agency has an emergency procedure. This includes telephone numbers of fire, police, and rescue squads. It also includes a plan of whom to call during what emergency. It is your responsibility to be familiar with this plan and these telephone numbers.

As you make a decision about giving first aid, remember that the person is a whole unit and will react physically and emotionally to the emergency situation.

If you are faced with a situation where there is nobody else to help you or to send for help, take care of the person before you leave him to get help. If you are faced with an emergency situation where more than one person needs help, you will have to review the whole situation to decide who to help first.

### STEPS TO BE TAKEN IN AN EMERGENCY

Before you take any action, you must know the following:

- What is the problem or emergency?
- What must be done?
- What *you* are capable of doing.
- Can the person be moved?

Get the person to safe, firm ground away from danger of electrical shock, fire, or explosion. Do not move the person unless he is in great danger of further injury. Remember, you should do this without causing serious injury to yourself.

Do not leave a person who needs help. Have someone else call for additional help. If the person does not need immediate help to maintain his life, your responsibility is to prevent additional injury and to provide comfort and security until medical help arrives. Keep the person warm, comfortable, and safe. If he is on the floor leave him there until medical help arrives.

When a person is severely injured, he is treated according to common first-aid priorities (Fig. 20.1).

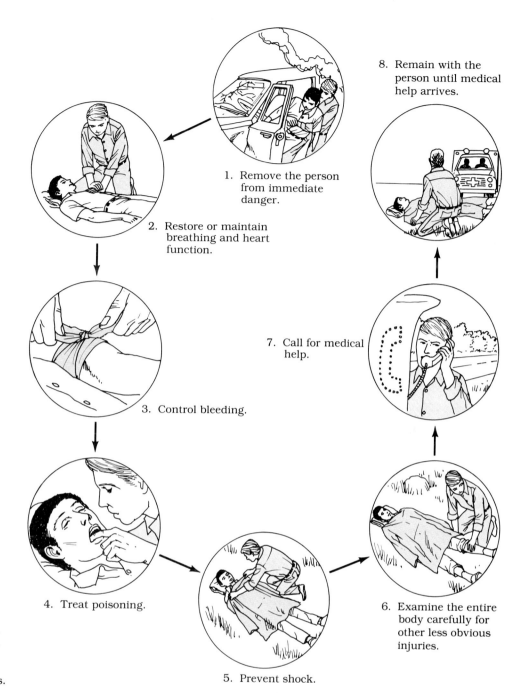

8. Remain with the person until medical help arrives.

1. Remove the person from immediate danger.

2. Restore or maintain breathing and heart function.

7. Call for medical help.

3. Control bleeding.

4. Treat poisoning.

6. Examine the entire body carefully for other less obvious injuries.

5. Prevent shock.

FIGURE 20.1 In an emergency common first-aid practices must be followed to ensure the safety of the person until medical help arrives.

# Section 2  Restoring Breathing

## Objectives: What You Will Learn to Do

- Demonstrate the proper technique for dislodging a foreign body in the airway.
- Demonstrate the proper technique for mouth-to-mouth resuscitation.

# Introduction: Restore or Maintain Breathing Function

Heart function and breathing function are related. When oxygen to the lungs is cut off, oxygen to the brain is also decreased. When this happens, cells that control heart function die and the heart becomes weak. As a homemaker/home health aide, you will only be concerned with restoring an open airway and restoring breathing.

You should carry a pocket shield so that if you have to perform artificial breathing, you will be protected.

When an object blocks air from getting into a person's lungs, it must be removed or the person will choke to death (Fig. 20.2).

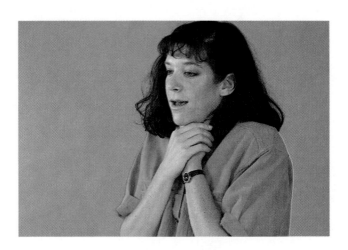

FIGURE 20.2  A blocked airway can threaten life and must be treated immediately.

## OBSTRUCTED AIRWAYS

A person's airway can be **obstructed** (blocked) by:

- Foreign matter in the mouth, throat, or windpipe, such as food, vomitus, blood, or a foreign object
- Unconsciousness, leading to relaxed muscles and the tongue falling back and blocking the airway

Children and adults are treated differently.
A person can have a:

Partial airway obstruction: Some air passes to and from the lungs, but the conditions must be improved. Snoring sounds, weak coughs, gurgling, or crowing sounds are signs of this. Also, if the lips, nails, tongue, and skin have a dark or bluish color, a partial obstruction might be the cause. *Do not interfere with the person if he is able to breath, cough, or speak.* Just call for help.

Complete obstruction: No air passes to and from the lungs. The person may be conscious or unconscious. The conscious person will not be able to speak or cough and may clutch his throat. He will become unconscious if the situation is not remedied. The unconscious person will have no chest movement.

## CHILDREN LESS THAN ONE YEAR OLD

Children and infants are treated differently than adults when they have difficulty breathing. *If the child or infant is breathing, speaking, or coughing, do not help, but call for assistance immediately.*

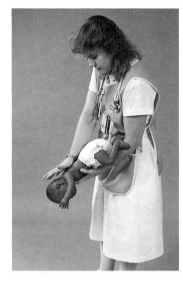

If the child or infant has had an infection, a high fever, or has taken medication and is having difficulty breathing, call for help immediately.

If the child or infant is unable to speak or cry and is conscious, act quickly to relieve the obstruction. Use a combination of back blows and chest thrusts on an infant. Do not use back blows on a child. Do not use abdominal thrusts on an infant, as this action can damage their under-developed organs. Back blows are quick, forceful blows between the shoulder blades used to dislodge objects when the person is an infant; chest thrusts are similar to the compressions given in CPR. Abdominal thrusts are performed on a child similar to the way they are used on adults.

*For the infant:*

- Call out for help.
- Turn the infant face down on your forearm and support his head in your hand. Rest your arm on your thigh for support and keep the infant's head lower than his body (Fig. 20.3).
- Deliver up to five back blows forcefully between the shoulder blades with the heel of one hand.
- Sandwich the infant between your arms and turn the infant over as you continue to support his head in your hands. Again, support him on your thigh.
- Provide up to five quick downward chest thrusts with two fingers in the same location as chest compressions (the lower third of the sternum, approximately one finger-width below the nipple line) (Fig. 20.4).
- Check the mouth. If you see the foreign object, use your little finger in a hooking motion to remove it. If you DO NOT SEE IT, DO NOT sweep the mouth.
- Open the airway and attempt rescue breathing. If no air enters, reposition the head and attempt to breathe again. If still obstructed, repeat these steps until the airway is clear (Fig. 20.5).

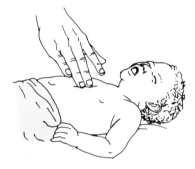

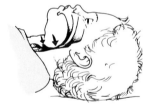

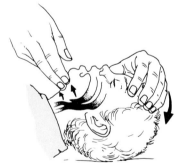

## ABDOMINAL THRUST

**Manual thrusts** are a series of quick movements to the upper abdominal area or chest area to force the obstruction to move. **Abdominal thrust,** also called the **Heimlich maneuver,** is used when the person cannot breathe, cough, or speak. Talk to the person as you are doing this. Tell him you are going to do the Heimlich maneuver to help him breathe easier. Do not use the Heimlich maneuver on pregnant women, infants, or small children.

*When the person is sitting or standing and conscious:*

- Stand behind the person and wrap your arms around his waist.
- Put the thumb side of one hand on the abdomen between the navel and the end of the breastbone (sternum). Do not actually touch the chest.
- Grasp this hand with the other hand and press it into the abdomen with a quick upward movement (Fig. 20.6).
- Repeat and continue this until the object is expelled. Each thrust should be separate and distinct.

*When the person is lying down and unconscious:*

- Position the person on his back. Open airway and attempt to ventilate. If no air enters, reposition head and attempt to ventilate again. If unsuccessful, perform the following steps.

FIGURE 20.6

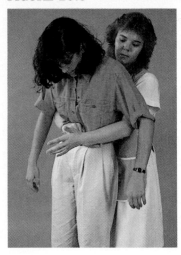

- Kneel astride the person at hip level.
- Put the heel of one hand on the abdomen between the navel and the end of the breastbone (Fig. 20.7).
- Put the other hand on top of this hand.
- Rock forward and push your hands upward. Repeat five times.
- Open the mouth and sweep it with one finger using a hooking motion. (Do not use finger sweeps in infants and children unless you see the object.)
- Attempt to ventilate. If unsuccessful, reposition the head and attempt to ventilate again.
- If unsuccessful, repeat sequence of abdominal thrusts, finger sweep, attempt to ventilate, reposition.

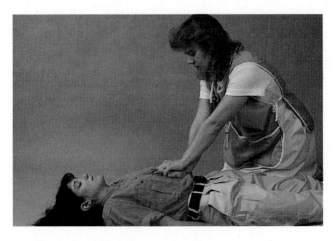

FIGURE 20.7

## CHEST THRUST

This is a useful procedure when the person in danger is large and your arms will not reach around his abdomen but will reach around his chest. It is used when the person is pregnant (Fig. 20.8).

*When the person is standing or sitting and conscious:*

- Put your arms around the person's chest.
- Put the thumb side of one fist on the breastbone (sternum) just above the lower end.
- Grasp this hand with your other one and push quickly directly backward.
- Repeat until airway is clear.

*When the person is lying down and unconscious:*

- Position the person on his back. Open airway and attempt to ventilate. If no air enters, reposition head and attempt to ventilate again. If unsuccessful, perform the following steps.
- Kneel beside him close to his chest.
- Place the heel of your hand just above the lowest end of the breastbone (Fig. 20.9).
- Put your other hand on top of this hand, and lean forward. As you do so, exert quick pushing pressure (Fig. 20.10).
- Give five chest thrusts.
- Open mouth and finger sweep.
- Attempt to ventilate. If unsuccessful, reposition the head and attempt to ventilate again.
- If unsuccessful, repeat until the obstruction is dislodged.

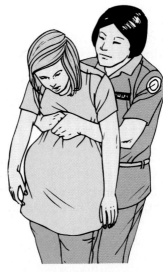

FIGURE 20.8 On large persons or pregnant women use the chest thrust to dislodge any obstructions.

FIGURE 20.9

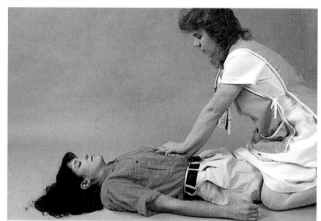

FIGURE 20.10

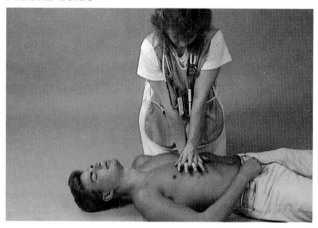

## FINGER SWEEPS

This is the removal of an object that you can see. There are some agencies that do not advise the use of this technique unless you can *clearly see the object* and the person is conscious. Check with your agency for their policy. *Call for assistance if the obstruction cannot be easily removed.* Never use this technique with a child less than eight years old (Fig. 20.11).

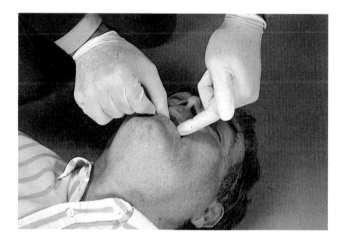

FIGURE 20.11

## MOUTH-TO-MOUTH VENTILATION (RESCUE BREATHING)

This is the exchange of air between you and an unconscious non-breathing person, or a person who loses consciousness while you are trying to dislodge an obstruction. If an obstruction is present, continue this process until help arrives. You must dislodge the obstruction first or you will not be able to ventilate the person.

- Check for response. If no response, call or send someone for medical assistance.
- Tilt the person's head back by putting one hand under his chin and lifting gently, and pressing down with the other hand on his forehead (Fig. 20.12a).
- With the fingers of the hand on the person's forehead, pinch his nose closed.
- Open your mouth and take a deep breath. (If you have a mouth shield always use it when giving mouth-to-mouth ventilation.)

- Cover his mouth with your mouth and breathe into the patient so the chest rises. Give two initial breaths, about 1½–2 seconds per breath (Fig. 20.12b).
- Lift your head and allow him to exhale passively (Fig. 20.12c). You should be able to see the chest fall.

FIGURE 20.12a

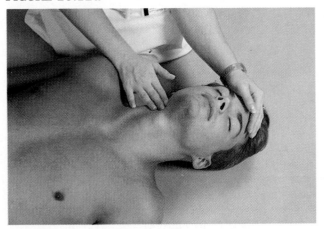

FIGURE 20.12b

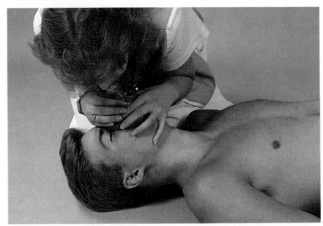

FIGURE 20.12c

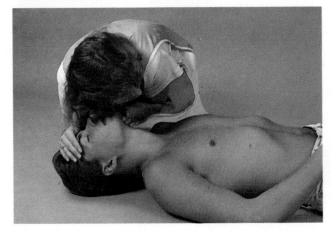

FIGURE 20.13

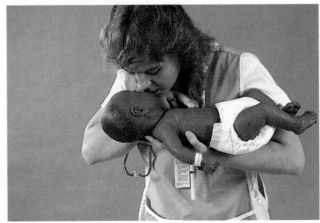

- Check pulse.
- If the airway is *not* obstructed and there is no pulse, continue mouth-to-mouth resuscitation until medical help or someone arrives who is qualified to administer CPR. Give 10–12 breaths per minute.
- Ventilating infants and small children: Deliver two slow initial breaths (1½–2 seconds per breath) with sufficient volume to make the chest rise. Then give a breath every three seconds. Do *not* hyperextend the neck (Fig. 20.13).

# Section 3 Stopping External Heavy Bleeding

## Objectives: What You Will Learn to Do

▨ Demonstrate the proper first aid for controlling external bleeding.

### *Introduction: Control External Bleeding*

**hemorrhage** excessive bleeding

Severe blood loss or **hemorrhage** leads to several effects on the body, including shock (see Section 5).

▨ Body cells are damaged due to lack of circulating oxygen.

▨ Blood pressure drops.

▨ The heart pumps faster in an attempt to circulate the remaining blood, but each heart beat is less forceful.

#### EMERGENCY PROCEDURE

**external** outside the body

**External** blood loss (bleeding outside the body) can come from an artery, a vein, or a capillary. Each of these must be controlled in the same way.

▨ Apply direct pressure over the wound (Fig. 20.14). Use any clean cloth. Keep pressure for 10 to 30 minutes while someone else calls for help.

▨ If possible, elevate the limb to decrease the blood supply (Fig. 20.15).

▨ Remain with the person until help arrives.

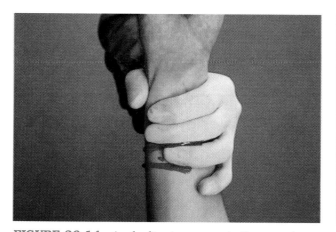

FIGURE 20.14   Apply direct pressure to the wound.

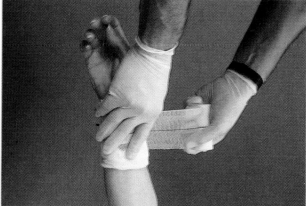

FIGURE 20.15   Cover the wound with a clean, dry cloth and elevate the limb if possible.

# Section 4 Poisoning

## Objectives: What You Will Learn to Do

- List the four kinds of poisoning.
- Discuss the first aid for a victim of poisoning.

## Introduction: Poisoning

**poison** substance causing illness or death when eaten, drunk or absorbed in relatively small amounts

A **poison** is any substance to which the body has a bad reaction. What is poisonous to one person may not be to another. Quick action and careful observation are necessary if poisoning or an overdose of medication is suspected.

- Look for a container that might have held the poison. Do not follow antidotes on the bottle. Call poison control.
- Check the mouth for chemical burns.
- Check the breath for odors.
- Gather as much information as possible about this incident before you act. A person can be poisoned by:
  a. Inhaling a poison through his mouth and nose
  b. Swallowing it
  c. Injecting himself or being injected (drugs, insect bites) with it
  d. Absorbing it through his skin

### EMERGENCY PROCEDURE

#### Swallowed Poisons

If the person is conscious and does not have convulsions:

- Dilute the poison with a glass of milk, not oil.
- Call the poison control center with as much information as you have. Follow their instructions.
- Save any vomitus.

If the person is unconscious:

- Do not give anything by mouth.
- Position the person on his side. If he vomits, it will drain out.
- Maintain a clear airway. If the person stops breathing, give mouth-to-mouth resuscitation. There are times when you should not perform mouth-to-mouth resuscitation due to the type of poison involved. If poison remains on the person's mouth or if you could be poisoned by fumes, do not give mouth-to-mouth resuscitation.
- Call for help and remain with the person until someone arrives.

#### Poisoning by Inhalation

Chemicals and gases can poison people and cause various reactions, such as irritations of eyes, throat, and skin; difficulty seeing, hearing, and speaking; hallucinations; fatigue; or collapse.

- If you can move the person to a safe area away from the poison, do so, but do not expose yourself to a hazardous environment.
- Send someone for help. Ventilate the area if possible.
- Loosen tight clothing around the neck.
- Call the poison control center.
- Keep the person warm and comfortable.
- Mouth-to-mouth resuscitation may be necessary if the person stops breathing. See Section 2 on how to restore breathing.

### Injected Poisons

- Insect bites can cause allergic reactions. If the person experiences difficulty breathing, tingling in the area of the bite, swelling, or redness, call for assistance immediately.
- If you suspect that someone has had a drug overdose, call for help. Do not leave him alone, and be alert for changes in his condition.

### Absorbed Poisons

- Some chemicals react violently with water. Powders should be brushed off.
- Call poison control.
- Poison ivy and related plants can cause irritation and rashes. Wash area and report to your supervisor.

# Section 5  Shock

## Objectives: What You Will Learn to Do

- Define shock.
- Demonstrate first aid for a shock victim.

## *Introduction: Shock*

**shock** state of collapse resulting from reduced blood volume and pressure usually caused by severe injury or emotional reaction

**Shock** is the failure of the heart and vascular system to pump enough blood to all parts of the body. There may be many causes for this such as loss of blood or heart damage, but the result is the same (Fig. 20.16).

### SIGNS AND SYMPTOMS OF SHOCK

- Eyes are dull and pupils wide.
- Face is pale; may be bluish in color. (Lips and nail beds will be dusky blue.)
- Person may be nauseated.
- Respirations are shallow, irregular, and labored.
- Pulse is rapid and weak.
- Skin is cold and clammy.
- Person is restless.
- Person is very weak and may collapse.

- Send someone for help. Talk to the person and make him comfortable until help arrives.
- Position the person with the head lower than the legs. Keep him warm. Blood loss makes the patient cold, so cover him (Fig. 20.17).

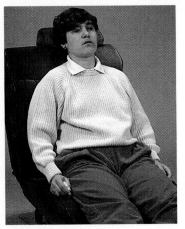

*FIGURE 20.16*

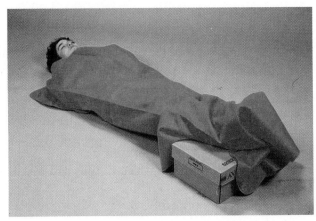

*FIGURE 20.17*

# Section 6  Burns

## Objectives: What You Will Learn to Do

- Demonstrate first aid for a victim of a burn.

### *Introduction: Burns*

**burn** injury to tissues caused by exposure to heat or to substances which stimulate the sensation of heat

A **burn** is tissue damage caused by excessive heat regardless of the source. The heat may come from fire, electricity, chemicals, the sun, or steam.

Burns may be caused by heat or chemicals. In both cases, however, damage to the skin and sometimes to various organs is the result. By acting quickly and correctly, you can prevent further injury.

Burns are usually labeled first, second, or third degree. First degree is the least severe burn, second degree causes blistering, and third-degree burns indicate near destruction of the body part.

The complications from burns are many. They include infection, shock, pain, loss of body heat and fluid, swelling of breathing passages, and death. All treatment for burns is aimed at preventing complications and speeding up the healing process.

### EMERGENCY PROCEDURE

#### *Small Burn Areas (First Degree—Reddening of Skin)*

- Do not remove clothing stuck to the burned area.
- Put the body part in cool water, if possible. Let remain for 2 to 5 minutes. Do not put ice on the burn.

- Cover the area with a sterile or clean cloth.
- Continue to put cool water over the dressing.
- Get medical help. Stay until someone arrives.

### Larger, Deeper Burn Areas (Second Degree—Blistering; Third Degree—Charred)

- Do not remove clothing stuck to the burned area.
- Check to see if the person is breathing. Resuscitation may be necessary.
- Keep the airway open.
- Stop the burning, if necessary, by dowsing with cool water.
- Cover the area with sterile or clean dry cloth or sheet.
- Do not wet the dressing. This will chill the person and cause shock.
- Get medical help. Stay until someone arrives.

### Chemical Burns

- Flush with water for at least 20 minutes.
- Wrap area with clean cloth or sheet.
- If patient complains of burning, flush again.
- Call for medical help.

## Section 7  Heart Attack

## Objectives: What You Will Learn to Do

- Define a heart attack.
- List the signs and symptoms of a heart attack.
- Demonstrate the proper first aid for a victim of a heart attack.

### Introduction: Heart Attack—Myocardial Infarction—Chest Pain

The heart is a muscle that has its own blood supply. Any damage to the blood supply may lead to damage to the heart muscle. This is a **heart attack** or **myocardial infarction**. Therefore, anyone who has any type of chest pain should seek medical attention immediately! Most heart attacks do not follow unusual physical activity but occur during sleep.

#### SIGNS OF HEART ATTACK

*Pain like a vise or a belt around the chest.* It may radiate to the jaw, neck, or inner left arm. Other symptoms of a heart attack are:

- Wet clammy skin
- Perspiration
- Pulse rate is rapid and weak
- Color is pale
- Generalized weakness
- Low blood pressure
- Shortness of breath
- Nausea
- Respirations are shallow and difficult

- If unconscious, check response. If no response, call for help.
- Restore breathing if the person has had a cardiac arrest. This is when the heart has stopped beating and there is no breathing.
- If conscious, help the client into a comfortable position. Loosen his clothing if it is tight. If he wants to walk around, tell him it is important to rest and remain quiet.
- Reassure him. Continue to talk to him. Tell him what you are doing. If he asks you if he is having a heart attack, tell him that this could be many things, but it is safest to treat it as though it were a heart attack.
- Do not give him anything to eat or drink.
- If he stops breathing, start mouth-to-mouth ventilation.

# Section 8  Stroke/Cerebrovascular Accident

## Objectives: What You Will Learn to Do

- List the signs and symptoms of a CVA.
- Demonstrate the proper emergency care for a victim of a CVA.

### Introduction: Cerebrovascular Accident

When a blood vessel to the brain is damaged and a part of the brain no longer has its own blood supply, it dies. This is called a **stroke, cerebrovascular accident,** or CVA, as discussed in Chapter 19. If you suspect that your client is having a CVA, treat him as though he were.

**stroke** cerebrovascular accident

**cerebrovascular accident** a blockage of a blood vessel within the brain leading to death of brain tissue

### SIGNS AND SYMPTOMS

- Headache
- Change in state of consciousness or orientation
- Difficulty breathing
- Difficulty with speech or vision
- Paralysis in an extremity
- Seizure
- Unequal pupils

### EMERGENCY PROCEDURE

- Provide ventilations if needed.
- Call for help.
- If conscious, assist the client into a comfortable, safe position. Position paralyzed extremities in proper body alignment.
- Be sure that the client can spit out his saliva. If he is lying down, position him on his side for drainage.
- Do not give him anything to eat or drink.
- Remain with him and reassure him that help is coming.

1. Review some of the incident reports that your agency has had in the last several months. Were they emergency situations? Would you have acted in the same manner?
2. Discuss your feelings about giving mouth-to-mouth resuscitation. Review your agency policy as to when it is done and when it might not be done.

# Glossary

A glossary is a list of words and their definitions. All new words used in this book are defined here. Many of the words are familiar to you, but they may have been used in this book with new health-related meanings. These words are included here, too.

**abdomen**   the region of the body between the chest and the pelvis

**abdominal thrusts**   quick movements in the abdomen to remove a foreign body from the airway

**abduction**   to move an arm or leg away from the center of the body

**abrasive**   substance used to rub or scrape away another substance

**abuse**   any act that causes another harm; using a substance to excess

**abusive**   insulting or mistreating

**acetone**   a chemical found in urine

**active motion**   movement performed consciously by oneself

**activity tolerance**   the most activity the client will be able to perform on a given day

**acute**   state of illness that comes on suddenly and may be of short duration

**adduction**   to move an arm or leg toward the center of the body

**administer**   to give a client medication without his assistance

**adrenal glands**   two small endocrine glands located above the kidneys

**affected**   refers to the body part that is damaged by the disease process; involved

**aggression**   an act of hostility; an unprovoked attack

**aging**   to get older

**aging process**   changes in the body caused by growing older

**airway**   the passage by which air enters the lungs

**align**   to put the body into its proper anatomical position

**alveoli**   microscopic air sacs in the lung where oxygen passes into the blood in exchange for waste products

**Alzheimer's disease**   a form of irreversible mental deterioration

**ambulate**   to walk

**ambulatory**   able to walk

**amputation**   the removal of a body part through accident or surgery

**anaerobic**   growing in the absence of oxygen

**anal**   pertaining to the anus

**anatomical position**   person standing facing you, feet together, palms forward, head up

**anatomy**   the study of the structure of the body

**anemia**   decrease in red blood cell count and/or hemoglobin content of the blood

**anesthesia**   drug causing loss of feeling or sensation in a part or all of the body

**angina**   brief, temporary chest pain resulting from a decrease in oxygen to the heart

**ankylosing spondylitis**   an arthritis-type disease that affects the spine and/or shoulders and hips

**aneroid sphygmomanometer**   blood pressure measuring device with a dial

**anterior**   located in the front

**antibiotic**   drug that prevents disease-causing microorganisms from multiplying

**antisocial behavior**   acts that are harmful to the welfare of people

**anus**   opening of the rectum onto the body surface

**aorta**   major artery that carries blood away from the heart

**appendix**   slender growth attached to the large intestine

**aphasia**   loss of speech or language abilities due to injury to the brain

**apical**   refers to the apex of the heart

**arteriosclerosis**   "hardening of the arteries" due to thickening of the blood vessel walls

**artery**   blood vessel that carries blood away from the heart

**arthritis**   disease characterized by inflammation and destruction of the joints

**asepsis**   free of disease-causing organisms

**aspirate**   to remove material from a body cavity; to draw material into the lungs from the mouth

**atherosclerosis**   increased formation of fatty deposits and fibrous plaques, resulting in decrease of the lumen of the blood vessel

**atria**   the two upper chambers of the heart

**atrophy**   decrease in size of a muscle or tissue

**aura**   sensation before an epileptic seizure

**auricles/atria**   two upper chambers of the heart

**autonomic nervous system** part of the nervous system that carries messages without conscious thought

**axillary** area under the arms; the armpits

**bacteria** microorganisms that may or may not be pathogens

**base of support** part of the body that bears the most weight

**bath blanket** thin cotton blanket used to cover the client during a complete bed bath

**bed cradle** frame placed over a body area to hold bedclothes away from the body part

**bedpan** container into which a person defecates or urinates while in bed

**bedsores** decubiti

**bell** the cone shaped end of a type of stethoscope that is placed on the body

**benign** nonmalignant

**bile** substance needed for digestion that is secreted by the liver and stored in the gallbladder

**biopsy** examination of tissue taken from the body

**bladder** membranous sac that serves as a container within the body such as the urinary bladder which holds urine

**blood** fluid that circulates through the heart, arteries, veins, and capillaries. It carries nourishment and oxygen to the tissues and takes away waste matter and carbon dioxide

**blood-borne pathogens** those disease-causing entities transmitted through contact with blood

**blood pressure** force of blood on the inner walls of blood vessels as it flows through them

**blood pressure cuff** a sphygmomanometer

**blood vessels** the tubes that carry the blood throughout the body

**body alignment** arrangement of the body in a straight line, placing of body parts in correct anatomical position

**body language** gestures that function as a form of communication

**body mechanics** proper use of the human body to do work, to avoid injury and strain

**bony prominences** areas of the body where the bones are close to the skin surface and subject to decubiti

**bowel movement** the expulsion of feces from the rectum through the anus

**brain** main organ of the central nervous system, found in the skull

**bronchi** two main branches of the bronchial tree that lead to the lungs

**burn** injury to tissues caused by exposure to heat or to substances which stimulate the sensation of heat

**burp** the release of air from the stomach through the mouth

**bursa** sac of fluid within a joint capsule that provides lubrication for joint movement

**calculi** stones, usually found in the kidneys and/or gallbladder

**calibration** graduations on a measuring instrument

**calories** unit for measuring the energy produced when food is oxidized in the body

**capillaries** minute blood vessels which connect arteries to the veins

**carbohydrate** one of the basic food elements necessary for the body to function properly. It includes all sugars and starches.

**cardiac** refers to the heart

**cardiac arrest** absence of heart motion

**cartilage** tough connective tissue that holds bones together

**cast** rigid dressing molded to the body to give support and proper alignment

**case manager** coordinates care for the clients with all caregivers

**catheter** a tube used to remove body fluids from a cavity

**catheterization** insertion of a catheter into a body cavity, usually done under sterile conditions by a nurse or a doctor

**cell** basic unit of living matter

**cell membrane** thin layer of tissue surrounding the cell contents

**center of gravity** point at which, when held, you will have the greatest control over an object

**centigrade** measurement of temperature using a scale divided into 100 units or degrees. In this system, the freezing temperature of water is 0° centigrade, written 0°C. Water boils at 100°C. Also referred to as Celsius.

**central nervous system** part of the nervous system made up of the brain, nerves, and the spinal cord

**central venous lines** intravenous lines in place, surgically, in large veins of the body

**cerebral** pertaining to the cerebrum or brain

**cerebrospinal fluid** fluid secreted by cells in cavities within the cerebrum. It circulates through the membranes that cover and protect the brain and spinal cord.

**cerebrovascular accident** a blockage of blood vessel within the brain leading to death of brain tissue

**cervix** the narrow lower end of the uterus

**chemotherapy** the regime of taking drugs to treat a malignancy

**Cheyne-Stokes** a type of noisy breathing alternating with periods of no breathing; usually precedes death

**chronic** state of disease that lasts a long time

**chronic obstructive pulmonary disease** refers to diseases that cause permanent damage to lung tissue, including emphysema, asthma, and chronic bronchitis

**circulation** continuous movement of blood through the heart and blood vessels to all parts of the body

**circulatory system** organs of the body concerned with circulation

**circumcision** removal of the foreskin of the penis by a surgical procedure

**clean** uncontaminated by harmful microorganisms

**clean-catch** urine specimen obtained, following the careful cleansing of the urinary meatus and surrounding area, into a sterile container

**clockwise** the direction in which the hands of the clock move

**closed bed**   bed made with the bedspread in place

**clot**   semisolid mass of blood

**collateral circulation**   circulation taken over by smaller blood vessels after obstruction of the larger ones has occurred

**colon**   large bowel

**colostomy**   surgical procedure that creates an artificial opening through the abdominal wall into a part of the large bowel through which feces can leave the body. Can be temporary or permanent.

**coma**   state of deep unconsciousness caused by disease, injury, or drugs

**commode**   a portable frame, with a pan or pail, into which clients urinate or defecate

**communicable**   spread from one person to another

**communication**   exchange of information

**compliance**   following a prescribed routine

**complete bath**   bathing of a person usually in bed, to include all body parts

**complication**   unexpected condition occurring during the course of an illness or disability

**concentration**   accumulation or collection of particles; close attention

**congenital**   physical or mental characteristics present at birth

**congenital anomaly**   a deviation from the normal present at birth

**congestion**   unusually large amount of blood or fluid pooled in a body part

**connective tissue**   tissue that connects, supports, covers, ensheathes, lines, pads, or protects

**consistency**   the firmness felt when touching something

**constipated**   having hard, difficult to expel bowel movements

**contagious**   readily transmitted by direct or indirect contact

**continuous**   uninterrupted; without a stop

**contract**   get smaller

**contracture**   abnormal shortening of tissue, such as a muscle

**contraindication**   condition that forbids the use of a particular treatment or drug

**convulsion**   a seizure

**coronary**   pertaining to the heart

**counterclockwise**   in the direction opposite to that in which the hands of a clock move

**credential**   a letter or certificate indicating that a right or privilege has been attained or that a position of authority may be exercised

**crisis**   a serious or crucial time that requires action to avoid a material change to be suffered

**cross-infection**   infection by a new or different microorganism from a visitor or health team member

**cubic centimeter**   a unit of measure used in the metric system

**cyanosis**   blue or gray color of the skin due to lack of circulating oxygen

**cystitis**   inflammation of the bladder

**daily ability level**   the capability of the client to perform an activity on a given day

**daily living skills**   those tasks done each day to meet a person's basic needs

**death rattle**   noisy breathing of a dying person

**deceased**   dead

**decubitus ulcer**   bedsore; open wound caused by lack of blood supply to an area usually located on a bony prominence

**defecate**   to have a bowel movement

**defense mechanism**   a thought used unconsciously to protect oneself against painful or unpleasant feelings

**deficit**   lack of

**deformity**   distortion or malformation

**dehydration**   condition in which the body has less than normal amount of fluid

**dementia**   loss of mental powers

**denial**   refusals to believe or accept reality

**dentures**   false teeth

**dependent position**   part of the body that is hanging downward unsupported

**depression**   low spirits that may or may not cause a change of activity

**dermis**   the skin in general; specifically the second layer of skin

**developmental disability**   any condition that interferes with the normal development of a person

**diabetes mellitus**   condition that develops when the body cannot change sugar into energy

**diabetic acidosis or coma**   hyperglycemia: an excess of circulating sugar in the blood

**diagnosis**   identification of the disease producing a specific condition

**diaphragm**   muscular partition between the chest cavity and the abdominal cavity; also the flat end of a type of stethoscope that is placed on the body

**diarrhea**   abnormally frequent discharge of liquid fecal matter

**diastolic blood pressure**   the pressure in the blood vessels measured when the heart is relaxed

**digestion**   process by which food is mechanically and chemically changed into forms that can enter the bloodstream

**digestive system**   group of body organs that carry out digestion

**dilate**   expand; get bigger

**dirty**   contaminated by harmful microorganisms

**disability**   partial or complete loss of the use of a part or parts of the body

**disc**   round piece of cartilage between the vertebrae

**discharge**   termination of service; abnormal material excreted from the body

**discipline**   a system of rules

**discoloration**   change from normal color

**disinfection**   process of destroying most disease-causing organisms

**disposable equipment**   material that is used one time only for one client and then discarded

**distended**   swollen, stretched out, enlarged

**dominant**   stronger half of a pair

**dorsal**   back of an organ or the body; posterior

**dorsiflexion**   to bend backwards

**double bagging** technique of putting contaminated material into two plastic bags for protection

**drainage** discharge from a sore, wound, or body part

**draping** covering a client or parts of the client's body with a sheet, blanket, bath blanket, or other material

**draw sheet** small sheet made of plastic, rubber, or cotton placed across the middle of the bed to cover and protect the bottom sheet and assist in moving the client

**dressing** bandage for an external wound

**dry shampoo** product used to clean hair without water

**duct** passage for fluids

**duodenostomy** an opening into the duodenum

**duodenum** first part of the small intestine

**earmold** an impression of the ear used with a hearing aide

**edema** abnormal swelling of a part of the body caused by fluid collecting in that area

**ejaculate** to discharge fluid suddenly, especially the discharge of semen from the male urethra

**ejaculatory ducts** part of the male reproductive system

**emaciation** wasting away of flesh caused by disease or lack of food

**embolus** a clot carried by the circulatory system from its place of formation to another site usually causing an obstruction

**embryo** human being during the first 8 weeks of its development in the uterus

**emergency** a sudden unexpected crisis, injury, or illness

**emesis** vomitus

**emesis basin** kidney-shaped basin used to collect material the client spits out or vomits

**encrustation** drainage from the body that has formed a crust

**endocrine glands** ductless glands in the body that secrete hormones into the blood

**endometrium** lining of the uterus

**enema** introduction of fluid, through a tube into the rectum to cleanse or introduce medication

**environment** surroundings affecting the development of an organism

**enzyme** substance manufactured by the body that stimulates certain chemical changes

**epidermis** outermost layer of skin

**epididymus** organ attached to the testes

**epiglottis** small piece of tissue which sits on the larynx

**epithelium** tissue cells composing skin, lining the passage of the hollow organs of the respiratory, digestive, and urinary systems

**esophagus** muscular tube for the passage of food, which extends from the back of the throat (pharynx), down through the chest and diaphragm into the stomach

**ethics** system of moral behavior and beliefs

**evaporate** to pass off as vapor, as water evaporating into the air

**excreta** urine and feces; waste matter from the body

**excrete** eliminate or expel waste matter from the body

**exhale** to breathe out air in respiration

**expectoration** coughing up matter from the lungs, trachea, or bronchial tubes and spitting it out

**expiration** act of expelling air

**expressive aphasia** difficulty communicating in writing and orally

**extend** to straighten an arm or leg

**external** outside the body

**extremities** arms, legs, hands, and feet

**facilitate** to make easier

**Fahrenheit** system for measuring temperature. In the Fahrenheit system, the temperature of water at boiling is 212°F. At freezing it is 32°F.

**fallopian tubes** also called the oviducts, through which an egg travels from the ovary to the uterus

**family** a group of people bonded together and working to meet the needs of all members

**family dynamics** the ways in which family members interact and get along with each other

**fanfold** method of arranging bed linens so that the cover and bedspread are folded at the foot of the bed out of the way

**feces** solid waste material discharged from the body through the rectum and anus; also bowel movement, fecal matter

**feedback mechanism** process whereby the output of a system is fed back into the system (input) to change the way the system works or what it produces

**fertile** the period of the month when a woman is able to conceive

**fertilization** union of male and female cells; conception

**fetus** developing infant in the uterus, after the first two months

**fever** condition when body temperature is above normal

**fibrous** composed of thin thread-like structures

**first aid** emergency treatment given for injury or illness before regular medical treatment is available

**flammable** substance that will burn quickly

**flatus** intestinal gas

**flex** to bend

**flexion** to bend a joint

**fluid balance** relationship of intake fluid with excreted fluid output

**fluid intake** liquid taken into the body

**fluid output** liquid excreted by the body

**food groups** the division of nutrients into categories of dairy products, vegetables, fruits, meat and fish, and bread and cereal products

**foot board** a flat piece of wood or cardboard placed at the end of the bed, under the covers so that the client can rest his feet flatly against it

**foot drop** a contraction of the foot due to a shortening of the muscles in the calf of the leg. The foot falls forward and cannot be held in proper position.

**force fluids** extra fluids taken in according to doctor's orders

**foreign body**   object that does not belong in the place it is found

**Fowler's position**   when the head of the bed is at a 45° angle

**fracture**   break

**friction**   rubbing of one surface against another

**functional**   able to be used

**functional limitations**   the inability to perform a task due to the deficit of a body part

**gallbladder**   organ attached to the liver in which bile is stored

**gastrointestinal**   refers to the digestive system

**gastrostomy**   an opening into the stomach

**gatch handle**   apparatus used to manually operate a hospital bed

**genital**   refers to the external reproductive organs

**geriatric**   refers to persons over 65

**germ**   any microorganism, especially those causing disease

**germicide**   chemical used to destroy germs

**gestation**   time from conception to birth

**gland**   organ that produces a chemical used by the body

**glucose**   sugar

**gout**   the buildup of uric acid crystals in the blood and joints

**graduate**   container used to measure substances

**grand mal seizure**   type of epileptic seizure

**guarding belt**   device placed around the waist, used to assist a client during ambulation

**gums**   firm flesh covering the jaws on the inside of the mouth and surrounding the bases of the teeth

**hallucination**   mental delusion or impression not based on reality

**hearing aid**   mechanical device used to help a person perceive sounds

**heart**   four-chambered, hollow, muscular organ in the chest cavity, pointing slightly to the left, that pumps blood throughout the body

**heart attack**   layman's term referring to damage to the heart; a myocardial infarction

**Heimlich maneuver**   a system developed by Heimlich to remove a foreign body from the airway

**hemiplegic**   one who is paralyzed on one side of his body

**hemorrhage**   excessive bleeding

**hemorrhoid**   swelling of a vein near the anus

**hereditary**   characteristics passed from parent to child

**homeostasis**   stability of all body functions at normal levels

**hormone**   protein substance secreted by an endocrine gland directly into the blood

**hospice**   program of care that allows a dying client to remain at home and die at home while receiving professionally supervised care

**Hoyer lift**   mechanical device, like a swinging seat, used for lifting a client

**hyperalimentation**   process of giving nutrients directly into the blood stream

**hyperextension**   beyond the normal extension

**hyperglycemia**   excess of sugar in the blood

**hypertension**   high blood pressure

**hypoglycemia**   deficiency of sugar in the blood

**hypotension**   low blood pressure

**hysterectomy**   removal of the uterus

**ileostomy**   surgical procedure that makes an artificial opening through the abdominal wall into the ileum, through which waste material is discharged

**ileum**   the last portion of the small intestine

**illness**   deviation from the healthy state

**improvise**   to make do with the tools or equipment at hand; to use an item for a task for which it was not originally designed

**impulse**   stimulus that travels along nerve tissue and causes activity in the body

**incident**   any unusual event such as an accident or condition

**incontinence**   the inability to control one's bowel movements or urination

**indicated**   treatment that is accepted as correct in a particular case

**infection**   condition in body tissue in which pathogens have multiplied and destroyed many cells

**inflammation**   reaction of the tissues to disease or injury. There is usually pain, heat, redness, and swelling of the body part.

**inflexible**   unbending, rigid

**inhale**   to breathe in air in respiration

**insulin**   hormone produced by the pancreas that is needed for the metabolism of sugars and starches

**insulin reaction or shock**   hypoglycemia due to too much insulin in the blood

**intake**   all substances ingested by the body, sometimes refers only to fluid consumed

**intermittent infusion**   alternating, stopping and beginning again

**intravenous therapy**   giving of fluids or medication directly into the vein

**involuntary**   action taken without conscious input

**involved**   body part undergoing therapy or part of a disease process

**irrigate**   cleanse or wash with water or fluid

**jejunostomy**   an opening into the jejunum

**jejunum**   second portion of the small intestine

**job description**   written document listing the parts of employment, such as the tasks one is responsible for

**joint**   part of the body where two bones come together and there is movement

**ketoacidosis**   a condition characterized by a large amount of ketone bodies in the urine

**ketones**   chemical compounds sometimes found in urine

**kidney**   organ lying in the upper posterior portion of the abdomen that removes wastes from the bloodstream and discharges them in the form of urine

**labored**   difficult

**large intestine**   lower part of the gastrointestinal tract consisting of the ascending colon, transverse colon, descending colon, rectum, and anus

**larynx**    area of the throat containing the vocal cords

**level of ability**    amount of activity a client is capable of

**ligament**    a tough band of tissue connecting bone to bone

**liquid**    substance that flows freely, like water

**liver**    body's largest gland located in the upper left quadrant of the abdominal cavity, which helps process some waste products

**lubricant**    substance used to make a surface smooth and moist

**lumen**    inside passageway of a vessel or tube

**lungs**    primary organs of breathing

**lymph**    clear colorless fluid carried by an independent system of vessels that returns the fluid to the heart

**malignant**    cancerous

**manual thrust**    a quick movement of the hands to remove an obstruction of the airway

**meatus**    opening of the urethra to the outside of the body

**mechanical lift**    machine used to lift a client from one place to another

**medication**    substance or preparation used in treating a disease

**membrane**    thin layer of tissue

**meninges**    three membranes that protect the brain and spinal cord

**meniscus**    disc of cartilage between two bones at a joint that reduces wear on the ends of the bones

**menopause**    period of life in the female, usually between 45 and 50, when menstruation stops; change of life

**menstruation**    cyclical discharge of blood from the uterus

**mental disability**    the temporary or permanent disruption in the ability of a person to function satisfactorily in a society

**mental health**    the ability to function satisfactorily in a society; a sense of well being

**mental illness**    *see* mental disability

**mercury**    chemical used as part of a sphygmomanometer to indicate blood pressure

**metastisis**    the spreading of cancer within the body

**metric system**    a method of measuring temperature, length, and volume of fluid that is based on the decimal system

**microorganism**    living thing so small it can be seen only through a microscope

**mineral**    natural substance neither animal nor vegetable; one of the nutrients necessary for proper bodily function

**minimal assistance**    least amount of help necessary for a client to function safely

**mitered corner**    folding the bedding at the corners when making a bed so that the sheet is tightly stretched with no wrinkles

**modified**    changed

**mouth-to-mouth resuscitation**    emergency technique used to introduce air into lungs that are not breathing on their own

**motivation**    that which makes a person want to do something

**mucus**    sticky substance secreted by membranes in the lungs, nose, and parts of the rectal and genital areas

**muscle**    tissue composed of fibers with the ability to elongate and shorten causing joints and bones to move

**muscular system**    group of organs that allow the body to move

**myocardial infarction**    death of a part of the heart due to blockage in a blood vessel

**necrosis**    death of a cell from disease or injury

**need**    requirement; a lack of something

**nephron**    function unit of the kidney that filters out those substances the body does not need and reabsorbs those that it does

**nephrostomy**    incision into the kidney with drainage to the outside of the body

**nerve impulse**    regular wave of negative electrical impulses that transmit information along a neuron from one part of the body to another.

**nerves**    bundles of neurons held together with connective tissue. They go to all parts of the body from the central nervous system, that is, from the brain and spinal cord.

**nervous system**    group of organs that control and stimulate the activities of the body and the functioning of the other body systems

**neuron**    nerve, including the cell and the long fiber coming from the cell

**newborn**    baby in the first month of life

**nonfunctional**    having no use; not able to be used

**nonjudgmental**    accepting communication without stating a personal opinion

**nonsterile**    not subjected to the sterilizing process and therefore possibly having pathogens

**nourishment**    process of taking food into the body to maintain life

**nutrients**    food substances that are required by the body to repair, maintain, and grow new cells

**nutrition**    that which nourishes; food

**obese**    very fat

**objective reporting**    reporting exactly what you observe

**observation**    gathering information about a client

**obstetrics**    branch of medicine dealing with pregnancy, labor, and the immediate postpartum period

**obstructed**    blocked

**occupational therapist**    trained person who assists people with performing their daily living tasks

**occupied bed**    bed containing a person, the process of making a bed with a person in it

**ointment**    substance applied to the skin for healing purposes

**omit**    leave out

**open bed**    bed with the top sheet and bedspread folded so as to give the client easy entrance

**oral**    pertaining to the mouth

**oral hygiene**    cleanliness of the mouth

**organ**    several types of tissues grouped together to perform a certain function

**organism** living thing

**oriented** realization of one's position in relation to time, place, and person

**orthopedics** medical specialty that covers the treatment of broken bones, deformities, or disease that attacks bones, joints, or muscles

**osteoarthritis** the most common type of arthritis

**ostomy** artificially created opening through the abdominal wall that provides a way for the intestinal organs to discharge waste products

**output** material discharged from the body; may refer only to fluids

**ovary** one of a pair of organs in the female that produce mature eggs and the primary female sex hormones, estrogen, and progesterone

**overdependence** too reliant upon something or someone

**ovulation** period of time in which the ovum is pushed out from the surface of the ovary and usually picked up by the oviduct

**ovum** egg

**oxidation** process by which food is combined with oxygen to form energy

**oxygen** a colorless, odorless gas making up about one-fifth of the air we breathe. It is essential for life.

**pacemaker** electrical device used to stimulate the heart

**palpate** to examine by touch

**pancreas** large gland that secretes enzymes into the intestines to aid in the digestion of food. It also manufactures the hormone insulin.

**paralysis** loss of the ability to move part or all of the body

**paraplegic** one who is paralyzed in half of his body, usually the lower half

**parenteral** method of giving substances to the client other than by mouth

**partial bath** washing part of the client's body

**passive motion** movement of a body part accomplished by external force rather than by the client

**pathogen** disease-causing microorganism

**pediatric** referring to children

**penis** male sexual organ; urine is also ejected through the penis

**perineal care** cleansing of the perineal area

**perineum** area between the anus and the external genital organs

**peripheral line** intravenous lines in place in the upper extremities

**peristalsis** movement of the intestines that pushes food along to the next part of the digestive system

**perspiration** body moisture given off during physical activity

**petite mal seizures** type of epileptic seizure

**phalanges** bones of a finger or toe

**pharynx** area behind the nasal cavities, mouth, and larynx that opens into them and the esophagus

**physical therapist** person trained to assist clients with activities related to motion

**physician** doctor, person licensed to practice medicine

**physiology** study of the functions of body tissues and organs

**pigment** that substance which gives the skin color

**pituitary gland** sometimes called the master gland; attached to the base of the brain and directs the flow of all hormones in the body

**placenta** oval, spongy structure in the uterus from which the unborn baby receives its nourishment. Sometimes called afterbirth, the placenta is discharged from the mother's body soon after childbirth.

**plaque** fatty deposits within the blood vessels attached to the vessel walls

**plasma** liquid portion of blood, or blood from which the red and white cells and platelets have been removed

**pleura** membrane lining the chest cavity and covering the lungs

**pleural cavity** chest cavity containing the lungs

**poison** substance causing illness or death when eaten, drunk, or absorbed in relatively small amounts

**pore** tiny opening through which fluids may be absorbed or discharged

**posterior** located in the back or toward the rear

**postmortem** after death

**postoperative** after surgery

**postpartum** following childbirth

**premature birth** birth of a baby before the normal gestation period is over

**prepuce** foreskin of the penis, often removed in an operation called a circumcision

**pressure sore** decubitus

**primary site** place of the original cancerous lesion

**principal care person** that person designated to be in charge of the client's care

**priority** giving something more importance than another

**prognosis** probable outcome of a disease

**projection** attributing to others those feelings and thoughts which are really one's own

**pronation** to bend downward

**prone** lying on one's stomach

**prostate** male gland behind the outlet of the urinary bladder

**prosthesis** artificial body part

**protein** one of the nutrients necessary to all animal life

**protocol** rules directing the actions of specific people

**protoplasm** refers to the cell body and the cell nucleus; living matter

**psychological** refers to all aspects of the mind such as feelings, thoughts, etc.

**pulling braid** a device used to assist a person in moving and/or sitting up in bed

**pull sheet** a sheet or piece of cloth placed under the client and used by the caretaker to facilitate moving the client in the bed

**pulmonary** refers to the lungs

**pulse** rhythmic expansion and contractions of the arteries caused by the beating of the heart

**punishment** action performed as the result of wrongdoing

**pus** a waste product of inflammation

**quadriplegia** paralysis of both upper and lower parts of the body

**radial pulse** throbbing felt at the inner part of the wrist

**radiating** spreading out from one place to another

**radiation therapy** the use of X rays to treat a tumor or a condition

**range of motion** exercises that take a body part through the entire ability of its motion

**rate** quantity of a thing being measured

**rationalization** the invention of a reason for a behavior that is really not accurate

**reagent** a substance used to measure or detect another substance

**reality orientation** a technique to orient people to their surroundings

**receptive aphasia** inability to understand stimuli due to a deficiency within the brain

**receptor organs** group of cells that receive and process stimuli

**rectal** having to do with the rectum

**rectum** lower 8 to 10 inches of the colon

**regression** reverting to an earlier, less mature behavior

**regulated medical waste** those waste products determined by law to be in need of special disposal

**rehabilitation** process by which people who have been disabled by injury or sickness are helped to recover as many as possible of their original abilities and live with the remaining disabilities

**reinfection** to become ill again with the same microorganism

**reproductive system** group of organs that carry on the creation of new life

**respiration** process of breathing; inhaling and exhaling air

**respiratory system** group of body organs that carry on the function of respiration. The system brings oxygen into the body and eliminates carbon dioxide.

**respite** temporary interruption of work

**responsibilities** those tasks one has to execute and for which one is held accountable

**restrain** limit or restrict

**restrict** limit or confine

**rheumatoid arthritis** crippling chronic disease of the joints

**rigor mortis** stiffening of a person's body and limbs shortly after death

**role** one's function

**rotation** movement of a joint in a circular motion around its axis. Internal rotation: to turn in toward the center. External rotation: to turn out away from the center.

**routine urine specimen** sample of urine obtained at any time during the day in a clean container

**safety razor** razor provided with a guard to prevent cutting the skin

**saliva** secretion of the salivary glands into the mouth. Saliva moistens food and is necessary for digestion.

**scrotum** pouch below the penis that contains the testicles

**secondary site** place in the body in which cancerous cells are found following the location of the primary site

**secrete** to produce a substance and expel it

**sediment** material that settles to the bottom

**seizure** convulsions or involuntary muscular contractions and relaxations

**self-inoculation** infecting oneself with one's own organisms

**semen** the fluid of ejaculation

**seminal vesicles** small glands in the male near the prostate and urethra where semen is stored before it is discharged

**sense organs** groups of tissue that make it possible for us to be aware of the outside world through sight, hearing, smell, taste, and touch

**shearing** the action of skin being moved in one direction while underlying tissue and/or bone is moved in another direction

**shock** state of collapse resulting from reduced blood volume and pressure usually caused by severe injury or emotional reaction

**signs** objective evidence of disease

**sitz bath** bath in which the client sits in a specially designed chair or tub with his hips and buttocks in water

**skeletal system** bones of the body which give the body shape and protection

**skeleton** bony support of the body

**skin** the largest organ in the body whose functions include protection from infection, temperature regulation, and removal of waste products

**small intestine** part of the gastrointestinal tract extending from the end of the stomach to the large intestine

**smooth muscle** appears smooth under a microscope; usually associated with involuntary actions

**socialization** learning to live together in a group with other human beings

**solution** liquid containing dissolved substances

**specific information** facts pertaining to a particular client or situation

**specimen** sample of material taken from the body

**sperm** male reproductive cell

**spermatic duct** tube containing sperm

**sphincter** ringlike muscle that controls the opening and closing of a body opening

**sphygmomanometer** apparatus for measuring blood pressure of which there are two types, mercury or aneroid; blood pressure cuff

**spinal cord** one of the main organs of the nervous system. The spinal cord carries messages from the brain to other parts of the body and from parts of the body back to the brain. The spinal cord is inside the spine (backbone).

**spleen** abdominal organ

**splint** a thin piece of wood or other rigid material used to keep an injured part, such as a broken bone, in place

**spontaneous combustion** process of catching fire as a result of the heat of the chemicals that are burning

**spore**  microorganism that has formed a hard shell around itself for protection. It can only be destroyed by sterilization.

**sprain**  to twist a ligament or muscle without dislocating the bones

**sputum**  waste material coughed up from lungs or trachea

**static electricity**  electrical discharges in the air

**sterilization**  process of destroying all microorganisms including spores; the process by which a person is rendered incapable of reproduction

**stertorous breathing**  respirations that have a snoring sound

**stethoscope**  instrument that allows one to listen to various sounds in the human body

**stimulus**  change in the external or internal environment that is strong enough to set up a nervous impulse

**stoma**  artificially made opening connecting a body passage with the outside

**stomach**  part of the digestive tract between the esophagus (food pipe) and the duodenum

**stool**  solid waste material discharged from the body through the rectum and anus. Other names include feces, excreta, excrement, bowel movement, and fecal matter.

**straight drainage**  method of collecting urine from a Foley catheter into a closed container

**straight razor**  razor without a safety guard, which protects the skin

**stretch receptors**  nerve cells that relay messages to the brain as the organ enlarges

**striated muscle**  appears to be lined under a microscope; usually associated with voluntary action

**stroke**  cerebrovascular accident

**subjective reporting**  giving your opinion about what you have observed

**substance abuse**  the use of anything, usually alcohol or drugs, to an excess and to the detriment of the person

**suction**  action or capacity for sucking up

**supination**  to bend upward

**supine**  lying on one's back

**support systems**  arrangement that gives aid and comfort to a person

**surgical asepsis**  completely free of microorganisms; as indicated, surgically clean

**surgical procedure**  repair to an injury or disease condition by making an incision into the body

**swab**  small piece of cotton used to apply a substance or to clean a body part

**symptom**  subjective evidence of a disease, disorder, or condition

**syringe**  instrument used for injecting liquids into body vessels and cavities or for drawing substances out of body tissues

**system**  group of organs acting together to carry out one or more body functions

**systolic blood pressure**  force with which blood is pumped when the heart contracts

**tact**  knowing the proper thing to say; a sensitive skill in dealing with people

**tactile**  pertaining to touch

**taut**  pulled or drawn tight, not slack

**temperature**  measurement of the amount of heat in the body at a given time. The normal body temperature is 98.6°F (37°C).

**tendon**  tough cord of connective tissue that binds muscles to bony parts

**testes**  pair of reproductive organs in the male that lie in the scrotum hanging from the perineal area, dorsal to the penis

**testosterone**  a male hormone

**texture**  arrangement of any substance; the feeling of this arrangement with one's fingers

**therapeutic**  an act that helps in the treatment of disease or discomfort

**therapist**  one who delivers a therapeutic action

**thermometer**  instrument used for measuring temperature

**thrombus**  blood clot that remains at its site of formation

**thymus**  ductless gland, part of the lymphatic system, located in the chest cavity just above the heart

**thyroid**  endocrine gland, located in the front of the neck. It regulates body metabolism. This gland secretes a hormone known as thyroxine.

**tissue**  group of cells of the same type

**tissue fluid**  watery environment around each cell that acts as a place of exchange for gases, food, and waste products between the cells and the blood

**tongue depressor**  flat blade-like instrument used to keep the client's tongue flattened during an examination of the throat and mouth

**toxic**  poisonous

**toxin**  substance that is toxic

**trachea**  organ of the respiratory system. It is located in the throat area. The trachea is commonly called the windpipe.

**tracheotomy**  surgical procedure to make an artificial opening in a person's neck connecting his trachea with the outside. This surgery may be necessary when the person's trachea above the opening is blocked and he cannot breathe.

**transmittable**  able to go from one person to another, as a disease

**trapeze**  metal bar suspended over the bed, used by a client to help him raise or move his body more easily

**trauma**  damage to the body caused by injury, wound, or shock

**Trendelenburg position**  bed is tilted so the client's head is about a foot below the level of the knees. This position is used to get more blood to the head and prevent shock. Also called the shock position.

**tub bath**  washing a person in a container that holds water

**tubule**  small tube

**tumor**  abnormal growth in the body

**umbilical cord**  long, flexible, round organ that carries nourishment from the mother to the baby. It connects the umbilicus of the unborn baby in the mother's uterus to the placenta.

**umbilicus**   small depression on the abdomen that marks the place where the umbilical cord was originally attached to the fetus; belly button

**unconscious**   not responding to sensory stimulus

**uninvolved**   body part that is not affected by the disease process

**unit pricing**   a system of showing the cost of food items in terms of common measurements such as ounces or pounds

**universal precautions**   those routine activities recommended to protect health care workers from contamination with blood and body fluids

**ureter**   tube leading from the kidneys to the urinary bladder

**ureterostomy**   an incision through the abdominal wall into the ureters resulting in drainage to the outside of the body

**urethra**   tube leading from the urinary bladder to the outside of the body

**urinal**   container into which male clients can urinate; women use female urinals

**urinalysis**   laboratory test performed on the urine

**urinary system**   group of organs that filter waste products from the blood, form urine, and discharge it from the body

**urinate**   discharge urine from the body; void; micturate

**urine**   liquid waste manufactured in the kidneys and discharged from the urinary bladder

**uterus**   expandable female reproductive organ in which an embryo grows and is nourished until gestation is complete

**vagina**   the birth canal leading from the cervix to the outside

**varicose veins**   abnormal swelling of veins

**vas deferens**   tubes carrying sperm from the testicles to the glands where they are stored in preparation for ejaculation

**vein**   blood vessel that carries blood to the heart

**ventricles**   lower two chambers of the heart

**vertebra**   one of the bones of the spinal column

**vertebral column**   back bone

**villi**   tiny fingerlike projections in the lining of the small intestines into which the end products of digestion are absorbed and distributed through the bloodstream

**virus**   a microscopic living parasitic agent that can cause disease

**visceral**   refers to the organs within the abdominal cavity

**vital signs**   temperature, pulse, respiration, and blood pressure

**vitamin**   substance found in food necessary in small quantities for proper bodily function

**void**   to urinate, pass water

**vomiting**   this occurs when the contents of the stomach are cast upward and outward through the mouth; throwing up

**vomitus**   material which is vomited; emesis

**womb**   uterus

# Index

Foley catheter, 296–297
Food, 159–72
    basic food groups, 159–62
    dying patient and, 90
    infant, 71, 75–76
    meal planning and, 163–64
    therapeutic diets, 168–70
Foot board, 157
Foot care, 195–97
Forcing fluids, 300–301
Foreskin, 79
Formula, infant, 75
Fracture, 97

**G**
Gastrointestinal system, 106–108, 112
    aging and, 51
Gastrostomy, 336
General mood, 23
Genitalia, 109–11
    aging and, 52
Geriatric client, 48–59
    safety precautions for, 149
    skin care of, 189
Gland:
    Cowper's, 111
    prostate, 111
Glass thermometer, 272–73
Glucose:
    blood, 356–58
    liver and, 107
    urine, 338
Gout, 362
Gown and mask, 125–26
Grand mal seizure, 337
Gravity, center of, 174–75
Grooming, 263–64
    hygiene and, 12–13

**H**
Hair, 96
    care of, 215–20
Handwashing, 116–18
Head raising, 186
Hearing loss, 254–56
Heart, 102–104
    aging and, 51
    maintaining function of, 378
Heart attack, 104, 351–54
    emergency procedures for, 387–88
Heimlich maneuver, 379–80
Hemiplegic client, 262–63
Hemorrhage, 359, 383
Hemorrhoids, 108
High calorie diet, 170
High protein diet, 170
Hip, 238
Homemaking:
    bedmaking, 136–47
    cleaning and, 129–36
Hormones, 101–102
    aging and, 52
    sex, 109, 111
Hospice, 5
House cleaning, 129–36

bathroom and, 133–34
cleaning products and, 130–32
dusting and, 132
floors and, 135
laundry and, 134–35
pests and, 135–36
washing dishes and, 132–33
Hygiene, personal, 12–13
Hyperalimentation, 347–48
Hyperglycemia, 357
Hypertension, 287, 350–51
Hypoglycemia, 357–58
Hypotension, 287
Hysterectomy, 110

**I**
Illness, 37–40
Incidents, 12
Incontinent client, 300
Indwelling catheter, 299–300, 322–27
Infant, 61–84
    bathing of, 79–82
    burping of, 76
    characteristics of, 62
    circumcision and, 79
    diapers and, 78
    feeding of, 71–75
    medication and, 83
    safety and, 82–83
    stool of, 77
    umbilical cord care and, 78–79
    urine specimen from, 310–11
Infarction, myocardial, 351–54
    emergency procedures for, 387–88
Infection control, 114–27
    disinfection and sterilization and, 118–20
    handwashing and, 116–18
    medical asepsis and, 114–18
    transmittable disease and, 120–124
Infusion, 329
Inhalation, 106
    poisoning by, 384–85
Injected poisons, 385
Instructions, 10–11
Insulin, 356
Intake and output sheet, 295
Intestine, 106
Intravenous therapy, 328–330
Involuntary muscles, 98
Involved side, 179
    positioning client on, 181
Irregular respiration, 285
Isolation techniques, 124–26

**J**
Jejunostomy, 336
Joints, 98, 234
    arthritis and, 361–62

**K**
Ketoacidosis, 357
Ketostix test, 342
Kidneys, 108
Kitchen safety, 150–51

Knee, 238
Kubler-Ross, Elisabeth, 86

**L**
Labored respiration, 284
Language therapy, 250–52
Large intestine, 106
Laundry, 134–35
    infection control and, 123–24
    occupational therapy and, 265
Legal aspects, 11–12
Leg bag, 326–27
Leg raising, 238
Leisure activities, 267
Licensed practical nurse, 6
Licensed vocational nurse, 6
Lift, mechanical, 241–42
Ligament, 98
Lips, 256
Liquid formula, 75–76
Liquids, flammable, 151
Listening skills, 18
    dying client and, 87–89
Liver, 104, 106
Log rolling, 185
Low calorie diet, 170
Lungs, 105–106, 367–68
    aging and, 51
Lymph system, 95, 102–105

**M**
Male genitalia, 24
Male reproduction, 111
Malignancy, 362–64
Manual thrust, 379–80
Mask, oxygen, 320
Mattress stain, 131
Meal preparation, 167
    occupational therapy and, 265
Mechanical lift, 241–42
Medical asepsis, 114–116
Medicare, 5
Medications, 316–20
    geriatric client and, 57
    infant or child and, 83
Menopause, 110
Menstruation, 110
Mental changes in aging, 52–53
Mental health, 41–43
Menu planning, 163–64
Mercury:
    sphygmomanometer and, 287–88
    thermometer and, 271
Metric system, 294
Microorganisms, 114
Midstream clean-catch urine specimen, 307–308
Mobilization, 257
Mood of client, 23
Mouth care, 200–204
    dying client and, 90
Mouth-to-mouth ventilation, 381–82
Movement, 234
Multiple Sclerosis, 369